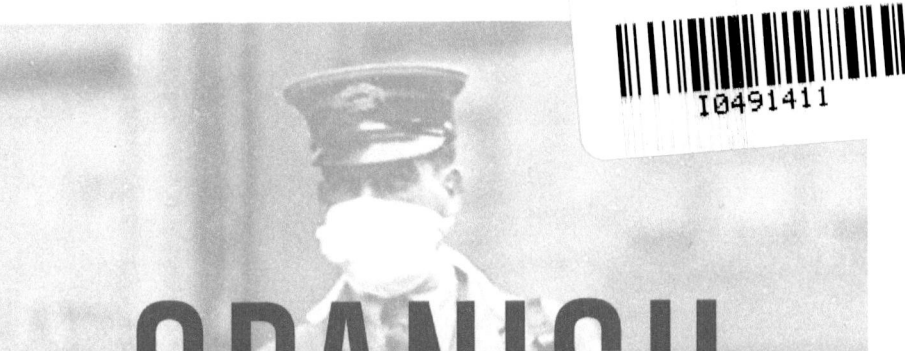

SPANISH INFLUENZA

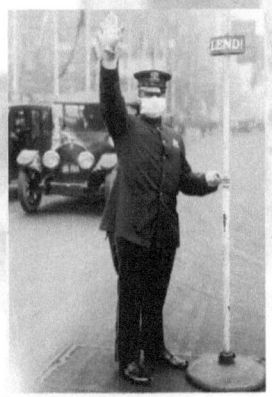

THE STORY
OF THE
EPIDEMIC
THAT SWEPT
AMERICA
FROM THE
NEWSPAPER
REPORTS
OF 1918

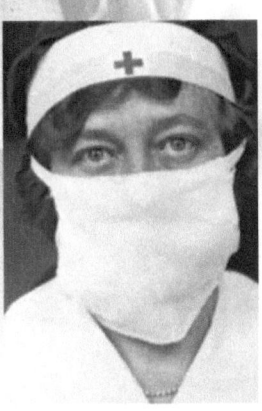

KEN ROSSIGNOL

KEN ROSSIGNOL

SPANISH INFLUENZA – THE STORY OF THE EPIDEMIC THAT SWEPT AMERICA FROM THE NEWSPAPER REPORTS OF 1918

By Ken Rossignol
Copyright Kenneth C. Rossignol 2020
ISBN: 9798654536792
The Privateer Clause Publishing
THE CHESAPEAKE TODAY LLC
Ken@theprivateerclause.com

DEDICATION

Dedication
To the many brave men and women who act quickly to aid those in distress
due to virus even at the risk of their own lives.

CONTENTS

SPANISH INFLUENZA – THE STORY OF THE EPIDEMIC THAT SWEPT
AMERICA FROM THE NEWSPAPER REPORTS OF 1918

ACKNOWLEDGMENTS

The various newspapers from which this information has been compiled
are attributed throughout this book.
Thanks to the Library of Congress and the Taxpayers of the United States
who fund this excellent organization which provides such a fine repository
for the tradition of news journalism in America.

INTRODUCTION

As many readers may have learned, modern references to the Spanish
Influenza of 1918 make various representations as to the virulence, the
spread, the affect and results of the world-wide epidemic that hit during
the last year of the Great War. The purpose of this book is to provide
the reader with a clearer understanding of the events of that era, based
on facts provided in 1918 rather than concoctions of those events in
2020 and beyond.

This telling of the story of the Spanish Flu of 1918 is best told and
understood from the newspaper reports of publications large and small
from every corner of the United States. The news reports have been
picked at random with an emphasis on selecting news articles that told
of effects in the rural, small towns, cities, army camps, navy yards, with
armed forces deployed at sea and in France as well as on Indian
Reservations. Many specific lives and deaths are related that reveal
much about life during the epidemic; and vaccines quickly developed
and used to inoculate hundreds of thousands of people.

There is no attempt here to provide a summary or interpretation for the
reader – read these reports which were produced solely for the
information of their readers by newspapers in 1918 and 1919 – and
make up your own mind.

The largest number of news stories are contained in the Fall section, as that is simply where the random selection process revealed.

NOTE TO THE HYPERSENSTIVE READER: Some of the language and terms regarding the origin of the term "Spanish Influenza", ethnicity and race were those used in 1918-19 and have not been modified to prevent the 21st Century reader from going into shock or apoplexy. **Proceed at your own risk**.

1 CHAPTER NAME

PART ONE
Spring of 1918

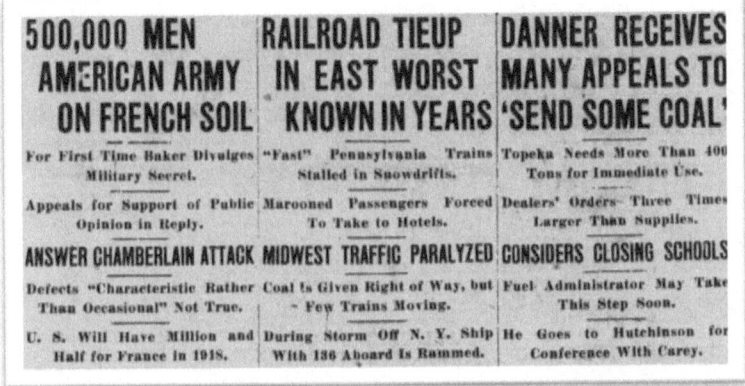

Topeka, Kansas – On January 28, 1918, in the *Topeka State Journal* on
the front page, there was little news being reported of the spread of the
Spanish Influenza.

Discussion of schools being closed was due to storms shutting down
railroad traffic and thus backing up orders of coal for heating schools.
The cold snap had temperatures that day at four degrees.

Fast passenger trains were stalled in the mountains with passengers being shuttled off to hotels in Altoona, New York, while ships collided off of New York.

A half-million American soldiers had arrived in France to pursue the Hun army, and a headline next to the war news blared out the possibility that undesirable pool halls in Topeka, Kansas, may have to close due to trouble in the river district.

Troublemakers were using the pool halls as headquarters for loafing as Americans were digging in to conserve raw materials, save scraps for recycling, raising money for Liberty Bonds, and young men signing up for service in the Army and Navy.

A mention was made of the army camps in Kansas that day regarding snowfall hampering marching. Reports of the terrible epidemic of flu killing up to 600,000 Americans with Kansas figuring as a hotspot in the early months had yet to develop. Still, by years end, the war would be over in Europe, and with multiple developments of vaccine, the decline of dreaded influenza would be at hand.

FEW GET TO LAWTON
Doniphan Officers Try to Keep Soldiers Away from Town.

THE TOPEKA STATE JOURNAL

Camp Doniphan Ok., (Jan. 8, 1918) – The town of Lawton has been practically quarantined by the military authorities so far as the soldiers are concerned. Not more than 5 percent of the command will be allowed to visit the town at any one time. This means that one man can visit Lawton only once every twenty days.

 The medical authorities at camp reported a number of cases of infectious diseases in Lawton. And the division surgeon believes that many cases of diphtheria and measles in the camp have been contracted in Lawton. The stringent quarantine order was issued to reduce the cases of sickness in camp to the lowest possible number and to keep it down.

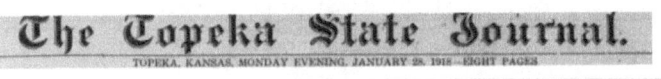

TOPEKA, KANSAS, MONDAY EVENING, JANUARY 28, 1918—EIGHT PAGES

BIG LINER GOES DOWN
Stayed Afloat After Hit by Torpedo,
But Efforts to 8ave Her Fail.

TOPEKA STATE JOURNAL

London, (Jan. 24, 1918) — The Cunarder Andania, reported yesterday to have been torpedoed but not sunk, went to the bottom in spite of efforts to get her into port, according to Information reaching the Associated Press today.

The Andania was torpedoed off the Ulster coast on Sunday morning. Press dispatcher from Belfast said it was believed no deaths resulted from the explosion. The Andania, 13.405 tons, was built in 1913 and has made many trips between British and American ports.

200 IN LIFEBOATS, LAND
Crew Also in Boats — Suffered Extremely from Weather

A Coast Town in the County of Antrim, Ireland, Jan. 28. More than 200 passengers and members of the crew of the Cunard liner Andania were landed here Sunday afternoon. Most of the crew were in a pitiable condition. Some were clad lightly and had suffered severely from their exposure in the lifeboats. Many were wrapped in blankets. Two babies were carried ashore by the sailors.

It was reported here that the explosion of the second torpedo had killed five stokers. Rescue of so large a number was explained from the fact that at the moment of the attack, the crew was preparing for boat

3

drill. The submarine which hit the Andania was twice seen, once twenty yards distant and again fifty.

Haste Caused Camp Illness, Says Gorgas

Surgeon General Tells Senate Hurried Mobilization Overcrowded Men

~~~~

Agrees Rush Was Necessity, However Emphasis Laid on Need of Observation Camp for All Recruits

NEW YORK TRIBUNE

Washington, D.C. (Jan. 26, 1918) – From Surgeon General Gorgas, the Senate Military Committee today sought light upon the health and sanitary conditions in the army, resuming its investigation suspended a few days ago to present the reorganization legislation about which centers the committee's controversy with the Administration. General Gorgas reiterated statements, made in his official reports to the department after a tour of inspection, that the crowding of men into cantonments and camps not ready to receive them was largely responsible for the epidemics of disease which have raged at some of the posts. He agreed with other officers who had preceded him on the stand, however, as to the necessity for hurried training.

"Wouldn't it have been better to have waited until the cantonments were ready, "asked Senator Frelinghuysen.

"From a physical standpoint, yes." the general replied, "but I think the training of these men should not have been delayed."

Conditions Now Improving

Hospital construction was stopped last summer, that barracks might be erected faster, he explained, and no camp hospital is complete now, though, sanitation conditions are improving, as shown by recent mortality reports.

General Gorgas emphasized the need for observation camps, the establishment of which is being considered, saying much sickness could have been avoided had there been such places where men reporting at a camp could be kept fourteen days.

While he said men should be dressed in warm clothing, the general told the committee he did not consider clothing shortage as an important factor in the pneumonia epidemic, explaining that control or avoidance of the germ was the principal point to be considered.

General Gorgas said he did not lack authority and had not been interfered with. He said he was not consulted in the selection of campsites, but that, except Camp Funston, Kansas, all were admirably located from a sanitation standpoint. Hospital plans are drawn by his department, he said, but under a plan of decentralization, he had nothing to do with selecting the place in the camp where hospitals were to be located.

Says Coordination Is Lacking

Senator Wadsworth suggested that lack of central power could be held largely responsible for overcrowding and inadequate clothing supplies. He said lie had been informed that the War Department expected to send the National Guard to France before winter, but bad not cooperated with the Shipping Board to the extent of requisitioning tonnage to send it across.

Questioned about hospital ships, General Gorgas said the question had been taken up by him seven or eight months ago, and that he was expecting a decision every day. He had been told it had

been decided that the navy would control these ships. It takes from two to three months, he said, to rent a transport so that it can be used for a hospital ship.

The general described the extensive plans being made for army hospitals outside the camps. It is hoped, he said, to provide 100,000 beds, and established hospitals have offered the department as many as 40,000 beds besides.

Physicians Called Ample

The 14,000 physicians in the service are declared, are ample to take care of the men now under arms, he said the army had the "cream of the profession," and when Senator Weeks suggested civilian doctors might have to help out, General Gorgas replied: "The shoe is on the other foot, as army doctors might be called upon to do the work of civilians."

Of the new Psychological Board, which is studying qualifications of officers and men, the general said he had little confidence in the system when first undertaken but now regarded it a really efficient asset to the department.

237 DEATHS IN ARMY
Slight Increase Over Previous
Week Due to Bronchitis and Influenza.

THE TOPEKA STATE JOURNAL

Washington (April 4, 1918) – The health of the army in the United States continues good, the war department announced today, although bronchitis and influenza complicated with pneumonia in many northern camps, increased the non-effective and death rates slightly over the preceding week. The total number of deaths reported was 237, of which 90 were among the regulars; 29 in the national guard and 118 in the national army.

MAD DOG AT WHITE HOUSE MAKES DASH AT SHEEP

White House policemen and secret service men were thrown into a near-panic yesterday when a mad dog slipped through the gates to the White House grounds and was making a wild dash for President Wilson's flock of sheep when stopped by a policeman from another part of the grounds.

The dog was said to have a well developed case of rabies, but was caught before any damage had been done.

SCHOOLS OPEN NEXT MONDAY

The Quarantine Regulations to Be Called Off Then.

PUPILS MUST ALL BE VACCINATED

County Health Officer Makes This Requirement Before They Enter School.

THE LIBERAL DEMOCRAT

Liberal, Kansas (April 25, 1918) – The closing order is to be called off in time to open school Monday morning unless further outbreaks of contagion occur, and this is not looked for by the County Health Officer and the physicians of the town.

The number of new cases has abated to the point where the authorities deem there is no further danger and have given permission to proceed with the schools.

The only stipulation is that pupils must either be vaccinated or show proof of successful vaccination within the past seven years.

There has been a wholesale vaccination among the children, and there is no kick in this ruling.

It would seem that all danger is past, and the prompt action of the health officials in causing the quarantine regulation is perhaps responsible for stamping out the spread of disease.

PART TWO
The Summer of 1918

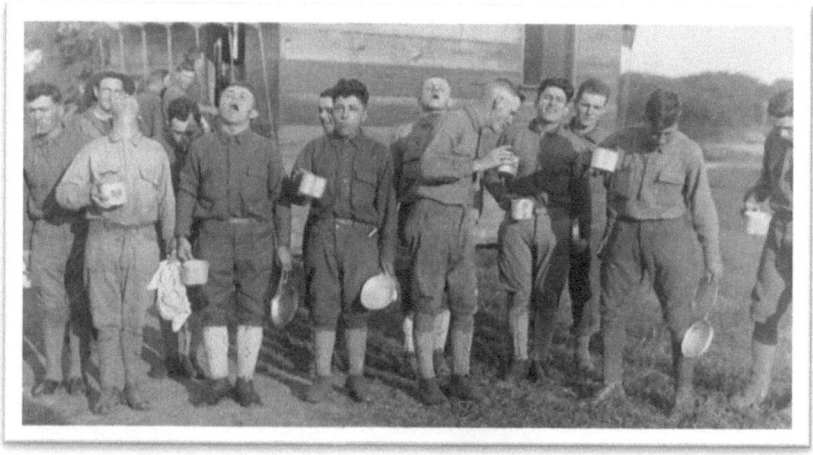

Soldiers at Camp Dix were gargling to ward off flu germs.

Going Forward to Camp Dix, N. J.

ST. MARY'S BEACON

Leonardtown, Md. - The following colored selects will entrain for Camp Dix., N. J. on or about August 22:

Moses Chas. Brooks, Park Hall

Wm E. Courtney, Hermanville
Geo. Arthur Scott, Beauvue
Richard Dade, Mechanicsville,
Wm. Arthur Bond, Morganza
Jos. McKeldry Jordan, Hollywood
Jesse Gant, Dameron
Wm. Briscoe Curtis, Blakiston
Chas. H. Jones, River Springs
Jas. R. Hungerford, Pearson
Alonzo Fenwick, Pearson

Jos. Hillery Neale, Leonardtown
George D. Forrest, Washington
Jas. Francis Barnes, Beachville
Lewis Grover Trent, Compton
J. Herman Cooper, Park Hall
Thomas Holly, Mechanicsville
Wm. Arthur Somerville, Compton
Joseph T. Edison, Pearson
Thomas Barnes, Drayden
James T. Dorsey, Abell
Jos. Lee Edwards, Hollywood
Ernest Barber, St. Mary's City
Harry Alex. Thomas, Hurry
Arthur Philip Thomas, California
Wilbur M. Smith, Ridge
James Gladden, Mullins, W. Va.
Harry Thompson, Washington
George Clayton, St. Geo. Island

To Go to Camp Sevier

The following colored registrants will go forward to Camp Sevier, S. C. on Thursday, August 1, 1918:

Charles H. Jones, Oakville
Robert J. Smith, Leonardtown

James H. Bond, Palmers
Henry J. Collins, Abell
John Henry Moore, Washington
Frank Alfred Armstrong, Ridge
Geo. A. Stephens, Baltimore
Benj. Jas. Gross, Piney Point
Jas. Lee Thomas (Jodie Bush) Leonardtown
Wm. A. Herbert, Loveville
John Holland Shaw, Clements
Benedict Brooks, Leonardtown
Sylvester Briscoe, Charlotte Hall
Wm. Howard Herbert, Morganza
Rodney Bowen, California
Jas. Leonard Bankins, Hollywood
John Wesley Jamison, Scottland
Geo. Arthur Scott, Beauvue

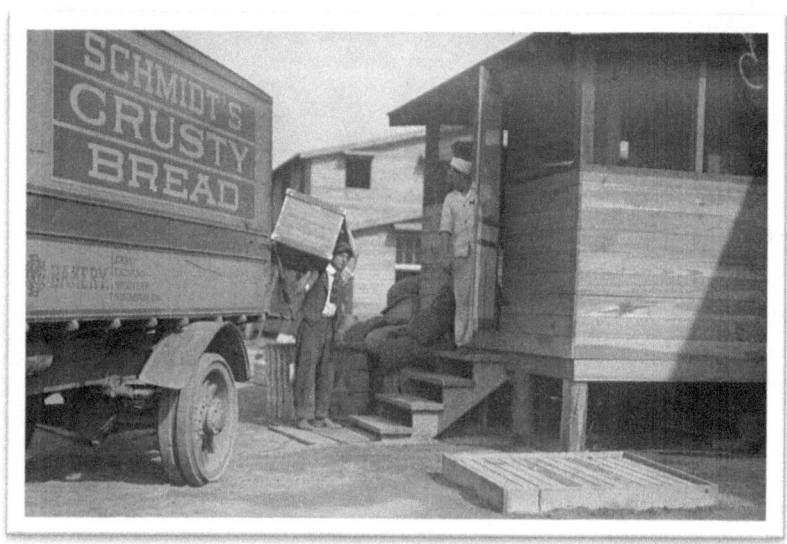

Schmidt's Bread delivery at Camp Meade in Maryland in 1918.
Library of Congress. Harris & Ewing

To Go to Camp Meade

Leonardtown, Md. (July 11, 1918)

The following have been selected to go to Camp Meade on or about July 22, 1918:

Richard S. Cusick, Oraville
Thos. Elmer Jenkins, Mechanicsville
Michael Kurtzman, St. Mary's City
Jas. Gustav Senner, Wash. State
Howard K. Purcell, Valley Lee
Clarence T. Taylor, Beechville
Robt. Irving Harrison, Chaptico
Wm. A. Owens, Dynard
Neal Fenwick, Leonardtown
Tony D. Delozier, Scotland
Manly Loundes Joy, Hollywood
Thos. Henry Fenwick, Scotland
*Bruce Johnson Quade, Hurry
*E. Burroughs, Oraville
(*) Alternates

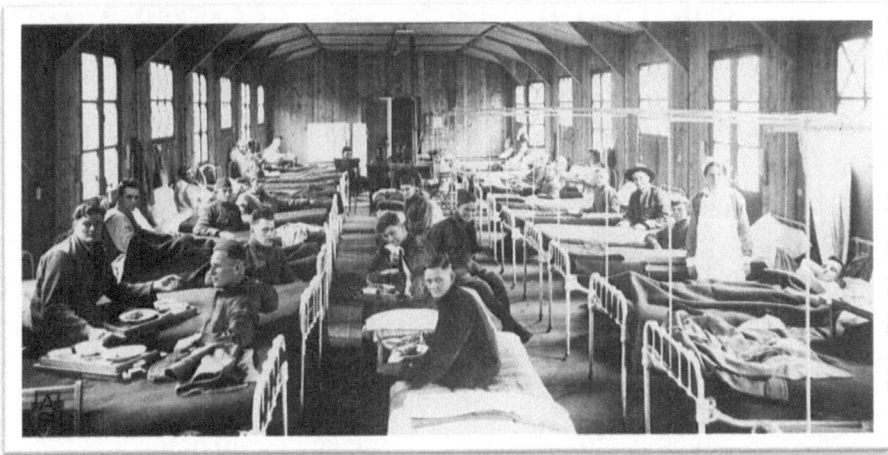

U.S. Army field hospital set up in France for treatment of flu victims.

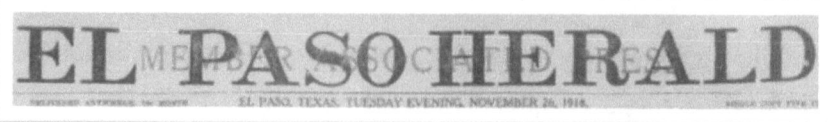

SOLDIERITIS IS LATEST
DISEASE OF EL PASO GIRLS

El PASO HERALD

El Paso, Texas (Aug. 16, 1918) – "Soldieritis" they named the new disease that appeared at the Union Station on Wednesday. A girl, about 15, was passing along the way to a train when a bunch of soldiers parted for her to go through. In the midst of them, she screamed and fell into the arms of one of them. Immediately, she revived, took two steady steps, repeated the performance, and then again. After the third act, the matron appeared and took her in charge. Scientists are looking for the germ and cultivating vaccine for securing immunity from the disease.

PUBLIC SCHOOLS TO OPEN SEPTEMBER 16TH

THE HERALD

New Orleans, La. (Sept. 5, 1918) – The public schools of New Orleans open for the term of 1918-1919 on Monday, Sept. 16, and Prof. J. M. Gwinn, superintendent of schools on Saturday sounded the warning that every child should be prepared to enter the schools at 9 a.m. that morning.

Prof. Gwinn, with the aid of the City Board of Health and the medical profession, has mapped out a program for the vaccination of pupils. A child who has not been vaccinated will not be permitted to enter the schools.

Physicians will be at McDonogh No. 4 school, corner of Alix and Bermuda Streets between 9 and 11:30 am on the following dates to vaccinate all children who are going to attend school:

September 9 and 10, for white pupils of the fifth district.

September 11 and 12, for colored pupils of the fifth district.

LARCENY OF CLOTHING

THE HERALD

New Orleans, La. (Sept. 5, 1918) – Lawrence Williams, who is known by the alias "Up Jump the Devil," was arrested by Corporal Hyde and Patrolman Hoffman at the head of Morgan Street, Friday, on a capias from the First City Criminal Court, where he is charged with the larceny of clothing, which he is alleged to have stolen while engaged in the pressing and cleaning business.

Part Three – Fall 1918
The Grip Tightens

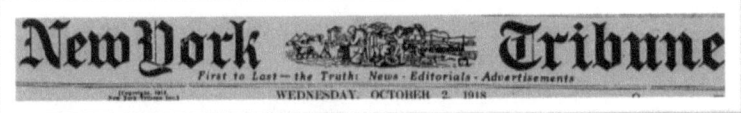

F. D. Roosevelt Has
Pneumonia After
Influenza Attack

Assistant Secretary of Navy Stricken on
Ship Returning from Europe

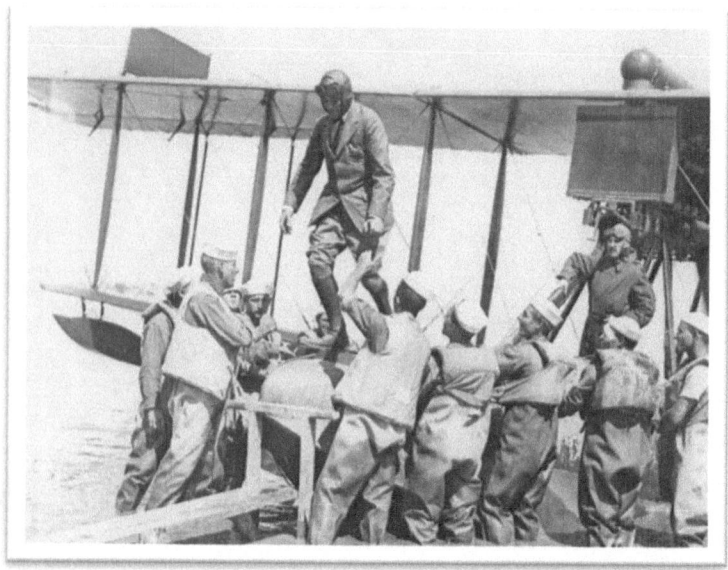

Assistant Navy Secretary Franklin D. Roosevelt debarks from a seaplane in France. *National Archives*

NEW YORK TRIBUNE

Sept. 20, 1918 – Franklin D. Roosevelt, Assistant Secretary of the. Navy, who has been in France and England, was taken yesterday to the home of his mother. Mrs. James Roosevelt, 47 East Sixty-fifth Street, suffering from pneumonia, following Spanish influenza. He was removed as soon as possible after the arrival at an Atlantic port of the government ship on which he was a passenger.

The case of pneumonia was said to be a light one, and Mr. Roosevelt's condition is not regarded as serious. He contracted influenza on the voyage, and his case is said to be one of several that developed on the trip from Europe. Mrs. Roosevelt said that her son's physicians expected a quick recovery. His return to Washington, however, will be delayed for several days.

Josephus Daniels. Secretary of the Navy, who announced in Washington the arrival of Mr. Roosevelt, made public at the same time a cable message to Mr. Roosevelt from Sir Eric Geddes, First Sea Lord of the British Admiralty. It was, in part:

"The spirit of comradeship between your navy in European waters and ours, both in administration and operation, has long been a source of pride to us. It is an additional satisfaction that you should have personally observed it and returned to the United States bearing witness to the sincerity of our brotherhood in arms and unity of purpose."

Dr. Royal S. Copeland, Health Commissioner, conferred yesterday in his office with transportation and theatrical men on an anti-sneezing campaign, which he intends to launch as a counteroffensive to Spanish influenza.

Those present offered cordial cooperation to prevent unguarded coughs and sneezes from spreading germs in public places, and "The Subway Sun" will issue an "extra" dealing with the matter. The following placard will be posted prominently:

"To prevent the spread of Spanish influenza, sneeze, cough or expectorate if you must, in your handkerchief. You are in no danger if everyone heeds this warning."

Forty-seven new cases of Spanish influenza had been reported yesterday to the Department of Health. Of these all but ten were positive, and the others were suspected cases. Five of the positive and the ten suspected cases were found in Manhattan, three in Queens, one in the Bronx, and twenty-eight in Brooklyn. Of those in Brooklyn, seven were private cases, and four were in hospitals, while seventeen were of men from ships and military camps.

Of the seventeen last mentioned, thirteen of the patients were taken from one vessel to the Kingston Avenue Hospital, and two of them have the complication by which the disease sometimes becomes fatal pneumonia.

Influenza Grips Thousands at Navy And Army Bases

AVER, Mass. (Sept. 14, 1918) – Five thousand soldiers at Camp Devens were under treatment at the base hospital today, a majority of them ill with influenza. Six deaths occurred overnight.

Lieutenant Colonel C. C. McCormack, the division surgeon, said the influenza epidemic was on the wane. New patients admitted yesterday numbered 600, while 500 were discharged.

NEWPORT, R. I., (Sept. 19, 1918.) – Influenza, which has been prevalent among the men in the Second Naval District, was on the wane today. Three deaths and new cases were reported, a decrease of 160 cases from yesterday. Nine hundred patients in the naval hospital here are about ready to be discharged.

GREAT LAKES, Illinois., (Sept. 19, 1918) – With about 1,000 cases of a mild form of influenza at the naval training station hire, the medical authorities said today the disease is under control.

Influenza Causes 48 Deaths In Day In New England

BOSTON, (Sept. 19, 1918) – Deaths from influenza and pneumonia in the twenty-four hours ended at 10 o'clock tonight showed a falling off in various sections of New England. In this city, seventeen deaths were reported, as against about twice that number yesterday forty-eight deaths were recorded New England to-day. There were more than seventy yesterday. Health authorities were inclined to the opinion that influenza and resulting pneumonia had run their course and that the fair-weather would prevent a further spread.

Spanish Influenza of 1918 Ignored, Engaged, And Defeated as World War Raged
NO SPANISH INFLUENZA HERE
Health Department Not Alarmed at Prospect of Outbreak

BALTIMORE SUN – Sept. 20, 1918

BALTIMORE, MD. – Health Commissioner Blake declared yesterday that the department felt no anxiety whatever as to any threatened outbreak of Spanish "flu" or any other form of infectious disease at this time. He said that so far as the department was aware, there was not a case of the "flu" in Baltimore.

Discussing the disease, which seems to have alarmed other large municipalities in the country, Dr. Blake went back to the epizootic in 1870. He said it first attacked animals, principally horses, and tied up the streetcar lines, then operated by horsepower.

It later broke out among humans, and caused considerable concern, having been followed by serious cases of bronchitis and pneumonia, many of the latter disease proving fatal.

"In 1890, we had another outbreak, similar to the one in France at the same time," Dr. Blake went on to say. "It was then called la grippe. Now comes along another outbreak, and we are asked to change the name of our old acquaintance and call it Spanish influenza because it started in Spain."

"Not a single case has been brought to the attention of the Health Department, and there is no special reason that I know of to fear an outbreak of this disease in our city. Of course, at this time of year, we expect, and do have many affections of the respiratory tract."

FLU BLOCKS SOUSA
FAMOUS BAND UNABLE TO
START ON LIBERTY LOAN TOUR

Chicago. (Sept. 22, 1918) – Because of the prevalence of Spanish Influenza at the Great Lakes Naval Training Station, the Liberty Loan campaign tour of Lieut. John Phillip Sousa and the Big Band schedule to star tonight has been canceled. It was feared the sailors might carry the disease into the civil communities. It is hoped to make the trip later.

Ravages in Army Camps

New York, (Sept. 22, 1918) - Spanish Influenza continued its rampage in army camps about New York today, although the city health authorities reported not a case had been discovered during the day among civilians.

A Camp Dix. N.J., 14 deaths resulting from the disease have been reported in the past 21 hours. A number of new cases were isolated, but camp physicians say the epidemic is under control.

Only one death was reported from Camp Mills today. Fifty-two soldiers suffering from the disease were removed to the base hospital.

Camp Devens Has 28 Deaths

Ayers. Mass. (Sept. 22, 1918) – Twenty-eight deaths among the soldiers at Camp Devens were reported by the army authorities today. With 200 fewer cases in the camp hospital, however, the authorities were confident that the disease was on the decline.

An order issued tonight made effective the quarantine declared by the town of Ayers against the soldiers at the encampment. Until further notice, no soldier will be allowed to go into the town without a written pass. The quarantine does not apply to officers.

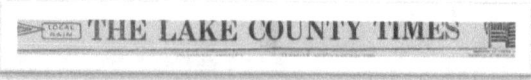

THE LAKE COUNTY TIMES
Hammond, Ind. (Sept. 24, 1918)

GOT THE FLU?
WHAT TO DO

Boston Health Chief Calls Rest, Sunshine, and Prophylactic Measure Important; Disease Raged in the 14th Century.

- Keep feet and clothing dry.
- Avoid crowds.
- Protect your nose and mouth in the presence of sneezers.
- Garble your throat three times a day with a mild antiseptic if only salt and water.
- Don't neglect a cold.
- Keep as much as possible in the sunshine.
- Don't get "scared."

It is found in the blood, though here it is comparatively inactive, and in enormous numbers, where it is coughed up to renew its pernicious work. This germ forms toxins or poisons which continue on the rampage long after apparent recovery.

It exerts such a general devitalizing effect on the tissues that other dangerous micro-organisms which ordinarily are held in check run riot, and catarrh, pneumonia, and similar conditions develop. It particularly attacks over-worked and weakened organs, such as the heart and lungs. For this reason, rest, nutrition, warmth, and tonics are important factors in its treatment.

There is no known serum or antitoxin that will make a person immune to Spanish Influenza. Salts of quinine, aspirin, and Dover's powder afford some relief, the doctors in Boston found.

Surgeon-General Gorgas of the Army advises the use of dichloramine as a nose and throat wash, but not one in a thousand druggists ever heard of it.

Measures of Precaution.

Precautionary measures are simple.

Keep away from Infected persons.

The sick should be separated from the healthy. Sputa should be received in vessels containing disinfectant.

Promiscuous spitting and coughing should be absolutely prohibited.

Antiseptic gauze masks should be worn, and great care exercised in handling clothing and all articles that have come in contact with the stricken.

Only by loyal and intelligent cooperation of the general public can the epidemic of Spanish influenza be prevented from spreading throughout the country and hampering our war work.

Do your bit.

BUY A LIBERTY BOND TODAY

MANY ILL IN HAMMOND

Hammond has been hit hard by the so-called Spanish Influenza though doctors say they see no difference between it and the old-fashioned grippe. A great deal of sickness is reported, and doctors are kept pretty well on the jump. The disease is highly infectious, and, in some cases, whole families are down with It.

No fatalities have so far been reported.

320 NEW "FLU" CASES THERE
BY UNITED PRESS

CHICAGO, Sept. 24 The Influenza epidemic at Great Lakes naval station is under control, according to a statement today from the Commandant Moffet's office.

During the last twenty-four hours, 320 new cases have developed as against 440 for the previous twenty-four hours, it was said. No figures were given out as to the number of men in the hospitals or the number of deaths.

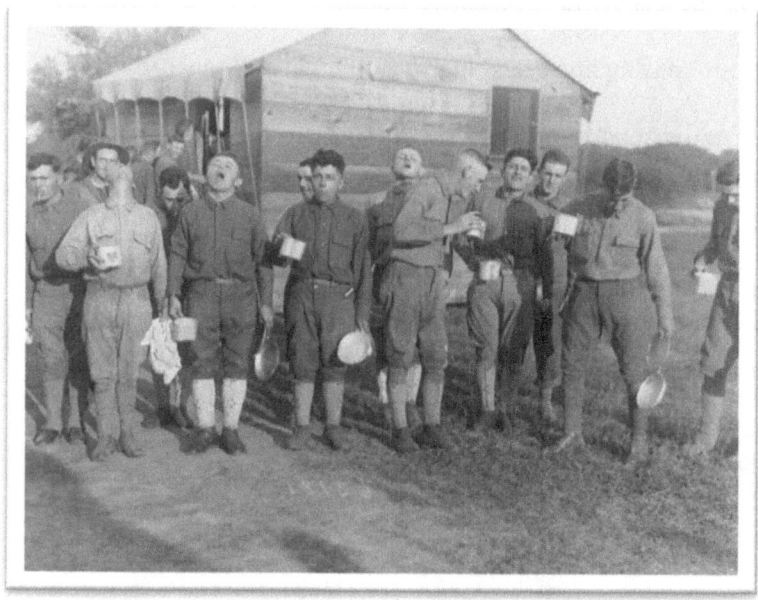

Soldiers at Camp Dix, New Jersey.

1,800 ILL FROM "FLU" AT CAMP DIX
BY UNITED PRESS

NEWARK. N. J. Sept. 24, 1918 – Eighteen hundred soldiers of Camp Dix were in the camp base hospital today, victims of Spanish Influenza. Of this number have developed pneumonia and are in a serious condition. Thirty-four soldiers have died.

EPIDEMIC SPREADS IN BOSTON
BY UNITED PRESS

Boston, Mass. (Sept. 24, 1918) – With the death toll from the epidemic influenza mounting steadily, the schools of Boston were closed at noon today until the disease is stamped out. There were approximately 100 deaths in the twenty hours ending today. Of them, seven were among men in the first naval district. Officials also reported seventy new cases among the sailors this morning.

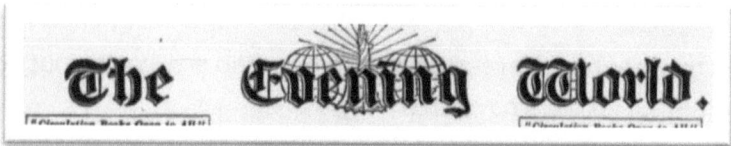

U. S. WILL FIGHT INFLUENZA
SPREAD AS WAR MEASURE

Nursing Units Operating Under Government to Be
Provided in Epidemic Areas.

BACILLUS IS ISOLATED.

Rome Surgeon Announced He Has Found Germ, While
Search Goes on Here.

NEW YORK EVENING WORLD

WASHINGTON, D.C. (Sept. 26, 1918) – Stamping out of Spanish
Influenza, which has extended to more than a score of army camps and
many sections of the country, has been recognized by the Government
as a war measure.

Medical and nursing units today were mobilized in communities where
the epidemic has gained considerable headway under the general
direction of a central committee representing the Public Health Service,
the army, the navy, and the American Red Cross.

Home defense units will be organized with such nurses as may be
spared from other duties, mid each unit placed at the disposal of the
central committee. Where local funds and buildings are not available,
these will be obtained by the Red Cross, which also will open emergency
hospitals.

ROME, (Sept. 26, 1918) – Prof Ciauri, director of the military hospital at
Cotrone, announced today that he had discovered and Isolated tho
bacillus of Spanish Influenza.

The disease, which was brought In by repatriated prisoners, Is raging throughout the country.

Dr. Royal B. Copeland, Health Commissioner of New York, said this morning that the Rome despatch was reassuring and that he believed Dr. William H. Park of the Health Department had made the same discovery.

"Dr. Parke has been working in the laboratory of the Health Department trying to discover the bacillus," said Commissioner Copeland. "I believe he has succeeded, but he has been too modest to announce the result of his work."

"I am agreed with Dr. Parke that influenza we find with us now is not entirely new in form but is just a special form of streptococcus not found in the old Pfeiffer bacilli or Influenza germ."

Dr. Parke, when seen this morning at the Board of Health Research laboratory, stated that he was devoting all his time to an attempt to isolate the bacillus of the new disease, but that be had accomplished nothing as yet. His research showed, he declared, that the bacillus of the ordinary Influenza was dominant in the disease

Mr. Copeland said that Spanish Influenza has not reached an epidemic stage in Ney York and that he has no intention of advising the closing of the schools.

One hundred and seventy-four new cases of Spanish Influenza for the twenty-four hours ending at 10 A. M today, as against 172 cases reported on the previous day, were announced by Health Commissioner Copeland.

The figures were given as follows Manhattan, 68 (35 men, 27 women) Brooklyn, 47 (29 men, 27 women), Bronx 45 (25 men, 20 women), Richmond 11 (6 men, five women), Queens (3 all women), making a complete total of 86 men and 84 women.

The largest number of cases reported from any individual district yesterday was from Hoboken, where there were 1,025 sufferers in the various military camps.

"1 do not think it necessary to close schools," Dr. Copeland said. "There is no epidemic in this city. Closing the schools would be evidence of hysteria rather than good judgment. The number of cases here is negligible when compared with the Immense population, and since the first of July, we have had less than 500 influenza victims, and a large proportion of these were soldiers and sailors."

A dispatch today to The Evening World from Syracuse, N.Y., says that there are 1,700 cases of Spanish Influenza at Camp Syracuse and that ten deaths have occurred from the malady in the last twenty-four hours. The dispatch declares that there is a serious shortage of medical attendants at the camp and that hospitals are overcrowded.

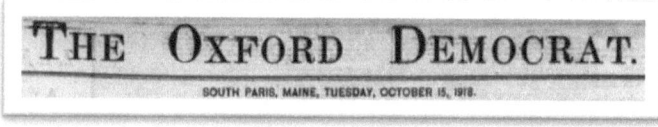

THE OXFORD DEMOCRAT.

SOUTH PARIS, MAINE, TUESDAY, OCTOBER 15, 1918.

Soldiers Die from Influenza.

OXFORD DEMOCRAT – (Oct. 1, 1918) – The epidemic of Spanish influenza, which is now raging so fiercely in many places in the country, especially in some of the cantonments, took a heavy

toll of our soldiers. Several Oxford County men have succumbed to it during the past week.

Private Cecil S. Brown of Norway died with pneumonia following influenza at Camp Devens Wednesday morning, the 25th. Mr. Brown was the son of Mrs. Ella (Myers) and the late Herbert O. Brown of Norway and was born in Bethel Jan. 18, 1893, coming to Norway fourteen years ago. He graduated from Norway High School in 1912, spent one year at the University of Maine, and then took the course in the law school of that institution, graduating in 1917.

After being admitted to the bar, he opened an office for the practice of law in Norway but was soon engaged as chief clerk of the Oxford County Local Board and continued in that work until early in September, making an efficient and courteous official. Being of draft age, he was examined and classified as qualified for limited or special service. Early in September, he went to Camp Devens, expecting to be inducted into the service for clerical work with local boards. Still, upon being examined, there was Inducted into the general service and assigned to the supply department.

He was a member of the Commercial Club and the Algonquin Tennis Club of Norway and several social organizations. '

He is survived by his mother and two sisters, Mrs. Arthur Parker of Norway with whom be lived, and Mrs. Elmer Parker of Bath. He Is also survived by three half-brothers and two half-sisters.

Mrs. Herbert Chapman of North Newry and Mrs. Nellie Wheeler of Lynn, Walter Brinck of Bethel and Percy, and Arthur Brinck of Newry.

Private Brown's remains were brought to Norway, arriving on Saturday, and the funeral was held at 1 o'clock that afternoon at the Norway Methodist Church, attended by Rev. H. L. Nichols, the pastor, Rev. M. O. Baltzer of the Congregational church participating in the service. Mr. Brown was a member of the Methodist Church. Burial was in Pine Grove Cemetery.

Private William Harvey Snow of Norway died early Tuesday morning at the hospital at Camp Devens. He was born in Norway, Maine, on Feb. 28, 1891, and was the son of Harvey Snow, who died some years ago. He was educated at Norway High School and worked aa shoemaker in that town until called into service June 26, 1918. He was a member of Norway Camp, Modern Woodmen of America.

He is survived by his mother, Mrs. George Currier of Norway; four brothers, Robert, and Roy, who are in the service overseas, Winnie of Bath, and Perley of Norway; and three sisters, Mr. Carl Pratt of Auburn, Mrs. Carl Robinson of South Paris, and Mrs. Thomas Corby of Lewiston.

The remains of Private Snow were brought to Norway, under the escort of a comrade, arriving on Friday, and the funeral was held at the Norway Baptist Church at 2:30 pm Saturday, attended by Rev. G. H. Newton, the pastor. Burial was in Rustfield Cemetery.

Corp. Verne Allie Thomas of Paris died at Camp Devens of pneumonia Wednesday, Sept. 25, after a brief illness. His aunt, Mrs. Bessie Walker of Lewiston, was summoned and went to Camp Devens on Sunday preceding. Corp. Thomas was born 28 years ago in Paris and has always lived there, except for brief absences at work elsewhere. He was the son of Jesse and Elizabeth Ella Thomas. He is survived by his father, who lives at Hicks Crossing, South Paris, and three brothers, Claude of Otisfield, Frank of North Hoosick, N. Y. and Alton, who now is overseas, going over in the regular army and now overseas. His mother is also living. He was called June 25th and went to Camp Devens on the 26th. His corporal's stripes were received shortly before he was taken ill.

The funeral of Corp. Thomas was held at 2 o'clock Sunday, at Spiller's undertaking rooms in Norway, attended by Rev. C. G. Miller. Burial was in Pine Grove Cemetery.

Charlie H. Rowe of Buckfield died at Camp Devens on Thursday. He was the oldest of eight children of Mr. and Mrs. Mordaunt L. Rowe and was 21 years of age. He went to Camp Devens on the third of September. The remains were brought to his home in Buckfield, where his funeral was held on Saturday.

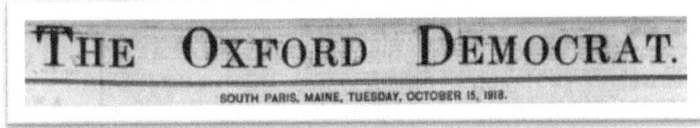

All Public Gatherings Suspended
SCHOOLS, CHURCHES, ETC.,
CLOSED BECAUSE OF INFLUENZA

OXFORD DEMOCRAT

Paris, Maine (Oct. 1, 1918) – By order of the local board of health issued Sunday noon, all schools, churches, theaters, and public gatherings are closed for the present week at least.

This is on account of what Is called the 8panish Influenza or grippe. The malady did not make its appearance here until later than in many other places, but it got a quick hold here. There are now said to be now fifty cases of it In South Paris, and three times as many in Norway.

The home visitation by the churches and Sunday Schools, which was set to begin at S o'clock Sunday afternoon, was necessarily postponed to some later date, though most of the workers had assembled at Deering Memorial Church before they knew of the closing order.

Among the affairs which will be postponed was the business lecture which was to be given by L. P. Zehring at Savoy Theatre Tuesday evening, and the district convention of the Knights of Pythias, which was to have been held with Craigie Lodge at Oxford on the same date.

Callup Deferred Due to Influenza Sweeping Army Camps

Oxford County Draft Notes.

OXFORD DEMOCRAT

Paris, Maine (Oct. 1, 1918) – Apportionment of the 861 men to be called in October from Maine for Camp Devens was announced Thursday. Oxford County's quota Is 51. This will more than exhaust the Class 1 men {remaining from all registrations previous to September, the number in that class supposed to be available now being 47.

These men were to have been called to entrain during the five days beginning Oct. 10 but owing to the prevalence of influenza at the army camps ol the country, the call will be postponed, and the date is not yet fixed.

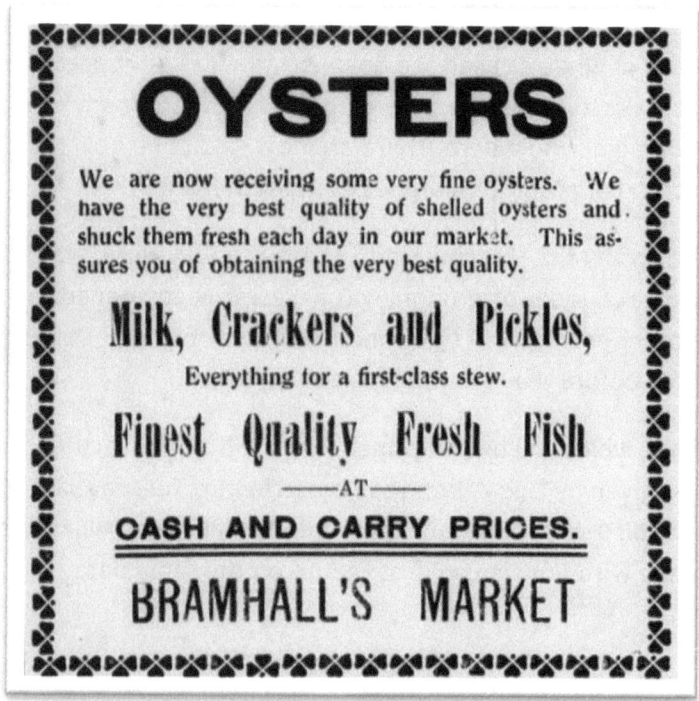

SPANISH INFLUENZA

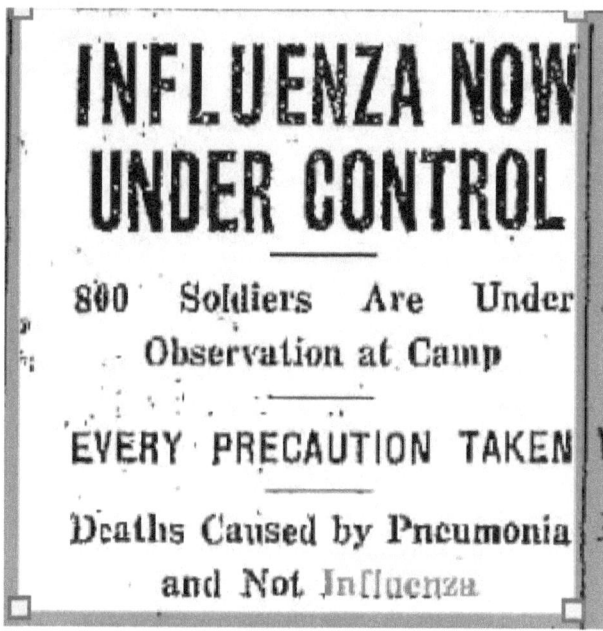

The Des Moines News

INFLUENZA NOW UNDER CONTROL

800 Soldiers Are Under Observation at Camp

EVERY PRECAUTION TAKEN

Deaths Caused by Pneumonia and Not Influenza

EVERY PRECAUTION TAKEN
Deaths Caused by Pneumonia
and Not Influenza

DES MOINES NEWS

Des Moines, Iowa (Oct. 2, 1918) – Medical officers at Camp Dodge believed Wednesday that that has the epidemic of Spanish Influenza well in hand.

Approximately 300 more soldiers have been placed in the base hospital for observation, bringing the total from Sunday up to 800.

Examination of more than half of this number has brought out only 181 cases of Spanish Influenza. An official report of this number has been sent to the surgeon general in Washington.

The fact that so many men are placed under observation shows that the precautionary measures medical officers say, which are being taken.

Lieut. Col. E. W. Rich, the division surgeon, issued a statement Wednesday, correcting the report made in his office by the base hospital that three deaths occurred from Spanish Influenza Tuesday.

Die of Pneumonia

"Further examination of these particular cases," Colonel Rich said, "shows death resulted from pneumonia and no evidence of the influenza was found, as was first reported."

A big force of medical officers and their assistants is working day and night in the base hospital laboratories, examining cultures from the throats of the men under observation, to determine which ones are infected with influenza.

Anti-Spitting Law

The City Council will be asked by Dr. W. C. Witte, city health officer, to enforce the anti-spitting ordinance to prevent infection from Spanish influenza.

Three cases of ordinary influenza or grippe have now been recorded, and every doctor in the city have been sent a personal letter by Dr. Witte asking him to report all cases immediately.

"Spanish Influenza has nothing to do with a bad cold," says Dr. Witte. "but it is a parasitic disease. It spreads swiftly because of the rapid incubation of the germ. It exerts such a general devitalizing effect on the tissues that other dangerous microorganisms run riot, and catarrh, pneumonia, and similar conditions develop."

Precautionary Measure

Simple measures of precaution by which it may be prevented as given by Dr. Witte, are:

- Keep away from infected persons.
- The sick should be separated from the healthy.
- Sputa should be received in vessels containing disinfectants.
- Promiscuous spitting and coughing should be absolutely prohibited.
- Antiseptic gauze masks should be worn by all attendants on a case.
- Public towels and drinking cups should be avoided and great care exercised in handling clothing and all articles that have come in contact with the stricken.

VACCINATION IS OPPOSED
Howe Presents a Petition Against Ordinance

DES MOINES, IOWA (Oct. 2, 1918) – The vaccination question was discussed pro and con in a heated argument of three hours duration before the city council Wednesday by Judge Howe, who presented a petition against it and Dr. W. C. Witte, city health officer, defending it.

The petition contained names of some of the Des Moines members of the American Medical Association, as well as citizens who oppose compulsory vaccination of school children.

According to testimony, two Des. Moines children have been made ill following vaccination.

Judge Howe presented as an amendment to the ordinance, clause now in effect in Cleveland, Ohio and Portland, Oregon, providing for exceptions to the compulsory rule excusing children whose parents submit, satisfactory evidence that they are opposed to vaccination on principle, or that the child is an unfit subject for vaccination.

The efficacy of vaccination was defended by Dr. Witte, and the city's legal right to make such action compulsory was asserted, as a war measure.

The matter was referred to the city's legal department for consideration.

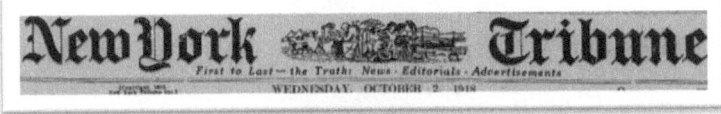

GOD BLESS YOU!

Two Habits Influenza Has Given Us

NEW YORK TRIBUNE

New York, N.Y. (Oct. 2,1918) – If you fall a victim of influenza and amid your sneezing exclaim, "God bless you!" after the manner of many persons who sneeze, you will unconsciously be repeating a prayer that had its origin in one of the earliest known epidemics of influenza. This epidemic visited the south of Europe in 491, and few persons escaped its ravages. Its symptoms were severe pains in the head and uncontrollable sneezing and yawning.

There were no health departments in those days to order sneezers to employ a handkerchief as a muffler to prevent the spread of the disease germs, but nevertheless, the sneezing was recognized as a peril. Upon one of the attacks of sneezing overtaking a victim, his solicitous friends would give vent to a pious "God preserve you!" or "God bless you!" And when the sufferer would find himself unable to control his yawns, he would make the sign of the cross in front of his mouth.

Gradually it became the practice for the sneezer himself to say, "God bless you!" or "God save us!" and from making the sign of the cross to evoke divine aid in stifling a yawn, he resorted to covering his mouth with his hand as a mark of politeness.

Anti-Influenza Serum Made In Tests Here

City's Scientists Develop Vaccine To Be Used as Preventative

Death Rate Jumps As Disease Spreads

Health Chief Reports 836 Cases in 24 Hours—175 Pneumonia Deaths

How Spanish Influenza Can Be Checked

Sneeze, cough, or expectorate (if you must) into your handkerchief. You will be in no danger if everyone heeds this warning.

By order of the Board of Health.

ROYAL S. COPE LAND,

President.

New York, N.Y. (Oct. 2, 1918) – An effective serum for the prevention of Spanish influenza has been discovered by the city's scientists, working under the supervision of Dr. William H. Parke, and preparations are underway for its manufacture in quantities. It will be distributed to physicians as fast as it can be made. This statement and a sudden increase in the number of new cases and death rates in New York featured the report of Health Commissioner R. S. Copeland last night.

The anti-toxin developed in the city laboratories is a product entirely independent of that announced as a discovery within the last few days by the Public Health Service at Washington.

Dr. Copeland yesterday sent a telegram to Surgeon General Blue, of the War Department, requesting details regarding the Washington serum and its use.

Not Designated as Cure

The New York anti-influenza serum, it is emphasized, is purely a preventive and is not for use as a curative treatment after the disease has developed.

No details have yet been given out as to the constituency of the vaccine or its methods of application, except that it is introduced as other preventative anti-toxins by inoculation.

A total of 836 new cases of influenza in twenty-four hours has not yet alarmed the health authorities. It is supposed that many of the cases reported yesterday should have been included in the Sunday report. The fact that no reports were filed on Sunday has often led physicians to delay in making statements, and Tuesday's figures have come to be recognized as containing cases that rightly belonged in earlier charts. The total cases of pneumonia for the twenty-four hours reached 130, while the deaths from influenza and both lobar and bronchial pneumonia totaled 122. Forty-seven of these were credited to influenza alone.

Still for Open Schools

"I am still of the opinion," said Commissioner Copeland, "that the schools should be kept open. The children are freer from the danger of infection in the schoolroom than in the streets. I have been informed by the management of the subways, elevated lines, and surface car lines that they are doing everything possible to cooperate with us, and unusually strict sanitary measures are in effect."

"I feel that the increase in the number of cases shown by the day's report is no cause for panic or hysteria. The figure is still small when compared to the city's population, and we must expect a gradual growth of the disease. This gradual growth, coupled with the fact that the majority of the patients who take care of themselves are fully recovered in three days, gives us ample opportunity to give treatment to all those afflicted.

"Our quarantine stations at the railroad terminals are proving an effective means of nipping the spread of influenza here."

Many Nurses Volunteer

The appeal for more nurses has met with gratifying responses. The Association for the Improvement of the Condition of the Poor has volunteered to look after many private cases in homes, and the Y. W. C. A. Training School for Nurses' Aids has offered to assist in the city hospitals where there is a shortage of both orderlies and nurses.

Recent autopsies are disclosing the fact that fully one-third of all the fatal cases of secondary lobar pneumonia here are induced by Spanish influenza. Dr. Parke reports that the pure influenza bacilli have been found in the lungs of those who have died of the lobar type of pneumonia within the last few days.

While the health authorities are making every effort to show a smiling face and a calm exterior while discussing the reassuring angles of the situation in New York, there is an undercurrent of apprehension.

Prospects Are Encouraging

The sudden jump in the number of new cases and deaths, while explained away to a large extent by the official view, does not serve to illumine the prospect for the immediate future.

It is very evident that the figures for the next few days will indicate definitely whether or not the disease is actually under control in New York or whether the city faces a disastrous scourge, such as that under which Boston and other Eastern cities have been

suffering for weeks.

Several interesting points in connection with the epidemic are shown by figures compiled in the offices of the Department of Health. The deaths from influenza and secondary pneumonia during the last week show a heavy mortality preponderance among males, 87 men to 9 women. In the grippe epidemic of 1916-18, the death toll was largely taken among females.

Men 15 to 45 Hit Hardest

The heaviest mortality is also found among persons between fifteen and forty-five years of age, in spite of the fact that between these ages, some 200,000 men have been removed from the city by the war. In influenza, the fifteen-to-forty-five rule is found to hold good in 70 percent of the deaths, and in pneumonia, the average is 95 percent.

The appearance of the disease so early in the season is without precedent. Grippe epidemics have never appeared here earlier than December and frequently not until March.

Commissioner Copeland has issued a direct appeal to the dispensers of drinks to use paper cups as a means of preventing the spread of the disease.

He strongly intimates also that he may find it convenient, if the appeal does not have the desired effect, to order paper cups used exclusively as an emergency measure.

Boy Scouts Are Helping

The Boy Scouts of America are contributing their efforts to the Health Department's fight by helping to enforce the anti-spitting section of the sanitary code. Cards are being printed bearing the words, "You are violating the Sanitary Code," and these will be placed in the hands of the scouts, who will hand one to every person seen expectorating on the sidewalk. This offense carries with it a maximum penalty of $250 fine or six months' imprisonment.

The 836 new cases appeared in the following boroughs: Manhattan, 378; Bronx, 143; Brooklyn, 204; Queens, 51; Richmond, 60. The pneumonia reports show the following division: Manhattan, 92; Bronx, 14; Brooklyn, 15; Queens, 6; Richmond, 3.

Chairman Charles B. Hubbell of the Public Service Commission yesterday forwarded a letter to the heads of all the city's transportation companies requesting them to give marked attention to sanitation in the care and conduct of their cars and also at stations. '

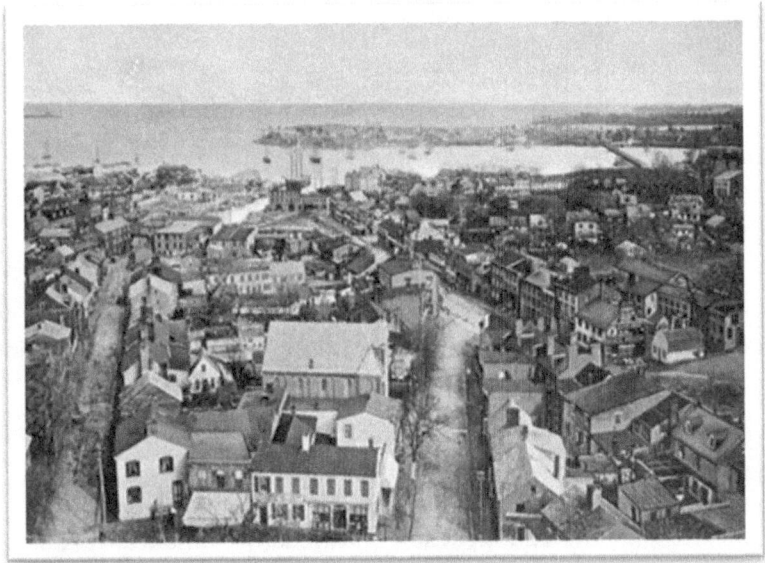

Annapolis looking towards Eastport.

MORE 'FLU' CASES; VICTIMS INCREASE
Each Day Finds New Case of Spanish Influenza Reported
in Town
WHO'LL BE THE NEXT?

Evening Capital

ANNAPOLIS, MD. (Oct. 2, 1918) – Another member of the Capital force has fallen by the wayside and is ill of "Flu." This makes the3 number out of this office five, but still, the Capital lives.

At the city post office, two of the clerks and carriers are victims of the disease. Mr. Alex Proskey is very sick at his home at West Annapolis.

Mrs. G. Wythe Munford has joined her husband, who has been ill for several days, with an attack of "Flu."

Mr. and Mrs. Harry M. Heidler and two children, of 131/2 Dean Street, are confined to bed with the Spanish Flu.

Mr. Eugene Igehart is a victim of the Flu.

Several members of the family of Mr. Vansant, Conduit Street, are sick with the disease.

Messrs. Nees, Melvin Cranford, Munford, Reese Abbott, and the janitor, Harrison Harried, all of the Capital Office, are confined to their respective homes ill from the Flu.

News has been received here of the slight improvement in the condition of Mrs. William Sullivan, wife of Ensign Sullivan, U.S.N., who has been critically ill of Flu in Boston, Mass., Mrs. Sullivan's sister, Miss Ella Small, are both sick with the disease.

Mr. William H. Small, the youngest son of Mrs. James Small, is very sick of Flu, at his residence on North Street, and Miss Mollie Miller, her niece, is confined to their room with an attack of Flu.

Mrs. Annie J. Munroe and daughter, Miss Mary, are victims of Flue.

Mr. John M. Green, the assistant cashier of the Annapolis Bank, is at home sick with influenza.

Three daughters in the family of Chief of Police O'Berry are ill of Flu.

Mr. Leonard A. Clark, of Dean Street, is another "Flu" victim.

Three other victims of the "Flu" are Wilmer, substitute carrier of the city post office, and his brothers, Robert and Carl Basil, sons of Mr. and Mrs. Frank N. Basil, West Street.

Mrs. C. H. Foster, wife Instructor Foster at the Naval Academy, is confined to her home by sickness. Her son Charles Pratt has been and is still sick.

Flu has made inroads on the force of the local post office. Superintendent of Mails, V. D. Russell, is ill of Flu. Temporary Carrier

Frank W. Basil is a victim, and even the post office janitor, Sam Peters, is down with the Flu. Special Messenger Stevens is also reported today another victim.

SPANISH "FLU" PUTS BAN ON ARMORY DANCE

Weekly Entertainment for Service Men at State, Amory is Called Off

Annapolis, Md. (Oct. 2, 1918) – The prevalence of Spanish influenza in the town and the restriction placed by reason of quarantine upon the servicemen, has caused the regular weekly dance at the State Armory, Bladen Street, to be called off tomorrow night.

There will consequently be no dance for men of the service given this week by the War Camp Community Service.

After careful thought and deliberation, this course was thought by the Hostesses; the Secretary, Mr. Roland, and the official committee, to be the proper one, and the action was taken to suspend dances until the contagion now prevalent throughout the city has subsided.

The calling off of the dance is a source of great regret to many but inasmuch as all medical authorities advise not mingling with the disease, it was deemed the best course, besides there are so many of the servicemen under the restriction that to give the dance would practically mean for the girls to dance with each other.

Tomorrow night's dance was the last to have been giving by the War Camp Community Service under the present committee and the present official Hostesses.

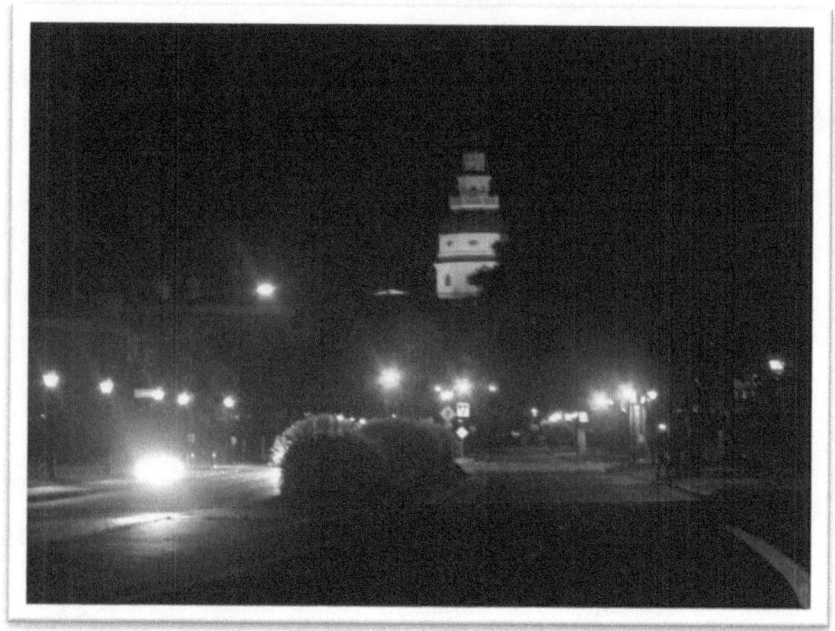

The Maryland State House is the oldest state capital building in continuous use in the United States. *THE CHESAPEAKE TODAY photo*

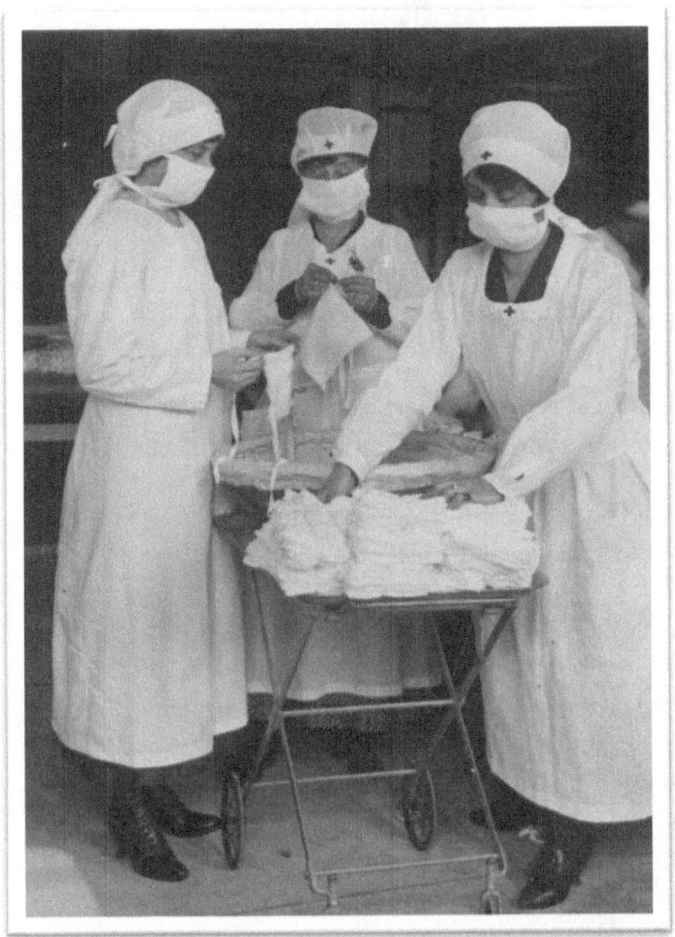

CRITICALLY ILL

Bradford, the elder son of Lieut. B. B. Bowie, U.S.N. and Mrs. Bowie, Conduit Street, near Gloucester, is critically ill of pneumonia, following influenza.

The younger son, Robert, is also seriously sick.

"FLU" CAUSES THE PUBLIC SCHOOLS TO BE CLOSED

Order Issued This Morning After Consultation with School Authorities and Health Officer

288 CASES IN THE GRAMMAR SCHOOL

Many Teachers Afflicted and Sick Pupils Cause Closing Of Schools For Few Days

Annapolis, Md. (Oct. 3, 1918) — With 288 cases of influenza in the Grammar school and a number among pupils in the High School, it was deemed necessary after a consultation between the County Board of Education, the Trustees, and the City Health Officer. Dr. William S. Welch to close the city schools for a few days.

No special date for the reopening was set, but it is hoped the schools may be open in at least a week.

For the past few days, the infection has been gradually spreading among the students of the school until yesterday, the number of children who were reported sick of the disease was alarming. Some classes were depleted to such an extent that only a handful was left. Many teachers in both the High and Grammar school were also sick, and it was impossible to secure substitutes.

In one class of 53 pupils, 46 were home ill with influenza. Accordingly, pupils who assembled at the school this morning were immediately dismissed and were told the school is closed until further notice.

Superintendent George Fox, when approached today on the subject, said he hoped the schools would be closed but for a few days, but as a precautionary measure and because of the depleted condition of the attendance, the closing was deemed expedient.

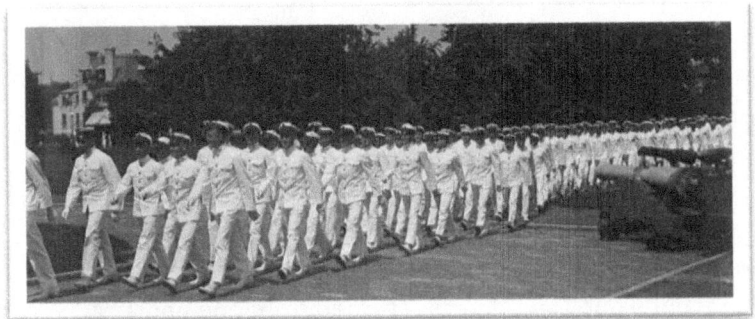

United States Naval Academy Graduates in 1917.

Photo by Harris & Ewing

MIDSHIPMAN McDUFFIE, CLAIMED BY DEATH
Member of the Third Glass a Victim of Pneumonia

Midshipman W A. McDuffie, a member of the third class at the Naval Academy, died at 8:30 o'clock. This morning at the Naval Hospital.

Death was due to pneumonia, following influenza. His is the first death in the regiment of over two thousand midshipmen since the "flu" made inroads here.

Midshipman McDuffie was a native of Columbus. Ga.

Funeral arrangements have not been completed, as the authorities at the Naval Academy are awaiting advice from his home.

The death of the young midshipman has cast a deep gloom over his comrades as the Academy.

LT. CHAPLIN EVANS, LAID TO REST
Funeral of Naval Academy Graduate, 1916,
Took Place at Alexandria, Va.

SAD CIRCUMSTANCES

Dying from pneumonia, following influenza, upon his return from overseas after an eighteen months' service, the death of Lieut. Chaplin Eppes Evans. U. S. N,, of Alexandria, Va., was surrounded by peculiarly sad circumstances.

His death occurred at Bridgeport, Conn., at 4.30 p. m. September 30, 1918, where he had been detailed for special work along submarine lines. Only recently had Lieut. Evans returned from one and a half years' destroyer duty in European waters when he was sent to New England, where "flu," in its worst form, is epidemic. He fell a victim and died in a few days following the attack.

Chaplin Evans will be remembered here as one of the most popular of the midshipmen at the Naval Academy during his four years' course. He was identified with the basketball squad, the varsity football squad, varsity crew, and boxing teams. He always took a prominent place in athletics and was the most popular midshipman. His death came as a great shock to his many friends here.

It is peculiarly sad, as Lieut. Evans was an only son, his father being an Army officer, now serving in Europe.
The funeral took place yesterday afternoon from St. Paul's Episcopal! Church, Alexandria, Va., the services, being conducted by the Rev. Sydney Key Evans. U. S. N., Chaplain of the Naval Academy.

PHOTO WITH EVERY DAILY TRIP
Commuters On Short Line Are Two-Faced. Say They Can Stand It If Conductors Can
LONG-SUFFERING ROAD

Oct. 3, 1918 Evening Capital

Everybody who travels on the Short Line, or at least everybody who commutes with a sixty-trip mileage book, between Annapolis and Baltimore, has had his or her picture taken.

Photographers have been almost as busy as the Draft Board, or the doctors, (the few of them who are left in town) attending cases of "Flu." The new order went into effect Tuesday, requiring photos to be pasted in mileage books.

It has been a case of "Look Pleasant Please," ever since the edict went forth that all commuters between the two cities on the Short Line had to present their photographs with each trip. There is a variety of styles In these photos. Some side faces, some three-quarter face, while others are full face pictures. But present your picture you must, if you would ride on the Short Line daily, and they do.

This state of affairs was brought about after the road had been victimized time without number by those who, desiring to get something for nothing, tore out the unused coupons of last month's trip book, and pasted in this months, or passed the book on to another making the trip back to Baltimore after they had arrived in Annapolis.

The long-suffering Short Line (if things can be long and short at the same time) could stand the deception no longer and took strenuous action by requiring a picture with every trip. Sounds like a cracker and cheese with every drink. The commuters say they can stand it if the conductors can. At any rate, every sixty-trip commuter is two-faced and shows both each time he rides on the Short Line.

SATURDAY'S GAME IS CALLED OFF

The football game scheduled for Saturday between St John's and Delaware College has been called off because of the quarantine existing at the local college. However, on the following Saturday, the ball will be started down the field in earnest. Twenty- five men even now are in St. John's moleskins, so it can be seen that Coach Wilson will have quite a formidable bunch ready for the initial fracas.

"FLU" ON INCREASE NEW CASES REPORTED

Many Events Called Off on Account of Infection.
Seems to be General Throughout City and County

ANNAPOLIS, MD. (Oct. 3, 1918) – Many new cases of Spanish influenza were reported today in the city and county. The infection, instead of subsiding, seems to be on the increase everywhere. At Camp Meade 1,756, cases are reported, and there have been many deaths. Last night over 100 coffins were shipped to the cantonment near Annapolis for dead bodies of Flu victims. The plague that had its inception in the New England States, where it has been most fatal, is spreading far and wide.

Every precaution should be taken to avoid its ravages.

A little child of Mr. and Mrs. Harry M Heidler, Dean street, is reported in a dying condition the result of pneumonia following the Flu.

Today, Mr. Holloway, State Supervisor of Schools in this county, was to come here for a trip through the county to inspect schools, but word came he is ill of Flu.

Mrs. Charles B. Abbott is a victim at her home on Conduit street.

Mrs. Keller is quite ill of Flu at the home of her mother, Mrs. Muhlmeister, West street.

Mrs. Joe Muhlmeister. of the county is reported seriously ill of influenza.

In one class of the Grammar school, nine pupils were stricken yesterday with the Flu.

Mrs. C. H. Foster, wife of Instructor Foster, of the Naval Academy, who has been nursing her son, Charles Pratt, ill of Flu, is now a victim of the disease.

Mrs. Waters Chaney, a stenographer in the office of Mr. W. G. Gott, is another victim of the Flu.

Miss Helen Hunter, one of the teachers in the Grammar school, is suffering from influenza.

Mr. F. S. Bullard. 16 Revell street is very sick of Flu.

Five in the family of Clerk of the Court, William N. Woodward, are victims of influenza.

Lieut. Commander James McDowell Cresap, U. S. N., is quite ill at his residence on Franklin street, another Flu victim.

Miss Sarah V. Sutherland, the Public Health Nurse, is a victim of Flu. Her patients are being sent to the Emergency Hospital.

Mrs. Nees, the wife of Mr. Benjamin Nees, of the Capital Office, is ill of influenza. Her husband has been sick for several days.

Mrs. A. Edward Dove is very ill at her home at Eastport, suffering from "flu." Mrs. Dove was formerly an assistant clerk in the office of the Capital.

Carrier boy Charles Johnson, of the Capital, is sick with the "flu."

MORE SCHOOLS CLOSED

Dr. J. J. Murphy. County Health Officer ordered the schools at Eastport, West Annapolis, and Linthicum Heights to be closed on account of the epidemic of Spanish influenza prevailing in the respective neighborhoods.

THE EVENING CAPITAL AND MARYLAND GAZETTE.
ANNAPOLIS. MARYLAND. FRIDAY. OCTOBER 4. 1918.

WOMEN WANTED TO MAKE MASKS
Twenty Thousand Influenza Masks
Asked for By the Red Cross

THE EVENING CAPITAL

Annapolis, Maryland (OCT. 4, 1918) – Twenty thousand influenza masks are needed immediately by the Red Cross for use at nearby camps. Hundreds of women are needed to make them.

The faster they are supplied, the more likelihood of checking the scourge, which is temporarily incapacitating thousands of Uncle Sam's fighting men.

The masks are being used not only for influenza sufferers but also for experimental purposes as a means of preventing the spread of the infection.

How much are you going to give
To this vital work today?

The workroom at the headquarters of the Hospital Supply Service, Druid Hill Avenue, and North Eutaw street Baltimore was open from 10 till five today and from 7.30 till ten this evening. The Eleventh Ward Community Workhouse, 916 North Charles Street. Baltimore will keep the same hours.

Drop whatever you are doing and enlist with the Red Cross. Lives hang in the balance while you hang back.

PRIVATE CONNOLLY, OF MEDICAL CORPS, DIES AT CAMP MEADE

First Annapolis Boy To Make "Supreme Sacrifice" Death Due to Pneumonia

CALLED TO COLORS ON LAST MAY 28TH

Member of Odd Fellows and Bricklayer's Union. Funeral on Sunday Afternoon

Private James M. Connolly, son of John W. Connolly, watchman at the Naval Academy, of 210 King George Street, died yesterday afternoon, October 3, 1918, at Camp Meade.

Death was due to pneumonia, following influenza, from which he had been suffering for about three weeks.

The young man, who was just 28-year- old, was called to the colors in the select draft that left here on May 28, 1918, for Camp Meade. He was later detailed to the Medical Corps at the cantonment and was expecting to go overseas in a short time. His father had visited him a few days ago, having been notified of the son's critical illness, but found his boy in a serious condition at that time.

The deceased lived with his father, his mother, having passed away some years ago. Besides his father, he is survived by a brother, John M. Connolly, of Albany, N. Y.

Young Connolly was before being drafted, employed as a bricklayer with the W. E. Feldmeyer Co., contractors, and had worked on Bancroft Hall. He was a member of Annapolis Lodge of Odd Fellows, and of the Bricklayers and Masons Union of this city, both of which organizations will attend the funeral which takes place on Sunday afternoon at 3 o'clock from his father's residence, 210 King George Street, the Rev. Dr. H. W. Burgan, of the First Methodist Episcopal church, of which he was a member, officiating.

The deceased is the first Annapolis boy, called to the colors, to make the "supreme sacrifice."

20,000 CASES THERE
In Philadelphia, the "Flu" Is Raging Without Check
THE TOPEKA STATE JOURNAL

Philadelphia, Penn. (Oct. 3, 1918) – City health authorities today appealed for the assistance of additional physicians and nurses to combat the spread of Spanish Influenza, which has crowded all private and public hospitals. Young doctors who have not practiced in Philadelphia but hold diplomas can be used in the present emergency and will be paid $75 a week. It is estimated there are 20,000 cases of influenza in Philadelphia.

First CLASSMAN VICTIM OF "FLU"
Midshipman H. F. Latta, Of Indiana, Died
This Morning at Naval Hospital
THIRD DEATH FROM "FLU"

Annapolis, Md. (Oct. 5, 1918) Midshipman H. F. Latta, a member of the First Class, Naval Academy, died this morning at 8:40 o'clock at the Naval Academy after an illness from Spanish Influenza, which developed into pneumonia.

Young Latta was a native of Goshen, Indiana, and is the third member of the regiment of midshipmen to die of the disease now prevalent throughout the United States.

Midshipman Latta was popular with his classmates and a great favorite with all who knew him. He had made many friends in the city who were shocked by his death.

Funeral arrangements await word from the young man's family.

It is probable the body will be sent to his home for burial, as in the other two of midshipmen who died the past two days, victims of the disease prevalent here and everywhere.

There are said, to be no other serious cases at the hospital at this time, and those existing are well in hand.

YOUNG MOTHER CLAIMED BY DEATH

Mrs. Newton Long, A Native of Annapolis, Passes Away
In Hagerstown

ANOTHER "FLU" VICTIM

Information was received here this morning by
telephone from Hagerstown of the death of Mrs. Mary Long,
wife of Mr. Newton Long, and daughter of Mr. and Mrs.
William R. Abbott, of Washington, formerly of this city.

Death was due to pneumonia, following influenza. The deceased was born in Annapolis and was about twenty-five years old. Besides her husband, she is survived by an infant a few months old, her parents and ten sisters and brothers. Her sisters are Mrs. Edward Farley, of Washington, Mrs. James Shehe, of Washington; Misses Katherine and Elizabeth and little Kenly Abbott and Mr. Francis Abbott, U. S. Navy; Private David Abbott, of the Army; Masters Ernest and Willis, are her brothers.

Mrs. Long was one of eleven children born to Mr. and Mrs. Abbott, and her death is the first among them. She was well known here, where she grew to girlhood and has frequently visited. She was a granddaughter of Mrs. William M. Abbott, this city, and Mrs. David O. Parlett.

Her death is peculiarly sad as she leaves a three-month-old infant. She was a graduate of the Washington High School and also Business College, and possessed of a pleasing personality, happy disposition, and noble character.

The funeral will take place on Tuesday from her late residence in Hagerstown.

HOLLADAY SCHOOL ORDERED CLOSED

As a precautionary measure against the spread of Spanish influenza, the Health officer has advised the closing of the Holladay School, a private institution, taught by Miss Lucy Holladay, and a corps of assistants.

While there are no cases in the school, it is deemed advisable to close the school during the prevalence of influenza, and there will be no session of the Holladay school next week.

Colored School
NOTICE!

Owing to the prevalence of influenza in Annapolis, the Health Department has ordered that the Colored Schools remain closed until further notice.

W. B. OVERTON, Principal

FEW WAR MOTHERS TO PARADE

But few- War Mothers were able to go to Baltimore today to participate in the parade in the interest of the Fourth Liberty Loan. This was due to so much sickness in the several families of the War Mothers, and the desire to run no risk by getting into crowds.

A few left names with Secretary Roland of the War Camp Community Service, out not so many as were expected.

NO INDOOR GATHERINGS

Through an order issued at the Naval Academy, there will be no indoor gatherings at the institution during the prevalence of influenza.

All services at the Chapel are suspended, all Y. M. C. A. meetings and everything of the nature of assembly indoors.

SPANISH INFLUENZA IS THREE-DAY FEVER CALLED THE "FLU"

The United States Public Health Service Issues Statement as To Causes of Disease
IS IT NEW? DOES IT COME FROM SPAIN?

Cover Up Each Cough and Sneeze.
If You Don't, You'll Spread Disease

The disease now occurring in this country and called "Spanish Influenza" resembles a very contagious kind of "cold" accompanied by fever, pains in the head, eyes, ears, back or other parts of the body, and a feeling of severe sickness. In most of the cases, the symptoms disappear after three or four days, the patient rapidly recovering; some of the patients, however, develop pneumonia or inflammation of the ear or meningitis, and many of these complicated cases die. Whether this so-called "Spanish" influenza is identical to the epidemics of influenza of earlier years is not yet known.

Epidemics of influenza have visited this country since 1647. It is interesting to know that this first epidemic was brought here from Valencia, Spain. Since that time, there have been numerous epidemics of the disease. In and 1890, an epidemic of influenza, starting somewhere in the Orient, spread first to Russia and thence over practically the entire civilized world. Three years later, there was another flare-up of the disease.

Both times the epidemic spread widely over the United States.

Although the present epidemic is called "Spanish influenza," there is no reason to believe that it originated in Spain. Some writers who have studied the question believe that the epidemic came from the Orient, and they call attention to the fact that the Germans mention the disease as occurring along the eastern front in the summer and fall of

1917.

There is as yet no certain way in which a single case of "Spanish influenza" can be recognized; on the other hand, recognition is easy where there is a group of cases. In contrast to the outbreaks of ordinary coughs and colds, which usually occur in the cold months, epidemics of influenza may occur at any season of the year; thus, the present epidemic raged most

intensely in Europe in May, June, and July. Moreover, In the case of ordinary colds, the general symptoms (fever, pain, depression) are by no means as severe or as sudden in their onset as they are in influenza. Finally, ordinary colds do not spread through the community so rapidly or so extensively, as does influenza.

In most cases, a person taken with Influenza feels sick rather suddenly.

He feels weak, has pains in the eyes, ears, head or back, and may be sore all over. Many patients feel dizzy, some vomit. Most of the patients complain of feeling chilly, and with this comes a fever in which the temperature rises to 100 to 104. In most cases, the pulse remains relatively slow.

In appearance, one is struck by the fact that the patient looks sick. His eyes and the inner side of his eyelids may be slightly "bloodshot," or "congested," as the doctors say.

There may be running from the nose, or there may be some cough. These signs of a cold may not be marked; nevertheless, the patient looks and feel very sick.

In addition to the appearance and the symptoms as already described, the examination of the patient's blood may aid the physician in recognizing "Spanish influenza," for it has been found that in this disease, the number of white corpuscles shows little or no increase above the normal. It is possible that the laboratory investigations now being made through the National Research Council, and they will furnish a more certain way in which individual cases of this disease can be recognized.

Ordinarily, the fever lasts from three to four days, and the patient recovers. But while the proportion of deaths in the present epidemic has generally been low, in some places the outbreak has been severe, and deaths have been numerous. When a death occurs, it is usually the result of a complication.

Bacteriologists who have studied influenza epidemics in the past have found in many of the cases a very small rod-shaped germ called, after its discoverer, Pfeiffer's bacillus. In other cases of apparently the same kind of disease, there were found pneumococci, the germs of lobar pneumonia. Still, others have been caused by streptococci, and by other germs with long names.

No matter what particular kind of germ causes the epidemic, it is now believed that influenza is always spread from person to person the germs being carried with the air along with the very small droplets of mucus, expelled by coughing or sneezing forceful talking, and the like by one who already has the germs of the disease. They may also be carried about in the air in the form of dust coming from dried mucus, from coughing and sneezing, or from careless people who spit on the floor and on the sidewalk. As in most other catching diseases, a person who has only a mild attack of the disease himself may give a very severe attack to others.

It is very important that every person who becomes sick with influenza should go home at once and go to bed.

This will help keep away dangerous complications and will, at the same time, keep the patient from scattering the disease far and wide. It is highly desirable that no one is allowed to sleep in the same room with the patient. In fact, no one but the nurse should be allowed in the room.

If there are cough and sputum or running of the eyes and nose, care should be taken that all such discharges are collected on bits of gauze or rag or paper napkins and burned.

If the patient complains of fever and headache, he should be given water to drink, a cold compress to the forehead, and a light sponge. Only such medicine should be given as is prescribed by the doctor. It is foolish to ask the druggist to prescribe and may be dangerous to take the so-called "safe, sure, and harmless" remedies advertised by patent-medicine manufacturers.

If the patient is so situated that he can be attended only by someone who must also look after others in the family, it is advisable that such attendant wear a wrapper, apron, or gown over the ordinary house clothes while in the sick room, and slip this off when leaving to look after the others.

Nurses and attendants will do well to guard against breathing in dangerous disease germs by wearing a simple fold of gauze or mask while near the patient.

It is well known that an attack of measles or scarlet fever or smallpox usually protects a person against another attack of the same disease.

This appears not to be true of "Spanish influenza." According to newspaper reports, the King of Spain suffered an attack of influenza during the thirty years ago and was again stricken during the recent outbreak in Spain.

In guarding against the disease of all kinds, the body must be kept strong and able to fight off disease germs. This can be done by having a proper proportion of work, play, and rest, by keeping the body well clothed, and by eating sufficient wholesome, and properly selected food. In connection with diet, it is well to remember that milk is one of the best all-round foods obtainable for adults as well as children. So far as a disease like influenza is concerned, health authorities everywhere recognize the very close relation between its spread and overcrowded homes. While It is not always possible, especially in times like the present, to avoid such overcrowding, people consider the health danger and make every effort to reduce the home overcrowding to a minimum. The value of fresh air through open windows cannot be overemphasized.

Where crowding is unavoidable, as in streetcars, care is taken to keep the face so turned as not to inhale directly the air breathed out by another person.

It is especially important to beware of the person who coughs or sneezes without covering his mouth and nose.

It also follows that one should keep out of crowds and stuffy places as much as possible, keep homes, offices, and workshops, well aired, spend some time out of doors each day, walk to work if at all practicable—in short make every possible effort to breathe as much pure air as possible.

"Cover-up each cough and sneeze,

If you don't, you'll spread disease."

TODAY'S CASUALTY LIST

HICKORY DAILY RECORD

Hickory, North Carolina (Oct. 7, 1918) – Total Number of casualties, including those announced Sunday, but not those announced today, were 40,671. In the number 7,990 were killed in action including 291 lost at sea; 2,586 died of wounds 1,992 died of disease, 960 died of an accident and other causes; 21,922 wounded in action; 5,221 missing in action, including prisoners.

The two lists issued today contained a total of 744 names, and Sunday's list contained 761 names.

The following are reported from North Carolina:

Killed in action: Lieut. Daniel C. Culbreth of Thomasville; Prlv. Fred Mathis of Parish.

Died of wounds: Privates Charles C. Riddle of Candor and Clarence L. Waters of Cherryville.

Wounded severely: Corporals Marshal L. Parsons of Norwood, Isaac C. Phillips of Bear Creek, Chatham County; Mechanic Walter C. Fitzgerald of Thomasville; Privates Gilbert E. Swindell of Thomasville, Hobert M. Flynn of Winston-Salem, Robert J. Hensley of Nealsville, Jesse D. Watson of Loray Substation, Gastonia, William A. Brown of Robersonville, John F. Hiatt of Thomasville Willie F. Croker of Ashboro.

Missing in action: Private William H. Leonard of Marshville, Jesse D. Grisdale of North Charlotte, John E. Wood of Sandy Ridge, Bennet Cornelius of Thomasville, Haymore Westmoreland of Thomasville, Walter L. Smith of Winston-Salem, Roscoe Brooks of East Durham.

HOWARD BOYD VERY ILL WITH INFLUENZA

A telephone message from Fishburne Military Academy yesterday announced that Howard Boyd, one of the Hickory boys in school there, had developed peritonitis and was being taken to the hospital at Staunton for an operation. Albert Miller was out of danger, and George Smith and Louie Whitener were reported to be doing nicely.

Miss Jo Moore, who has been attending King's Business College at Charlotte, has returned home for two weeks while the school is closed on account of influenza.

TWO MILLS CLOSE ON ACCOUNT DISEASE

The A. A. Shuford Mill Company and the Highland Cordage Company in Highland closed down on account of influenza. There are about 40 cases among the employees of these plants, Secretary A. A. Shuford said, but conditions are much better in West Hickory. Only five girls reported at one of the mills in Highland.

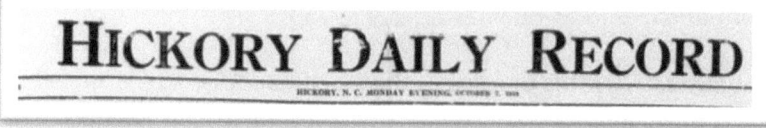

COUNTY IS PUT UNDER STRICT QUARANTINE

HICKORY DAILY RECORD

Newton, N. C. Oct. 7, 1918) – There was a slight increase in the number of influenza cases today, and Newton will quarantine all cases. The county board of commissioners today, in special session, took drastic action in the following order:

"Be it ordered by the board of commissioners that Catawba County, owing to the epidemic of grippe and Spanish influenza now prevalent that all schools, moving picture shows, fairs, circuses and other public gatherings, including church services, and Sunday schools are prohibited for a period of 14 days or longer as the situation might demand.

"Each physician is ordered to personally quarantine and placard each case for a period of 14 days, using white paper or cardboard with the words grippe or Spanish influenza written thereon.

"For violation of any of the above order, the person or persons will be prosecuted under Sections 9, 10, 14 and 15 of Chapter 52, Public Laws of North Carolina), session of 1911.

OSBORNE BROWN

Chairman Board of County Commissioners

CITY HAS QUARANTINED FOR SPANISH INFLUENZA

Schools, Churches, Theatres And All Public Meeting Places Closed Until Danger Passes —Fair This Year to Be Held on November 12

HICKORY, N. C. (Oct. 7, 1918) – President Clark announced this

afternoon that the fair dates had been changed to November 12-15 and that the institution would be held then. By that time, the disease should have run its course, and everything is right again.

City council last night in special session took drastic action to stamp out Spanish influenza and Mayor Young today issued closing schools, churches, theatres, and all public places where people gather.

In the list is included the Catawba County Fair, for which entries had been made, and all preparations completed for opening tomorrow at noon.

The school bells did not ring this morning. The church bells, with one exception, did not ring last night, and children will be kept off the streets.

A large gathering of citizens was before council with one voice when they recommended that the city goes into its own quarters. Earlier in the day, instructions from the state board of health had been received by Mr. J. W. Shuford, and these were turned over to Mayor Young, who called the council together. Messrs. J. L. Cilley, Eubert Lyerly, F. A. Abernethy, and A. P. Whitener and City Manager Ballew were all present, and members expressed themselves freely. Several citizens spoke, including Mr. A. A. Whitener, who gave it as his deliberate judgment that the council could do nothing less than close up all public gathering places. Messrs. N. W. Clark, J. F. Miller, and one or two showmen were present and spoke. It was agreeable to them to close up, and they realize that their business was ruined for the time being. Mr. Miller would have preferred a little more time, but he took the verdict good-naturedly, and the thing is a fact.

An ordinance drawn and passed last night is published elsewhere.

The greatest regret is expressed because the fair cannot be held at this time. Every arrangement had been made for it to open tomorrow at noon, speakers had been secured, a Y. M. C. A. had been erected, and the exhibits were on their way. An amusement company was in the city ready to show. The fair will be held during the week beginning November 12.

City Manager Ballew was authorized to employ such additional help as needed to enforce the ordinance, and he will utilize the services of Superintendent Carver and Principal Rhinehart of the North School and Principal Ramseur of the colored school to see that the quarantine signs are properly placed and enforced. Chief Lentz is the quarantine officer for this city and suburbs.

Dr. George Shipp of Newton, county health officer, Dr. T. F. Stevenson, and Drs. Blackburn and Hunsucker all expressed themselves in favor of closing. It would appear that there are about 200 cases in this section. There are 30 cases at Lenoir College, but all the patients are doing well.

Mayor Young said that the council a week ago had started to quarantine for the disease, but instructions had come from the state board of health not to do so. The authorities had acted on that advice. The state board has revised its ruling., but this can be explained by the fact that the national health service, which is more in touch with the disease, did not recommend quarantine until last Friday. The state board of health, backed by the governor and the state superintendent of public instruction, now asks that schools close and that everything is shut tight until the epidemic is stopped.

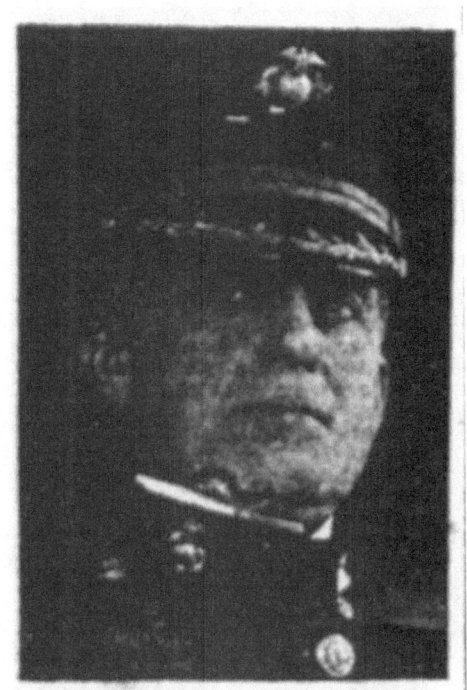

BRIG. GEN. C. A. DOYEN,
Commandant at Quantico Marine
Training Camp, Who Is Dead of
Pneumonia Resulting From
Spanish Influenza.

GEN. DOYEN IS INFLUENZA VICTIM

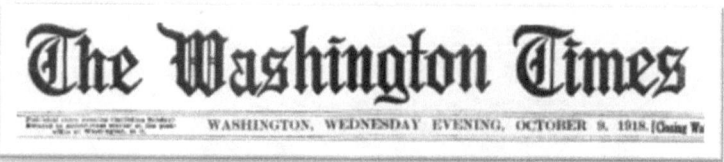

WASHINGTON, WEDNESDAY EVENING, OCTOBER 9, 1918. [Closing W

THE WASHINGTON TIMES
Washington, D.C. Oct. 7, 1918

The death of the first high military official In or near Washington as a result of the Spanish influenza epidemic is reported today from the marine corps training camp at Quantico, Va.

Brig. Gen. Charles Augustus Doyen, commandant of the camp, died at the Quantico base hospital at 9 o'clock last night.

He had been ill only a few days. Death was due to pneumonia, following an attack of Spanish Influenza.
General Doyen commanded the first regiment of Marines to go to France with General Pershing and was among the most famous officers of the Marine Corps.

Cadet In 1876

He was born September 3, 1859, in New Hampshire. General Doyen was appointed a cadet at the United States Naval Academy in 1876. He graduated in the class of 1881, having General Barnett, General Mahoney, and General Lauchheimer, of the Marine Corps, as classmates.

On July 1, 1883, General Doyen was commissioned a second lieutenant in the Marine Corps, and during his thirty-five years' connection with the marines served at every Marine Corps post in this country as well as in foreign lands. He saw service on many ships of the Navy and was close friends of Admiral Sims, commander of the American naval forces in European waters.

General Doyen received his commission as captain on June 2, 1898. He served during the entire Spanish-American War, being in command of the Marines on the St. Paul.

Becomes Colonel

In 1909, General Doyen was commissioned Colonel, and in May 1917, he was designated to command the first regiment of Marines to go to France. This regiment landed in France on June 27, 1917, and was quickly followed by a second regiment, the two forming the Fourth Marine Brigade, Second Division, American Expeditionary Forces. This brigade was part of the regular American Army and was among the very first to get into the fighting.

While in France, Colonel Doyen was promoted to be brigadier-general, receiving his commission on October 3, 1017, with rank as of March 26, 1917. He was subject to a survey of medical examiners in May 1918 and returned to the United States to become commandant of the Marine Corps training camp at Quantico, Va., which office he held at the time of his death. General Doyen made his home at Annapolis with his wife.

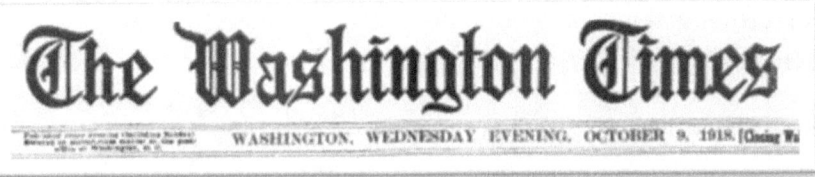

The Washington Times

WASHINGTON, WEDNESDAY EVENING, OCTOBER 9, 1918.

DISTRICT CHURCHES AND PLAYGROUNDS ORDERED CLOSED

The Commissioners today closed all churches and playgrounds in the District in the fight against the Spanish influenza epidemic.

The Commissioners issued an order that "all church services be omitted until further action by the Commissioners," because "indoor assemblages constitute a public menace."

Here is the official text of the Commissioners' order:

"Whereas the epidemic of influenza in the District of Columbia by its rapid spread threatens to impair the effectiveness of the machinery of the Federal Government, and, whereas, the Surgeon General of the United States Public

---

Washington, D.C. (Oct. 4, 1918) – The Commissioners today closed all churches and playgrounds in the District in the fight against the Spanish influenza epidemic.

The Commissioners issued an order that "all church services be omitted until further action by the Commissioners," because "indoor assemblages constitute a public menace."

Here is the official text of the Commissioners' order:

"Whereas the epidemic of influenza in the District of Columbia by its rapid spread threatens to impair the effectiveness of the machinery of the Federal Government, and, whereas, the Surgeon General of the United States Public Health Service and the Health Officer of the District of Columbia hare advised the Commissioners of the District of Columbia that Indoor assemblages constitute a public menace at this time, therefore, be It ordered by the Commissioner of the District of Columbia that all church services be omitted until further action by the

Commissioners.

The Commissioners today arranged for the closing to the public of the Congressional and Public libraries and the Corcoran Gallery of Art. Persons in the employ of the Government engaged in war work will be admitted to these buildings.

All Theaters Closed.

The closing of churches and playgrounds followed close on the order of the Commissioners shutting the doors of all theaters, motion picture houses, and dance halls. With the schools already closed, the Commissioners virtually have eliminated all public assemblages in the District.

Although no official statement has been made, it is understood that temporarily open-air meetings in the interest of the fourth Liberty Loan are to be permitted.

The number of cases of influenza reported to the District Health Department today is far in excess of the number reported on any previous day since the epidemic got a foothold,

but this Increase probably was due largely to the fact that more physicians are responding to the appeal of Commissioner Brownlow to make prompt report of all cases to the Health Officer

An order was issued today by the District Health Department compelling all nurses to report the name, age, sex, and color of persons having the disease. The nurses are required to sign their names to the report.

Only five more deaths among the civil population In the District were reported today. They are George Davis, colored, twenty-seven years old, Freedman's Hospital; Roy R. Painter, 235 H Street Northeast, eighteen years old; Catherine Semitone, twenty-seven years old, of 415 Twelfth

Street, Northeast; Edward J. Brown, of 827 Fourth Street, Northeast; and Joseph Garvey, twenty-four years old, of 6307 Blair Road.

Commissioner Brownlow today requested that all dances in homes and private establishments be stopped. He asks the cooperation of the young people in the city in carrying out this part of the program to prevent the spread of Influenza.

The "Daredevils," a vaudeville performance now being given at the American League Palk, has been ordered discontinued. Health Officer Fowler and Commissioner Brownlow decided that there was danger of spreading the disease at the assemblies at the park even though the performances were being given in the open air.

Commissioner Brownlow said today that he has the cooperation of the managers of all theaters In Washington and that they have heartily endorsed his action.

Mr. Brownlow said:

"I have received many telephone calls from theatrical managers, and they have all given hearty endorsement to my plan to check the spread of Influenza. While they realize they will have a great financial loss, they do not hesitate. In co-operating to the fullest extent with all orders."

Commissioner's Order.

Fifty-five moving picture houses seating 30,000 people, and eight theaters running vaudeville, music, drama, and burlesque seating about 12,000 patrons have closed their doors.

The order which closed theater movies and dance halls follow:

"Whereas the epidemic of influenza in the District of Columbia by its rapid spread threatens to impair the effectiveness of the machinery of the Federal Government, and whereas the surgeon general of the United States Public Health Service and the Health Officer of the District of Columbia have advised the Commissioners of the District of Columbia that the keeping open of the theaters and motion picture houses and like places of amusement constitute a public menace at this time; therefore be It ordered by the Commissioners of the District of Columbia that all theaters, motion picture houses, and dance halls be closed from and after 12 o'clock midnight of this day. October 3, 1318. and remain closed until further ordered by the Commissioners.

The Police Department will see that this order Is carried out, and all violations will be promptly reported.

Schools in the District, both public and private, still remain closed. The possibility of opening within the next ten days is slight. A meeting held yesterday of the high school and normal school principals and school officials resulted in the sending of a letter to the Commissioners recommending the closing of movies, theaters, and dance halls. The letter was sent by Superintendent of Schools Ernest L. Thurston, and follows:

Thurston's Letter.

"At a conference with the entire group of school officers, directors, the principals of high and normal schools, held to consider the situation created by the closing of the schools on account of the Influenza epidemic I was requested to convey' to you the unanimous feeling of the education administrative authorities that the closing of the public schools be Immediately followed by the closing of all other places of public assembly. Including theaters, motion picture houses, etc. The school officers are of the opinion that many of the school children released from school in order to reduce the danger from contagion will be exposed to contagion at other places of assembly, and because of the time at their disposal may be the freer to attend such places.

From school standpoints, a very general restriction of the public assembly will result in an earlier reopening of educational facilities."

Ninety-three Policemen III

Ninety-three members of the Police Department were off duty today because of Illness. Police officials stated that a number of the men were suffering from severe colds, while a few displayed symptoms of Influenza. Eighteen soldier-police and two chauffeurs are Included in the list.

The number of sick men, police officials stated, is not large enough to interfere seriously with the work of the department, although the list is more than fifty above the average.

More than fifty names are contained in the sick list of the Fire. Department. Seventeen of the men are suffering from Influenza. Sir of the twenty-four members from engine company No. 21 and No. 9 truck, a double company, quartered on Lanier Street, are said to be suffering from the plague.

"The number of sick men Is greater than the average," said Chief Wagner today, "but there Is no Immediate cause of alarm. Several of the men are off because of sickness In their families."

223 Car Men Sick.

Reports received from the two streetcar companies In the District show that 223 men are today at their homes suffering from Influenza. The Washington Railway and Electric Company reports 135 men are at home sick with the flu, and the Capital Traction Company, 88 men sick.

With this number of men absent from work, eighty cars are put out of running, and the number of cars is reduced at least 5 percent.

Little effect upon the schedules of the cars has been noted, however. Officials of the two companies report that the staggered method of opening Government departments and stores offsets the reduction in the number of cars used.

Commissioned Brownlow told *The Times* today that despite present conditions, better service is being given on the streetcars of Washington.

"The idea Is excellent," he said, "and it has had a wonderful effect upon the car service in the District."

To Inspect Restaurants

Drastic sanitary measures to combat the spread of Spanish Influenza in the District were undertaken today by officials of the Public Health Service in cooperation with officials of the District Health Department

The Public Health Service has called upon its various stations for providing assistance for Washington. Experts formerly stationed at places in the East have been brought here to take part In the fight against the epidemic.

Inspection of all restaurants and soda fountains will begin at once.

Ten Inspectors from other stations and all the Inspectors of the District Health Department and the Public Health Service will be furnished automobiles to facilitate transportation to points in the District. Restaurants will be ordered to take additional sanitation precautions, and particular attention will be paid to soda dispensaries and drug stores to prevent drinking utensils from becoming a dangerous medium of contagion.

Dr. H. S. Mustard, of the Public Health Service, has been placed In charge of the war of extermination for the Public Health Service and will coordinate its efforts with those of the District Health Department. The District Commissioners, and the Red Cross.

To Isolate Case.

The first point of attack after the sanitary zone has been placed in operation will be the Isolation of dangerous cases and a method of preventing persons not literally 111, but Infected with the disease germs from spreading It.

To complicate matters for the office under Dr. Fowler District Health Officer, two cases of smallpox have been reported among the colored population of the city. The first was reported Wednesday. Thursday, the second case was reported. There Is no immediate danger of an epidemic Dr. Fowler said.

The first case was reported from 1801 Vermont Avenue Northwest and the second from 1602 Thirteenth Street Northwest.

In the hospital being equipped today In the Ralston building, 602 F Street Northwest, treatment will be given civil employees of the Government and the District. The hospital will consist of about 100 beds, thirty-five in the building in C02 F street, formerly occupied by Annex No. 15 of the Shipping Board, and sixty-five in the Ralston building. The former Is a two-story brick structure and the latter four stories, with a court in the center.

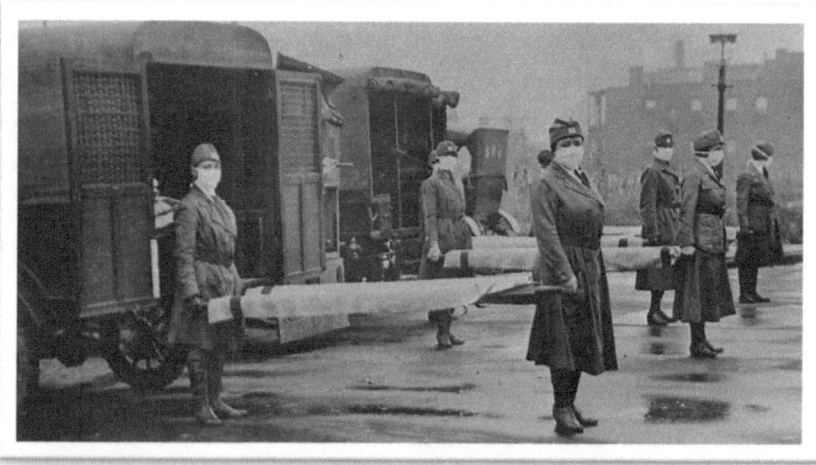

Red Cross motor corps in St. Louis on duty in Oct. 1918.

Red Cross Assisting.

The Red Cross is furnishing a large part of the equipment for the hospital and has agreed to furnish as many nurses as are available. The hospital is to be under the direction of the Public Health Service.

Asked as to the appropriation of $1,000,000 by Congress to fight the spread of the pandemic, Dr. Rupert Blue said that a large part of it Is being spent in an educational campaign. No part of the appropriation is allotted to any specific use, or to any specific part of the country. Itis available for districts needing money to fight the disease but will be spent at the direction of the Public Health Service as officials deem most expedient.

The opening and closing hours of two more departments, the Interstate Commerce Commission and the office of the Director-General of Railroads, were changed today.

Clerks in both departments now will report at 9:30 in the morning and quit at S at night instead of observing their old hours, which were 9 to 4:30.

1,500 Cases Dally.

An average of 1,500 cases of Influenza has been treated daily for the last five days at the Army Medical Dispensary. Of this number, the dally number of home cases, cases in which the doctor or nurse must visit the patient, have been 300. All of these cases are from some of the different Government departments.

Sixty-five nurses and doctors have been kept busy for twelve hours a day for the last five days treating Government employees who are sent to them for treatment.

Chief clerks of the various Government departments are expected to be ordered by the Public Health Service to keep all paper drinking cup holders well filled, or, in case glasses are used, to see that they are well sterilized. An old regulation provides that each Government employee must provide his own drinking cup. This rule has not been enforced, and the Government provides paper drinking cups.

No estimate as to the number of war workers who are incapacitated from influenza has as yet been compiled. Still, unofficial statements have It that at least 900 clerks for the last five days have been sent home dally with symptoms of Spanish Influenza. Of this number, 65 percent have colds that are likely to develop into influenza. The rest either have influenza or are on the verge of pneumonia.

ALEXANDRIA LISTS 2,000 GRIP CASES

More than 2,000 cases of Spanish influenza have been reported In Alexandria, Va., according to figures issued today by the Public Health Service. Two hundred new cases of the plague were reported to the health authorities yesterday.

The death record, officials stated, has been comparatively small. Five deaths have been reported since the disease was first discovered two weeks ago.

All schools and theaters In Alexandria and surrounding territory have been closed until the epidemic is checked.

Several cases have been reported at the Alexandria Shipbuilding Company's plant.

Fifty cases of Spanish Influenza were reported today In Alexandria County, according to Dr. H. C. Corbett, secretary to the health board Ballston and Clarendon are the most seriously affected.

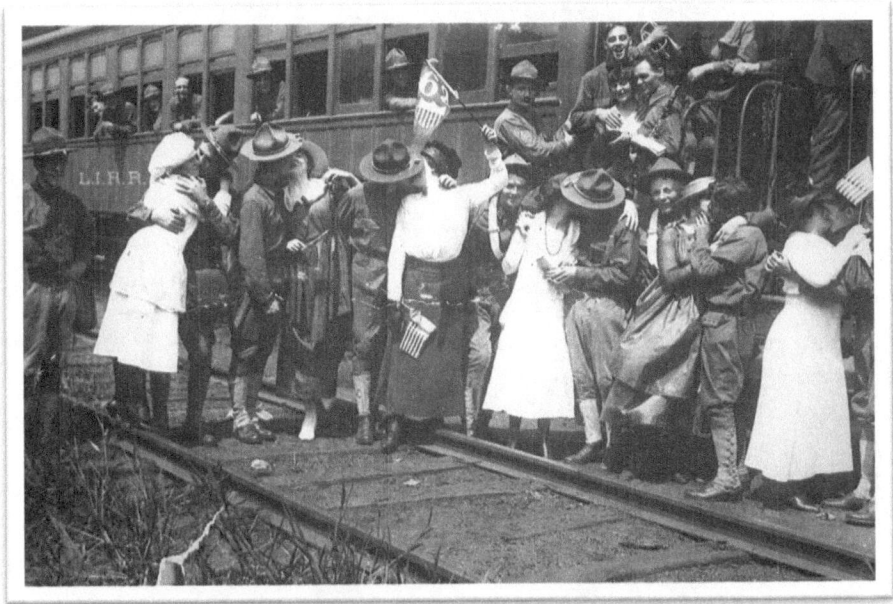

Nurses give a sendoff to troops in 1917.

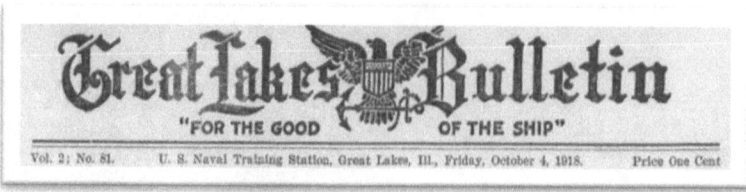

INFLUENZA IS NOW PRACTICALLY WIPED OUT

Only Twenty-Six New Cases Reported Yesterday

GREAT LAKES BULLETIN,

FRIDAY, OCTOBER 4, 1918 – The daily health report of Captain William A. Moffett, Commandant, shows that only twenty-six new cases of influenza had developed during the twenty-four hours ending at ten a. m. Thursday morning, a decided drop in the number of new cases from the previous twenty-four hours when fifty new cases were reported.

The report shows that 154 men were discharged to duty during this period and leaves 1,245 men still on the sick list.

The day's report would have been a remarkable one had it not been for eighteen cases which were brought here by men off ships.

The men had been on for a cruise of several weeks. The eighteen cases brought here are in addition to the twenty-six reported on the Station.

Yesterday's report shows that Spanish influenza has been practically wiped out here. Occasionally cases are expected to be brought here by men from other places, Station authorities announced, but despite these, the disease Is now practically wiped out.

Interesting Statistics

Some interesting statistics regarding the effect Spanish influenza has on civil and military life were given out yesterday by Lieutenant-Commander Mink.

In civil life, from forty to sixty percent of the population usually contracts the disease, Lieutenant-Commander Mink said. In comparison, in military life, only twenty percent of the men become victims.

This is attributed to the fact that men in the Navy and Army are more careful and better informed. They know how to use drinking cups, use the nasal spray, and to protect themselves in various other ways.

Better Informed

"It has become an established fact," said Lieutenant-Commander Mink, that men in service are better informed and that they are better practitioners. It has also been established that generally speaking, men are of a much higher standard so far as health is concerned after they have been in training a few months than they were when they entered service."

There were about 9,000 cases of influenza on the Station, Lieutenant-Commander Mink said, which is about twenty percent of the men here. At Camp Logan, there are about 2,000 men, and 500 of them contracted the disease, he said.

Figures regarding Spanish influenza in Germany were also given out by the senior medical officer. They are taken from German statistics. According to these, about forty-two percent of the population of Berlin contracted the disease. In Paris, sixty-four percent of the population was affected.

Army Percentage Low

In the German army, only eleven percent of the men fell victim, Lieutenant-Commander Mink said, which is another proof of the fact that the disease affects civil populations more than it does men in military life.

Regarding the meningitis situation on the Station, the senior medical officer said there was no cause for alarm. Only a few cases have developed in the last few weeks, he said, which is considered remarkable because a disease wave such as the one which swept the Station is invariably followed by some other malady.

175,000 CASES OF INFLUENZA IN U.S.

NEW YORK, Oct. 4, 1918 – Spanish Influenza, sweeping through big cities of the country as well as army camps, has brought suffering to more than 175,000 soldiers and civilians, reports from all sections showed today.

Death is occurring at the rate of one in each twenty-seven cases, according to unofficial estimates.

Here are unofficial reports showing total cases and deaths among civilians up to last night.

City	Cases.	Deaths.
NEW YORK	4,853	223
Boston	30,000	1,912
Burlington. Vt.	47	7

Springfield. Mass	690	28
Brockton. Mass	6,500	165
Bridgeport	203	10
Fitchburg. Mass	2,000	99
Findlay. Ohio	600	28
Cleveland	60	0
Wilkesbarre, Pa	50	5
Allentown, Pa	50	2
Scranton, Pa	90	2
Syracuse, N. Y.	736	8
Newark, N.J.	1,434	20
Schenectady, N.Y.	54	9
Westfield, Mass	129	7
New Haven	42	6
Philadelphia (24 hours)	711	145
Elizabeth, N. J.	1.200	(?)
Baltimore, Md.	2,500	25
St. Paul, Minn.	67	1
Milwaukee, Wis.	338	15
Racine, Wis.,	200	8

Oklahoma City	5,000	6
Dallas, Texas	143	1
Grand Rapids	6	1
Nashville, Tenn.	1,000	4
Memphis	2,000	4
Richmond, Va.,	1,029	25
Pensacola, Fla.	1,000	78
New Orleans	100	1
Birmingham, Ala	731	0
Durham, N. C.	200	0
Lancaster, Pa.	731	5
Kansas City	600	1
Chicago	1,349	102
Dayton, Ohio	27	2
Montreal, Canada	150	1
Wilmington, Del.	12,000	163

27 DEATHS IN DAY HERE FROM SPANISH.GRIP ARE REPORTED

FREIGHT SERVICE INTO WASHINGTON CRIPPLED

PASSENGER TRAINS MAY BE CURTAILED

Washington, D.C. (Oct. 5, 1918) – Twenty-seven deaths from Spanish influenza among the civil population of Washington were reported to the District Health Officer today. This is the largest number reported on any one day since the epidemic gained sway, the largest number previously reported in one day having been eleven, and the average deaths about four or five.

Freight service into Washington is crippled, and passenger service is threatened with curtailment by the spread of Influenza among railroad workers.

The closing of George Washington University, where 2,500 men and women are studying, is under consideration, and a decision whether the big institution will be closed or remain open will be reached by the university authorities within a few hours.

Plan Open Air Meetings.

The pastors of Washington churches, ordered by the Commissioners to hold no services indoors, have made plans to hold open-air services throughout the city if the weather Is favorable.

The deaths reported today are as follows: Thomas M. Corkklll, forty years, Providence Hospital; Nannie M. Smith, twenty-three years, 1330 Massachusetts Avenue Northwest, Gladys Turner, nineteen years, Garfield Hospital; Lula K. Hixon, twenty-four years, 635 A Street Southeast; Albert Gaff, one year, 143 N Street Southeast (colored); William J. Smith, twenty-eight years, 22 Bates Street Northwest, Mary B. Collins, forty-four years, K Street Northeast; Biaglo Kelling, twenty-eight years, George Washington Hospital, Margaret Shorter, twenty-seven years, 3517 Tenth Street Northwest. Ethel Harris, thirty years, H street northwest; John T. Langley, three years, K Street Southeast (colored); Susie Harris, thirty-five years, Washington Asylum Hospital (colored); Genevie Kundru, twenty-one years, Sibley Hospital; Henry Sage, thirty-four years, Casualty Hospital; Marcel Jaray, twenty-nine years; Annie Thornton, thirty-year (colored); Annie K. White, thirty-four years; Charles C. Lukner, thirty-five years, Ilene Meinberg, twenty-eight years; Annie Chapman, twenty years (colored). Helen North, twenty-seven years, Herman Hogan, thirty-four years; Caroline Virginia Poole, thirty years. Martha Taylor, forty-nine years, (colored) George J. Moody, twenty-four years; Leslie W. Cox, twenty-five years.

SENATOR KING ILL OF SPANISH INFLUENZA

URBANA DAILY COURIER

Washington, Oct. 5, 1918 —Senator King of Utah is ill with Spanish influenza. He has been confined to his home since Sunday. His condition Is not serious.

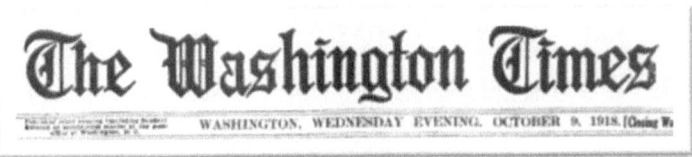

32 GRIP DEATHS

WASHINGTON TIMES

Washington, D.C. (Oct. 7, 1918) – Thirty-two additional deaths and 656 new cases of Spanish Influenza were reported to the District Health Department today. These figures convinced health officials that the epidemic rapidly is approaching its "peak. "

The report of 656 new cases of the disease is the largest in any single day since the epidemic started. Saturday 276 new cases were reported and on Sunday 279, making the total for the three days 1,211. This represents only the number of cases among the civil population officially reported.

Names of Victims
The thirty-two whose deaths were reported today follow

Helen W. Kirley, 27 years old, 1330 12th St. NW;

Frances Raetry, 22, Kendall House, 14th St.;

Walter W. Ballard Jr., #1 Hotel Powhatan;

Ira Z Myers, 30, 923 6th St. NW; Grace M. Lee, 15,

Casualty Hospital;

Sarah E. Smith, colored, 40, 345 V. St.;

Lucille Tawes, 22, Garfield Hospital;

Eleanore M. Kerr Hardman, 26, 118 7th St. SE;

Burney Cohen, 2, 409 H St. NW;

William E. Manweiller, 33, Casualty Hospital;

Nathaniel Gross, colored, 2, 810 New Hampshire Ave. NW;

Clinton H. Chapman, 28, 25 8th St. SE;

Pearl E. Evans, 42, Sligo Mill Road;

Alexander H. Summers, 34, 127 4th St. SE;

James Tamisica 23, Gallaudet College;

Julia A. Pitts, 22, 726 Maryland Ave. NE;

Anne R. Bray, 27, 116 5th St. NE;

Iris Lechisette, 21, Washington Asylum Hospital;

Thomas J. Kelly, 35, Georgetown University Hospital;

John S. Hutchinson, 26, Blue Plains;

Marion E. Farrow, 1242 D St. SE;

Ruth Rizer, 34, 1464 Belmont St. NW;

Anna E. Byrd, 32, 623 M St. NW;

George V. Minick, 25, Sibley Hospital;

Irvy L. Marshall, 36, 1204 C. St. NE;

John J. Lally, 34, Garfield Hospital;

John Meimberg, 23, Georgetown University Hospital;

Myrtle J. Jewell, 39, 809 6th St. NW;

Lee F. Lynch, 29, Walter Reed Hospital;

 Genevieve Knudsen, 21, Sibley Hospital.

MAYOR ORDERS CLOSINGS OF ALL PLACES OF ASSEMBLY

THE DAILY BANNER

Cambridge, Md. (Oct. 8, 1918) – Elsewhere in this issue will be found a notice from Mayor Orem, notifying all theatres, pool and billiard rooms, bowling alleys, churches, etc., to close at once, and giving notice that there will be no more public meetings of any kind in churches, halls, etc., until the Health authorities give permission for such. This notice, of course, refers to all church meetings, club meetings, lodge meetings, etc.

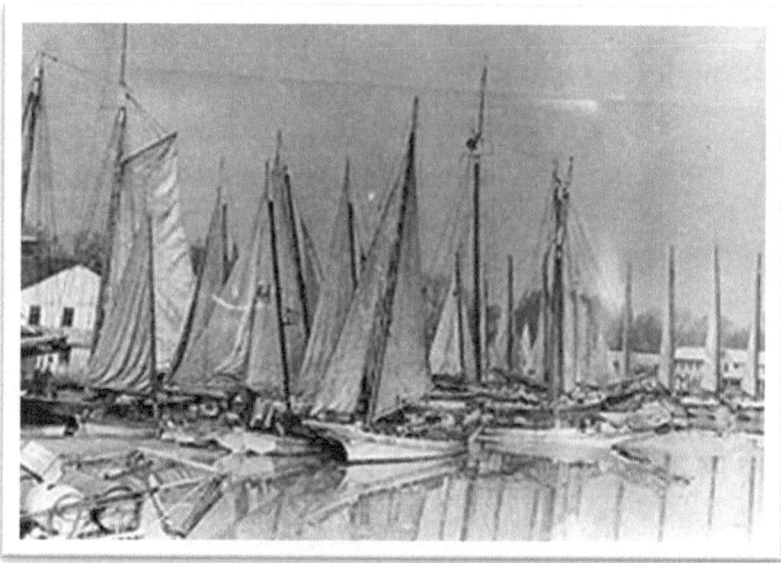

PUBLIC SCHOOLS CLOSED
ON ACCOUNT OF "FLU"

Dr. Guy Steele, Acting- Health Officer for The County, Advised to Close All Schools, Public Meetings, and Places of Public Amusements.

THE DAILY BANNER

Cambridge, Md. (Oct. 8, 1918) – Dr. Guy Steele, Acting Health Officer of this county, has received a telegram from Dr. C. Hampson Jones, Acting Secretary of the Maryland State Board of Health, advising that Surgeon General Rupert Blue, United States Army, suggests that the public schools, public places of amusement and public meetings be closed on account of the Spanish Influenza, which is, at this time, raging all through the Eastern section of the country.

This suggestion, coming from the highest authority in the United States, the Surgeon General, means that the necessary steps for the closing of such places will be taken at once, in fact, the county school authorities have already closed all the schools in Cambridge and have sent notices to the rural schools to do so immediately upon receipt of such instructions.

It is expected that the local authorities, Mayor Earle W. Orem, and Dr. E. E. Wolff, co-operating with the National and State authorities, will take steps at once to see that such places as coming under the scope of the suggestion are promptly closed. The telegram follows:

Dr. Guy Steele,

Cambridge, Md.

You are advised as Acting Health Officer of Dorchester County that Surgeon General Blue suggests discontinuance of all public meetings, the closing of public schools, and places of public amusements. —C. Hampson

Jones, Acting Secretary.

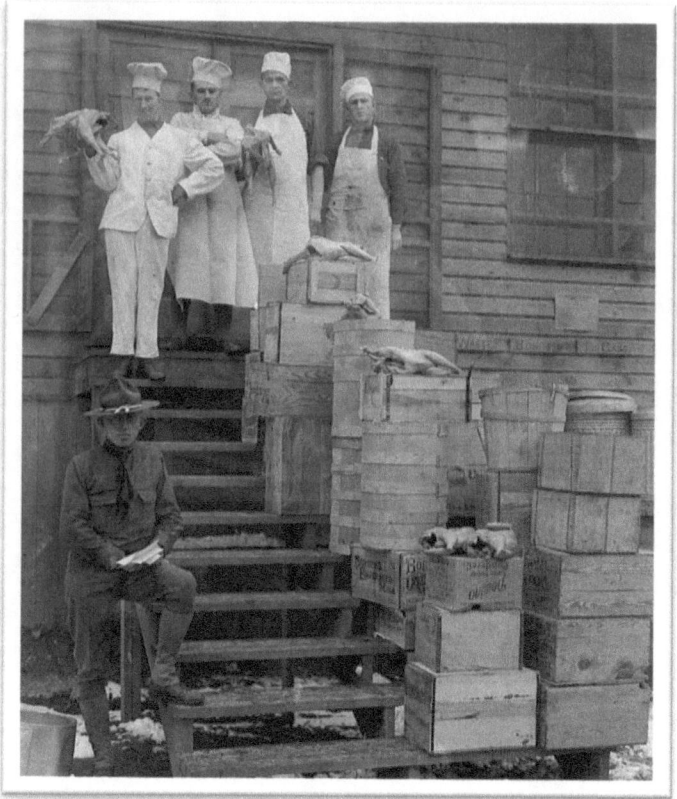

Ready to cook up a mess hall full of food at Camp Meade, Md. 1918, Harris & Ewing

ANOTHER DORCHESTER MAN DIES AT CAMP

George Edward Meredith, Son of The
late Pritchett and Mrs. Meredith,
Dies at Camp Pigeon, Near Wilmington.

Cambridge, Md. (Oct. 8, 1918) – Mrs. Pritchett W. Meredith, Race Street, this city, has been notified by the military authorities that her son, George Edward Meredith, died at Camp at Pigeon Point, near Wilmington, yesterday, as the result of an attack of pneumonia. It is presumed that Mr. Meredith was attacked first by Spanish Influenza, which quickly turns to pneumonia.

The deceased soldier was thirty-one years of age and left Cambridge on April 29th. He has two other brothers in the service, Clarence, who is in the service in France, and Eustace, who is at present ill at Camp Meade.

He is survived by his mother, five sisters and five brothers, who are: Miss Hilda, of Bonwell, S. C.; Mrs. Thurman Shorter and Mrs. Albert Smith, of near Cambridge; Misses Ruby and Modell, of Cambridge; Sergeant Clarence Meredith, in France, in the Twenty-Third Engineers; Private Eustace. Meredith, of Camp Meade; James Meredith, of Bristol, Pa.; Isidor, who is a student at Charlotte Hall, and Arnold, who resides at home. Owing to the impossibility of learning when the body will be sent home, no funeral arrangements have been completed at this time.

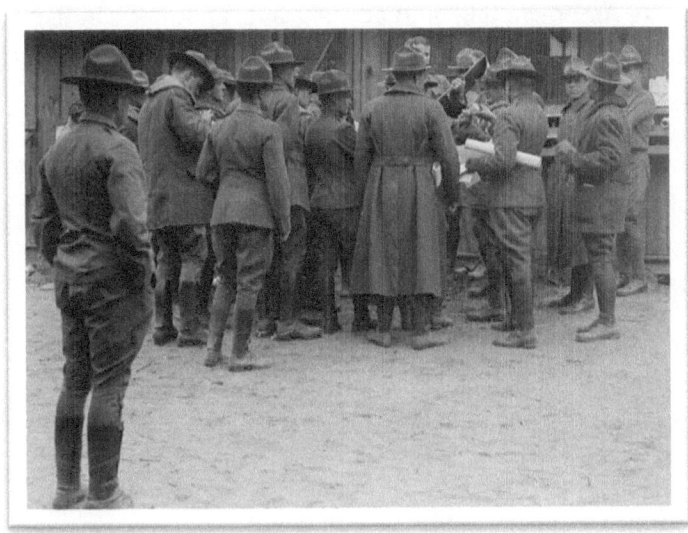

Mail call at Camp Meade, Md. in 1917. Photo by Harris & Ewing

CAMBRIDGE SOLDIER HAS MILITARY FUNERAL

Corporal Detailed from Camp Meade To Bring Remains Home and Attend Funeral
—G. A. R. Veterans Carry the Casket.

THE DAILY BANNER

Cambridge, Md. (Oct. 8, 1918) – The funeral of Private Earl Frampton, who died at Camp Meade last week, a victim of the Spanish Influenza, was attended by a corporal who was sent from the Camp. The corporal's instructions were to maintain military guard over the remains Saturday night and to attend the funeral services Sunday afternoon. The services were held at the home of the parents of the deceased soldier, on Trenton street, and were conducted by the Rev. W. E. Gunby, pastor of Zion Church. The casket in which the remains rested was draped with a large American flag, and at the grave, an American flag was placed in it. Local members of The John R. Kenly Post, Grand Army of the Republic, acted as pallbearers I

This young man was one of a large number of soldiers who have died at Camp Meade of Spanish Influenza. He bore a splendid reputation, being steady, honest, industrious, a dutiful son, and a good citizen. His family has the sympathy of the public in their great loss.

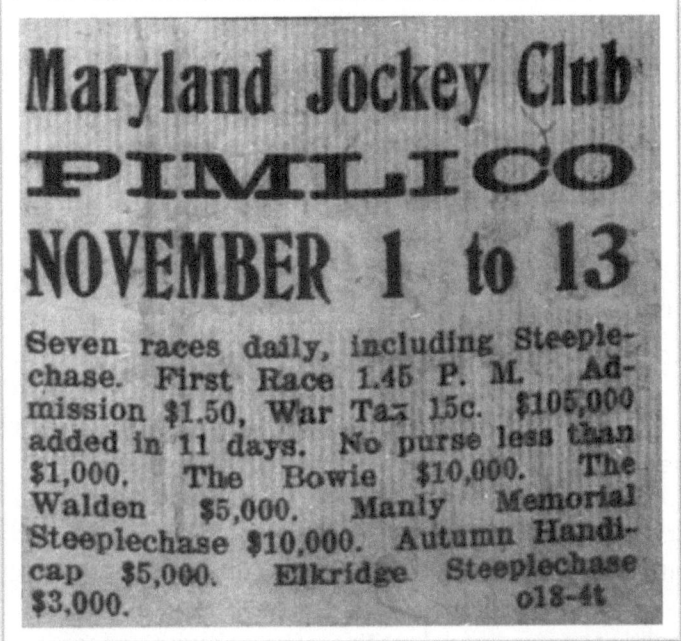

Maryland Jockey Club
PIMLICO
NOVEMBER 1 to 13

Seven races daily, including Steeplechase. First Race 1.45 P. M.   Ad-
mission $1.50, War Tax 15c. $105,000
added in 11 days. No purse less than
$1,000.   The   Bowie $10,000.   The
Walden $5,000.   Manly   Memorial
Steeplechase $10,000.   Autumn Handi-
cap $5,000.   Elkridge   Steeplechase
$3,000.   o18-4t

Pimlico Races Ready to Go

THE DEMOCRATIC ADVOCATE

Westminster, Md. (Oct. 18, 1918) – The Pimlico Autumn meeting, one of
the principal fixtures of the turf world, takes place November 1 to 13
with a brilliant program of seven races, including a steeplechase each
day.

Every stall has been engaged, and all the great horses in training will be
on hand to contest for the liberal purses amounting to $105,000 in
eleven days offered by the Maryland Jockey Club. The track is in fine
shape, and the steeplechase course, a popular landing place for
airplanes, is in tip-top condition.

On the Mend

Very few families in our community have escaped the flu. Some whole families are down at the same time. Although there are quite a number of cases yet, we are very glad to report that most all seem to be doing nicely and it is our sincere wish that all will soon be restored to their health again.

THE DEMOCRATIC ADVOCATE

SYKESVLLLE.

OCTOBER 18, 1918 – Mrs. Charles Thompson, of Baltimore, is visiting her parents, Mr. and Mrs. Charles Sullivan.

Mr. George Barnes, who Is working at Sparrows Point, spent the week's end at his home here.

Carolyn Bevard and Elizabeth Bennett, of Washington, spent from Friday until Sunday with their parents here.

Mrs. James Wheatly spent several days this last week with her son, James, at Camp Meade, who has been ill with pneumonia following influenza. Mr. Wheatly is much improved.

Mr. Walton Grant, brother of Mrs. Edwin Hood, who has been spending some time here, returned today to his home in Denton, Montana,

Prof. Unger, of Westminster, was seen on the streets of Sykesville today.

The order has not been given yet to open the schools. Quite a number around here have flu,d and the doctors have more calls than they can visit.

Mrs. Joseph Polishock is at a hospital In Baltimore for treatment.

Mrs. Knox is visiting her son, Mr. George Knox, at Statewood.

Mr. and Mrs. Richard Bennett, John and Lou Bennett, visited for several days last week Mr. Bennett's brother, Thomas Bennett, of Baldwin,

Harford County.

John Stem Bennett, who is in the aviation corps and who has been home on furlough, was called to report last Saturday.

Mr. Howard Hood arrived safely at his brother's, Mr. Edwin Hood, last Saturday, having just recently come from France. Mr. Hood returned because he was severely wounded, and he left one arm in France.

Jerold Neel, of Baltimore, spent last week with his aunt, Mrs. W. K. Marshall.

Miss Mary Hadley, of Portsmouth, Va., is visiting Miss Louise McDonald.

On account of the epidemic, the moving pictures will be postponed until further notice.

Miss Gengie Choate, of Baltimore County, has been visiting Mr. and Mrs. Pearce Prough.

We certainly missed having Sunday school and church services in our churches here last Sunday.

SHIPLEY.

Mr. Clarence Caples returned to Camp Meade Friday after spending several days with his mother and brother, who are on the sick list.

Mr. and Mrs. Joshua I. Logue have the sympathy of their many friends here by the death of their son, Winfield. He was a bright and pleasant little boy. The rest of Mr. Logue's children are very sick. It Is to be hoped they soon get well.

Those on the sick list are Mr. Robert Zahn, Miss Mildred Schneider, Master Rowe Davis, and others,

DETOUR.

On Friday morning, Jacob Myerly received word that his brother, Lem E. Myerly, of Baltimore, was very ill with pneumonia, which followed the flu. Mr. Myerly died on Saturday. His parents, Mr. and Mrs. James Myerly and Jacob Myerly, all of this place attended the funeral services at his home in Baltimore on Tuesday. ;

MILLERS.

Sherman, son of Mr. and Mrs. H. K. Miller, who we reported last week as being very ill with double pneumonia, died last Wednesday noon, aged 20 years, 11 months, and 13 days. The funeral was held on Saturday with services at home by Rev. Miller. Interment in the U. B. cemetery here. He is survived by his parents, three sisters and five brothers. Wink Brothers funeral directors.

Mrs. Belle Bortner was notified last week of the death of her daughter-in-law, Mrs. Annie Bortner, of Hanover, Pa. The funeral was held Monday at Hanover.

Mr. and Mrs. Thomas Martin was notified of the death of their daughter,

Mrs. Earl Murray of Baltimore died from pneumonia. We extend sympathy to all in their bereavement.

News is scarce owing to gasless Sundays and influenza.

SANDYVILLE.

There will be no services at Sandy Mount owing to the flu until further notice.

A large number of people in this community are suffering from flu, grip, and pneumonia.

Lottie Caple is very ill with flu and Bronchopneumonia.

PHYSICIANS HERE BUSY NIGHT & DAY

SCORES OF CASES OF INFLU-ENZA BUT NO PNEUMONIA.

AWFUL AT CAMP GRANT

Much Suffering From Wide-Spread Epidemic And Work Of Schools Hindered.—Sycamore Undertaker Called To Camp Grant By Telephone.

The True Republican

TRUE REPUBLICAN

SYCAMORE, ILLINOIS (Oct. 9, 1918) – Many scores of cases of the widespread epidemic of Spanish influenza, grip, or whatever it may be, are keeping Sycamore physician's busy night and day. One Sycamore physician was attending patients 22 hours in the 24 hours on Sunday.

Reports this Tuesday to the public health service showed the disease is spreading, and that the number of cases reported where it had been prevalent heretofore, is increasing. This, however, was not the situation in army camps, the number of new cases reported during the forty-eight hours ending at noon Monday showing a slight decrease.

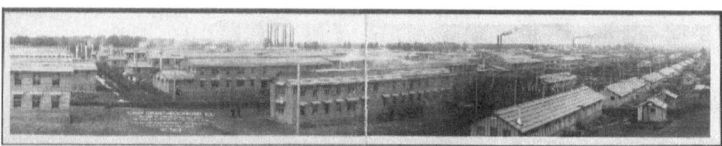

Camp Grant at Rockford Illinois in 1917

Pneumonia in the camps continued to increase, with 4,532 new cases and 1,388 deaths reported since Saturday.

Influenza cases reported from all camps since the disease became epidemic, Sept. 13, now total 167,000; pneumonia cases, 17, 102, and deaths 4,910.

Camps Grant, in Illinois, and Sherman, in Ohio, also reported increases in the number of pneumonia cases.

Capt. Hagadorn, commander at Camp Grant, issued orders Monday censoring not only the names of soldiers who are victims of- pneumonia but also the publication of the number of deaths resulting from the epidemic. Up to that time, the total number of deaths reported from pneumonia there was 535, and the surgeons on Monday feared the crisis had not yet been reached.

E. E. Johnson, the Sycamore undertaker, received a telegram from the Illinois State Undertakers Association stating that the government had appealed to the association to send a large number of undertakers to Camp Grant to care for the hundreds dead of influenza, and asking him to go. He immediately departed for that place, leaving here by automobile on Monday afternoon, and will "do his bit" for his country. It was reported that garages at the camps are filled with bodies.

The attendance at the Sycamore schools is largely reduced this week, only about half the pupils being in attendance in some grades, some of the little folks being sick, and others being absent because parents were afraid of them contracting the disease.

However, the disease in Sycamore has taken a light form, especially among children, and no serious cases have been reported of a large number of cases here. The contrast between the form of the disease outside and inside the army camps is puzzling physicians. In the camps, the mortality is terrible from pneumonia following influenza.

Over thirty of the nurses and many doctors are down with it, and many a kind woman from Rockford has gone to the camp to help win the war, for verily every boy who dies at the camp in their country's service is as much a hero as though he was killed in battle. Charles Rogers is recovering from an attack of influenza at Camp Grant, but the severest case of any of the Sycamore boys is that of James Malone, who was taken with it last Wednesday. His aunt and his uncle Will Murphy visited him last week and supposed all would go all right, but he has not been improving, and on Monday morning, Mr. Murphy and his mother and Mrs. Delana went to the base hospital and were allowed to see him. They were given some hope that day, but the two-former remained overnight, and in the morning, Mr. Murphy returned home, not having been allowed to see him, as they said he was much worse. Mrs. Murphy was allowed to remain with him at the hospital. Very little hope was given to them of his recovery.

****

Mrs. Margaret Onthank-West of Chicago passed Saturday and Sunday with her parents Mr. and Mrs. F. Onthank.

CAMP GRANT AND OUR SOLDIERS
News of Our Lads in Their Country's Service at the Numerous Cantonments and Somewhere Over There
TRUE REPUBLICAN

Sycamore, Ill. (Oct. 9, 19198) Special from Rockford Register Gazette— Stricken Camp Grant continues its grim, heroic fight against the deadly pneumonia invasion. With endurance almost superhuman, doctors and nurses are in a grapple with the malady which at 1 o'clock Friday had taken a toll of 234 lives. Camp Grant's medical men expressed fear that the list would mount to 250 by Saturday. Fifty-four deaths were reported Friday afternoon as occurring since midnight.

Up to Thursday at midnight, a total of 180 deaths had been officially reported as directly due to pneumonia complications following influenza. The base hospital reported 76 deaths yesterday for the 24 hours ending at midnight last night. Forty-three deaths were reported for Tuesday, but one of the numbers, it was officially announced, was not due to influenza.

Red Cross officials and volunteer workers from Rockford, assisting in the clerical work at the base hospital, are practically swamped by the vast amount of detail. The clerical staff is behind in its report, and it is with difficulty that information is obtained during the day on the exact number of deaths since midnight when official reports are made.

One hundred and ninety-three new cases of pneumonia were reported. A telegram was dispatched to the Western Casket company of Chicago by camp authorities relative to the handling of bodies, the number of which is said to have outgrown the capacity of the establishments of Rockford undertakers.

Sailor William Rissman of Hinckley died Friday of pneumonia, following an attack of Spanish influenza. He was granted a furlough to attend the funeral at Hinckley Tuesday of his nephew August Hartman, ten years old. He had suffered from an attack of influenza while at Great Lakes and had been in the hospital there but had improved and been discharged. He was taken with a chill Wednesday afternoon. His parents are Mr. and Mrs. Michael Rissman.

****

A letter received by his parents Mr. and Mrs. John M. Black from Harry Black on Monday told of the awful conditions prevailing in Camp Sheridan, Montgomery, Ala., because of the epidemic of Spanish influenza. He had been transferred from guard duty to hospital duty to assist in caring for the sick.

Will Organ, who is at Camp Grant, is with many other soldiers, assisting the nurses at the hospitals there in caring for the great number of patients suffering from influenza.

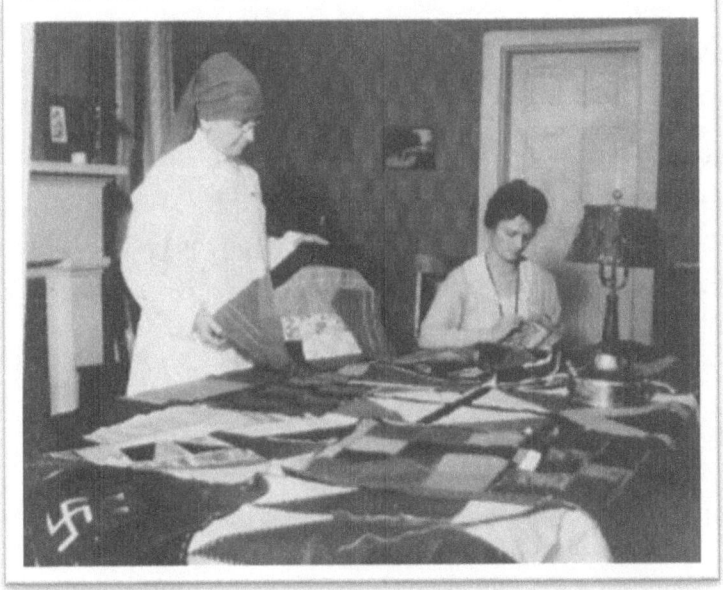

THE EPIDEMIC OF SPANISH INFLUENZA – has put a five week's stop to all Red Cross unit work in southern Ohio, so many Red Cross workers toiled for the cause in their homes. Mother and daughter secured a "patch" from each family free from the epidemic and worked them into the quilt shown, for the soldiers, at Miamitown, Ohio. – *National Archives. Photo by Felix J. Koch on Oct. 27, 1918.*

The Washington Times

WASHINGTON, WEDNESDAY EVENING, OCTOBER 9, 1918. [Closing Wall

FORTY DEATHS HERE IN DAY FROM INFLUENZA EPIDEMIC

PEACE NOW WRONG, SAYS LABOR HEAD

1,722 New Cases Reported in Last Twenty-four Hours. 5,176 Cases Since Saturday. Peak of Plague Not Yet Reached.

D. C. OFFICIALS TO HOLD BEN RUBIN

THE WASHINGTON TIMES
Washington, D.C. (Oct. 9, 1918)

Forty deaths among the civil population of Washington from the Spanish influenza epidemic were reported to the District Health Department in the twenty-four hours ended at noon today. This is the second-largest number of deaths reported in any twenty-four hours since the epidemic started.

New cases reported between 9 o'clock last night and noon today number 1,207. New cases reported between noon yesterday and 9 o'clock last night number 425, making the total number of new cases reported in the twenty-four hours ended at noon today 1,722.

A total of 5,722 new cases have been reported since Saturday, and

Health Department officials this does not represent the entire scope of the epidemic in Washington

Peak Not Reached.

Dr. William C. Fowler. District Health Officer today stated that the epidemic till is on the increase.

"The number of new cases reported still Is Increasing," said Dr. Fowler.

"I cannot predict when the epidemic will reach Its worst stage."

The epidemic has not yet even reached a peak, according to Dr. J. W. Schereschewsky, assistant surgeon general of the Public Health Service.

"We will know within two or three days whether the epidemic is to be kept under control by methods now in force, or whether much more drastic restrictions must be enforced," he said.

All Meetings Barred.

All outdoor public gatherings must be discontinued In the District. A formal order to this effect will be issued late today by Commissioner Brownlow.

"This order includes all indoor and outdoor services in churches," Commissioner Brownlow said. "No funerals or weddings will be permitted in churches, and no outdoor gatherings will be allowed. This means the discontinuance of all Liberty loan meetings. Therefore, I ask the people of Washington to buy more bonds. Don't let this epidemic lesson our bond sales."

Seventy-Five Die in Day at Meade.

The epidemic caused the deaths of seventy-live more soldiers In Camp Meade in the last twenty-four hours. A total of 2S9 new cases of pneumonia and of 166 new cases of Spanish Influenza is reported for the last twenty-four hours. The disease claimed the life of another Washington soldier today at Camp Meade. Capt. Edward C. Cissel of Company E., Seventeenth Infantry Regiment, died of pneumonia following Influenza.

Depleted staff at Washington hospitals today are coping with one of the most arduous tasks ever imposed upon local Institutions.

Two Physicians Succumb.

Two physicians and twelve nurses at the Emergency Hospital are suffering from Influenza, and the staff is depleted 15 percent. Dr. Noble B. Barnes and Dr. Charles King, members of the surgical staff of Casualty Hospital, were stricken with influenza last night, and five trained nurses iso are suffering from the disease.

Thirteen nurses at Georgetown Hospital are Influenza victims, and the nursing staff there is depleted by more than 10 percent. The hospital imported 45 new cases of Influenza today. The Homeopathic Hospital today, reports 14 nurses suffering from influenza, and an increase of more than 50 percent in the number of patients admitted to the hospital.

Two more nurses became ill today at the George Washington University Hospital, making a total of 16 nurses suffering from influenza.

SCHOOLS WILL REMAIN OPEN
Only Five Cases are Reported
Officially—Precautions to be taken.
GRAND FORKS HERALD

Grand Forks, N. D. (Oct. 9, 1918) – Preceding the regular meeting of the city council, a general conference with the health officer of the city was held last evening in the city hall. At the meeting, it was decided to close all public gathering places except the city schools, which are to remain open until further notice from the state.

Parents need not be alarmed and prohibit children from attending school as every precaution will be taken to guard against infection, and a report will .be made to authorities at the first Indication of sickness. The situation was viewed from every standpoint, and the parents of school children-are asked to co-operate with the school authorities and the city council in the steps taken.

DEATHS FROM INFLUENZA ARE LOWER IN NEW YORK

Camp Grant Reports Increase in Number of Cases New York,

New York (Oct. 9, 1918) – Deaths from Spanish influenza and pneumonia have decreased within the last 24 hours, and the number of new cases of pneumonia is considerably less, according to the report issued today by the department of health.

The death toll today was 124 from influenza and 166 from pneumonia as compared with 133 and 190 on Tuesday. New cases of pneumonia numbered only 212.

Camp Grant, Ill. (Oct. 9, 1918) —There were 107 deaths from pneumonia at Camp Grant during the 24 hours ending at midnight last night. There is now 1,500 pneumonia in the hospital. It was announced today. There were 188 new cases of influenza in the base hospital Monday and 171 new cases Tuesday.

Winona Fighting Epidemic

Winona, Minn., (Oct 9., 1918)—Organized effort to combat the increasing epidemic of Spanish influenza was launched here today. Dr. D. B. Pritchard, a city health officer, is chairman of a Committee of Red Cross workers who will, make a survey of the cases and employ sufficient nurses to handle the emergency. There are hundreds of cases here. Although several are serious, only one local death has been reported.

59 Deaths at Camp Taylor

Louisville, Ky., (Oct. 9, 1918)—Fifty-nine deaths from pneumonia and the admissions of 570 cases of Spanish- Influenza were reported today at Camp Zachary Taylor. Total deaths have been 230 with 9,082 patients, treated at the base hospital.

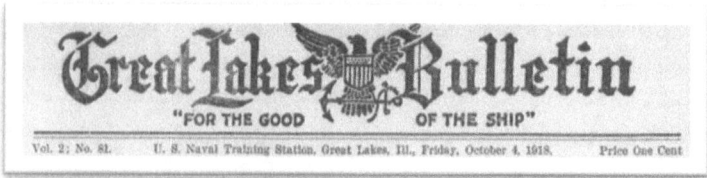

TAPS SOUNDED ON 1918 BASEBALL SEASON
Each Player Granted A Furlough of Ten Days
BY FRED II. YOUNG

Taps were sounded yesterday for the 1918 baseball season at Great Lakes when Lieutenant-Commander John B. Kaufman, Medical Corps, the athletic officer, announced that it had been definitely decided to call off the proposed western trip.

Each member of the team is to rate a ten-day furlough plus travel time as a reward for his services on the diamond this summer and most of the athlete's plan to shove off today.

It has been a great season for baseball on the Station, and it is doubtful if any service team in the country can produce as successful a record.

Then to Active Service

With the team disbanded, the players are now ready to go to sea or will be ready in a short time. They're on their way to the gun turrets, to the gold braid of commissioned officers or to the deck of an Atlantic fleet minesweeper.

At least ten of the players, who have helped carry the fame of Great Lakes to every section of the country, will enter the Seaman Gunner's school at Washington, D. C from which they will be graduated to the fleet.

These on Honor Roll

Verne Clemons and John Paul Jones, already first-class gunner's mates, will chaperone the party that sails out of here next month for Washington. These men are already experts in ordnance and have had several months of training in this line of warfare.

The other athletes transferring to the Seaman Gunner's School are Rube Erhardt, Billy Swanson, Bud Croake, Freddie Hoffman, Ray Neusel, Bill Fox, George -Cunningham, and Spencer Heath. Bill Johnson also plans-to shove off soon and may enter the same branch of service.

Several to Officer's School

Several of the members of the team have their hearts set on commissions and are already at work, preparing for

The DeKalb Daily Chronicle

SPANISH GRIP STILL WORKS IN THE CAMPS

THE DEKALB DAILY CHRONICLE By United Press

Washington, D.C. (Oct. 10, 1918) – Nearly 200,000 cases of Spanish Influenza in army camps have been reported to date, it was announced today.

Yesterday 13,605 were added to the list, making the total 198,799 reported since Sept. 13.

Among the camps with the largest number for the day is Grant, with 113. Pneumonia still claims the greatest number of victims among the sufferers.

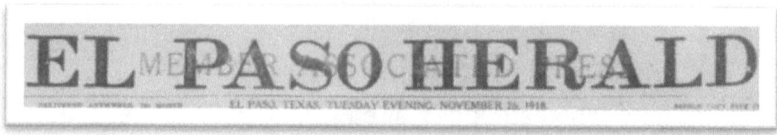

DIES TRYING TO SAVE SICK
Rev. R. A. Waltrip, Methodist Evangelist In Army 'Y,' Influenza Victim

THE EL PASO HERALD

El Paso, Texas (Oct. 10, 1918) – Rev. R. A. Waltrip died of pneumonia at a local hospital at 4 o'clock Wednesday afternoon, one hour after being admitted.

He was 37 years old. His wife and little daughter are In Hotel Dieu in a critical condition, suffering from pneumonia developed from influenza.

Rev. Waltrip had been engaged in army Y. M. C. A. work here for the past year. He was secretary of religious work at the remount building No—201, near Fort Bliss, during his first months here. At the time of contracting the illness, he was the general building secretary of Y. M. C. A. building No. 126 at Fort Bliss. He was a Methodist evangelist in the west Texas conference and had expected to be transferred to the Los Angeles district.

Works with Sick Till End.

Y. M. C. A. officials praise the work of the evangelist as being of the best.

When the influenza epidemic struck Fort Bliss, he stayed by the patient's night and day, endangering his own health unconsciously and, as a result, was himself stricken.

Rev. Mr. Waltrip is survived by his wife, three small children; two brothers, L. P. Waltrip, who is a professor in the public schools of Houston, Texas, and S. B. Waltrip, oi Mart Tex. The brothers were expected to arrive here Thursday. The body was prepared by Peak Undertaking company and will be shipped to Buffalo, Texas, the old home of Rev. Mr. Waltrip, and the two brothers will accompany it.

CORPL. C. E. DICKINSON DIES.
SON OF PIONEERS OF CITY

Charles Ernest Dickinson, aged 19, son of Mr. and Mrs. Fred P. Dickinson, died Thursday morning at the family home near the smelter, of influenza. The young man was born In Comanche, Texas, May 17, 1899, and had lived in El Paso all his life. Mr. and Mrs. Dickinson have been residents of El Paso almost continuously since 1888. The young man was a corporal and troop clerk in troop L. Third Texas cavalry. The funeral will be held Friday afternoon at 3 o'clock and will be private. Besides his parents, the deceased leaves two brothers, George, who is treasurer of the Crawford and Texas Grand theaters, and Fred P. Jr, who is in the navy, now located at Jersey City, N. J.

MRS. CLYDE WILSON FOLLOWS
HUSBAND TO GRAVE QUICKLY

News of the death, at Kokomo, Ind., of Mrs. Clyde Wilson, daughter of Mr. and Mrs. Fred Wright, 401 East California Street, El Paso, was received here Thursday. Mrs. Wright left here Sunday to be with her daughter, whose husband had died a few days before she expired.

Pneumonia Gets
Capt. J. D. Hess,
Veteran Of '98

Medical Officer, High Mason and Elk;
Was a Gallant Fighter at San Juan.

EL PASO HERALD – HOME EDITION

El Paso, Texas (Oct. 10, 1918) Capt. John D. Hess, medical corps, aged 41 years, died at the base hospital, Fort Bliss, Wednesday evening, after a week's illness of pneumonia. He was a recruiting officer and attending surgeon at the fort and had been here three months. His home was in Tokoa, Missouri. His mother, Mrs. Sarah E. Hess, and a sister were residing there. The mother was expected to arrive here Thursday, and the body, which is now at Peak's, will be accompanied by her back to Tokoa for burial.

Capt. Hess was a 32nd degree Mason, a Shriner, and an Elk. The Masonic relief board will have an escort join the military to accompany the body to the union depot. The date of shipment had not been decided Thursday at noon.

Capt. Hess was a Spanish-American war veteran. He participated in the attack on the blockhouse on San Juan Hill, Cuba. July 1, 1898, and was recommended for conspicuous gallantry shown in the encounter.

SPANISH INFLUENZA

BODIES OF AND WIFE
SENT TO SOCORRO RELATIVES

The bodies of Wm. B. Hill and wife, who died Sunday and Monday in local hospitals, were shipped Wednesday night to relatives in Socorro, N. M. Hill was a Paso del Norte bellboy.

MRS. HENRIETTA GOODLOE.

Funeral services for the late Mrs. Henrietta Goodloe, wife of Guy Goodloe, bookkeeper for the El Paso Printing Co.. were held Thursday afternoon at the chapel of Peak Undertaking Co. A short service was held at the grave. Rev. Ft. A. F. Upton presided. Mrs. Goodloe is survived, besides her husband and two little sons, by her mother, Mrs. Joseph H. Page; a brother, Joe Page, and a sister, Mrs. Paul Mattison. in El Paso, and two other sisters. Mrs. C. S. Turtle, Wichita, Kan., and Mrs. Evan Herd, Sanderson, Tex.

KATHLEEN DURHAM.

Funeral services for little Kathleen Durham, aged four, who died at the residence of her parents, Mr. and Mrs. J. S. Durham of 507 North Campbell street, were conducted Thursday afternoon at 2 o'clock from the chapel of McBean, Simmons & Hartford. Interment was in the Evergreen cemetery. Rev. Fuller Swift officiated.

ANTONIO MACIAS.

The funeral of Antonio Macias, aged 17, who died at his home, in Valverde addition, at 8:30 o'clock Wednesday night, was conducted Thursday morning at Peak's undertaking Chapel. Burial was in Concordia Catholic cemetery.

MRS. NETTIE RAY.

Mrs. Nettie Ray died Wednesday afternoon at 2M Mobile street. Her husband is very ill with influenza in the smelter hospital. The body is being held at the Peak undertaking house, pending word from relatives.

Mrs. C. M. HARLEY.

Mrs. C. M. Harley, aged 70, died Wednesday at noon at her residence, J1S East Missouri street. The body was shipped Thursday afternoon to relatives in Walterboro, S. C.

INFLUENZA AT STAND HERE

Believed New Cases Not Increasing; Deaths in Army and City Are 25.

The influenza epidemic, from reports, gathered Thursday, appears to be neither growing nor decreasing at El Paso. While the death toll of 15 in the last 24 hours is greater than that of the preceding day, the number of new cases has not increased.

The deaths are mostly cases seven days or more old. Ft. Bliss base hospital officials reported a total of 1369 cases received. 145 brought in during the 24 hours ending at 8 o'clock Thursday morning, 157 being discharged during that period.

Undertakers and Physicians Hard Pressed.

Undertakers in the city reported that night and day, and their telephones ring incessantly with calls from persons frantically seeking their assistance in securing doctors. Physicians often cannot be reached by telephone as they are out on calls most of the time.

Car Men Are Sick.

Traffic superintendent, H. S. Potter of the streetcar company, said that 35 carmen and three out of five inspectors were off duty on account of illness. He added that transportation superintendent Frank Scurlock and the majority of the company's office employees were ill also.

Soldier Dead, 18

Eighteen soldiers and seven civilians make up the death list of the last 34 hours. The soldier's dead are:

Capt. John D. Hess, medical corps, Johabea, Mo.

Pvt. Melvin H. Corbett. Medical Corps, Waco. Tex.

Pvt. Howard Fay. 82nd field artillery, Batavia. N. Y.

Pvt. Richard Wortham, 314th cavalry, Cicero. Ind.

Pvt. Raymond S. MacNeil, 214th cavalry. Quincy. Mass.

Pvt. L. Burnett, ninth engineers, Alcone, N. Y.

Pvt. Geo. Mansour, medical corps, Lowell, Mass.

Pvt. Wm. T. Hilt. 314th cavalry, Washington, Ala.

Pvt. Claude C Russell, medical corps. 3545 Memphis Street, El Paso.

Pvt. Amil R. Kickbush. Cavalry, unassigned, Firgrove, Mich.

Pvt. Thos. H. Bulkin, cavalry, unassigned, Scranton. Pa.

Pvt. Leonard Renis, seventh cavalry. Richmond. Ind.

Pvt. Mealude Baldez, medical corps, Gallup, N. M.

Pvt. John P. Carrol, cavalry, unassigned, Hart. Conn.

Pvt. Ed H. Taylor, medical corps, Ochiltree. Tex.

Pvt. Philip Smolders, 314th cavalry, Kalamazoo, Mich.

Pvt. Winfield Tucker, cavalry, unassigned, Hazlehurst, Pa.

Pvt. James Sweeney, ninth engineers, Lansford. Pa.

Civilians Dead, Seven.

The dead civilians are:

Rev. R. A. Waltrip. 1011 Nevada Street.

G. A. Gibson. Grant hotel.

Antonio Marcias, Val Verde addition.

Mrs. Nettie Ray. 2908 Mobile Street

Mrs. C. M. Harley. SIS East Missouri Street.

Florence Kathleen Burnham, 507 North Kansas Street.

Carl O. Waskey. 240 Porfirio Diaz Street.

ARMY AND NAVY JOIN IN PRESTON ROBERTS FUNERAL

A military escort and sailor pallbearers will accompany the body
of the late ensign Preston A. Roberts from the union station to the

Concordia cemetery Friday afternoon at 3:40 o'clock when it reaches here from Minneapolis, Minn., where young Roberts died a few days ago while attending navy medical school at the University of Minnesota. Chaplain J. M. Moose, seventh cavalry, will conduct service at the graveside. Mrs. Helen Roberts, the mother, will arrive with the body. At Minneapolis, a large number of naval students and friends escorted the body to the railroad station and offered profuse floral tributes.

Ensign Roberts was born and reared in El Paso. He recently worked for the Tuttle Paint and Glass company. He was the son of the late Ed C. Roberts, a pioneer. A brother, Maxey Roberts, is here from the Mare Island navy station to attend the funeral. A sister. Miss Helen Roberts lives here. The family home was at 911 North St. Vrain Street, in El Paso.

BODIES OF FIVE SOLDIERS
SHIPPED TO HOMES IN EAST

On Wednesday the bodies of the following soldiers who died of influenza and pneumonia were shipped by the Peak Undertaking Co. to the places designated:

Corp. Eugene L. Thornton, quartermaster corps, died Tuesday; body shipped to relatives in Lawnhill, Iowa accompanied by Pvt. Everett C. Tapp.

Pvt. Lawrence C Swift, Medical corps, died Wednesday; body shipped to relatives in Easton. Mass.

Pvt. Jos. Maretto, post bakery, died Sunday; body shipped to relatives in Rock Island, Ill., accompanied by Pvt. August A. Wisser.

Pvt. Chas. Graffonini, died Monday; body shipped to relatives in New Orleans, La., accompanied by Pvt. Wm. B. Rawlins.

Pvt. John Marik, died Tuesday; body shipped to relatives in Passaic N. J., accompanied by Pvt. Peter Mitchell.

NEW ASBURY PASTOR READY
TO GIVE AID IN SICKNESS

Rev. Hubert M. Smith, the newly appointed pastor of Asbury Methodist Church, said Thursday he would not be able to move into his parsonage at 3503 Hueco Street for a few days on account of illness in his family, his son. Guy Smith, having influenza.

Rev. Smith said, however, he is ready now to offer his services in cases of sickness or other matters demanding his attention. He still occupies the presiding elder's residence, 1107 East Boulevard: telephone 2009.

KIWANIS CALLS OFF.

There will be no meeting of the Kiwanis Club this week on account of Influenza. Secretary H P. Hadfield announced Thursday by card to members.

Flu May Close
Picture Shows
All Over U. S.

Picture Releases Discontinued Oct. 15th
Many New 'Flu' Cases.

New York, N.Y. (Oct. 1, 1918) – The National Association of Motion Picture Industries decided at a meeting here last night to discontinue all motion picture releases after Oct. 15 because of the epidemic of Spanish influenza. The embargo will remain in force until further notice.

Directors of the association were reticent regarding what occurred at their meeting. It was announced that a formal statement would probably be issued today. President Brady said the vote on the question of discontinuing releases was six to two. It was asserted, however, that the purpose was to close the motion picture houses of the country as a precautionary measure against influenza.

Proprietors of motion picture theaters seemed to be divided in their opinion as to the purpose of the drastic action proposed. Some of them asserted that it was a move on the part of the producers to hold back their feature pictures until attendance at theaters becomes normal, and they thus are enabled to obtain higher prices for their releases.

Hurting Bond Drive.

New York. (Oct. 10, 1918) – Hampered by the rapid spread of Spanish Influenza, which has seriously interfered with the Liberty loan campaign, the total of subscriptions in the Ni w York federal reserve district last night had reached only $378,163,700, or 21 percent of the $1,800,000,000 quota. The gain for the day was $40,960,050. New York city's total was $265,912,700, or 19.9 percent of its quota.

1004 Cases in Dallas.

Dallas, Texas (Oct. 10, 1918) All places of public amusement in Dallas will close today for an indefinite period upon orders Issued by the city commissioner, after the city board of health reported 1004 cases of Spanish Influenza In the city.

Maj. John O. McReynolds ordered Camp Dick placed under quarantine.

"Flu" Causes Bisbee Death.

Bisbee, Ariz. (Oct. 10, 1918) – The death of Frank Tracy, a miner, of pneumonia, following influenza, is the first in the epidemic of the disease now sweeping this district. Physicians here express the belief that the disease is now under control.

Closing Order at Tucson.

Tucson, Ariz. (Oct. 10, 1918) – Following the discovery of 2 cases or Spanish Influenza here, acting mayor Bernard issued a proclamation closing all theaters, schools, churches, pool halls, and other public places until further notice. There have been no fatalities.

Belen Issues Appeal.

Albuquerque. N. M Oct. 10. Belen, 30 miles south of here, reports between 200 and 300 cases of Spanish influenza there. There is only one doctor in the town, and he Is exhausted from constant attendance upon the sufferers. An appeal was made to the chamber of commerce here for physicians, and It was arranged for Albuquerque physicians to assist in giving the necessary medical attention.

5000 Monterey Cases.

Mexico City. (Oct. 10, 1918) – Five thousand cases of Spanish influenza have been reported in Monterey, and the disease is raging in the states of Nuevo Leon, San Luis Potosi, Coahuila, and Tamaulipas. In contrast, numerous cases have appeared in Saltillo, Torreon, and various other centers of population in the northern states.

Schools, churches, and other public meeting places are being closed.

Many New Army Cases.

Washington. D. C. Oct. 10. New cases of Influenza reported yesterday at array camps totaled 13,605, a slight increase over the number Tuesday. There also was an increase in pneumonia cases, with 2528 reported.

The 820 deaths made a total of 6543 in the camps since the epidemic started last month.

167 New Denver Cases.

Denver, Colo., (Oct. 10, 1918) – The health department at noon today had not received any reports of fatalities from Spanish influenza, but 187 new cases had appeared, bringing the total number to 845

Reports to the state board of health from Colorado counties showed little change except that from Rico, Dolores County. There is only one physician in Dolores County, and he is in a Denver hospital. Rico reported eight cases today. The Red Cross of Dolores county appealed to the state board for aid. The board will send physicians.

Influenza Slops Big Welcome to Potentate Jacoby at Albuquerque

Only informal greetings were extended to imperial potentate Elias J. Jacoby, of the Mystic Shrine, in Albuquerque. N. M- Thursday, on account of the city administration's request to suspend all public gatherings. A ceremonial by Ballut Abyad temple was called off. Mr. Jacoby arrived at Albuquerque early in the morning and was the guest of the Albuquerque Shriners during the day, and was met by nobles from Wichita, Kan., the next large city he will visit.

After witnessing a demonstration of artillery firing at the grounds near Fort Bliss Wednesday morning and an exhibition drill by troops of the Seventh cavalry, Mr. Jacoby was at luncheon at the Harvey house here and In the afternoon went to Juarez as the guest of Mexican consul general Andres Garcia and other Mexican officials. In the evening, the imperial visitor met Shriners at the Paso del Norte hotel and was again a guest at dinner at the Harvey house. He left for the north at 8:05 o'clock, accompanied by potentates J. C. Borrodaile. of Albuquerque, and Wyatt W. Evans, of El Paso.

In the trip to Fort Bliss, Mr. Jacoby Glover, Col F. W. Glover, chief of staff to Gen J. J. Hornbrook: Mayor Charles Davis. Mr. Evans, Mr. Borrodaile, and Lieut. C. W. Burk, representing Gen. Hornbrook.

INFLUENZA IN 77 COUNTIES IN TEXAS; SOME OFF ROADS

Austin, Texas (Oct. 10, 1918) – Reports received by the state health department indicate that Spanish influenza is prevalent in 77 counties in Texas, and in certain of these counties, it is epidemic. During September, reports were receiver from a total of 41 counties, and from October 1 to 5, 17 additional counties, while on Monday, reports were received from 19 counties, making a total of 77 counties in which this disease prevails at the present time.

The last reports received show that the disease is spreading in the western portion of Texas and away from the congested or thickly settled portions of the state.

WESTERN UNION SPECIAL

TELEGRAM TO BUREAU OF INDIAN AFFAIRS OFFICIALS

To WASHINGTON DC OCT 11, 1918

SUPT LAWRENCE KS

SPANISH INFLUENZA OF VIRULENT TYPE SPREADING OVER COUNTRY WITH ALARMING RAPIDLY MANY SUPERINTENDENTS REPORT SERIOUS CONDITIONS. INDIAN PUPILS AT OUR SCHOOLS AND INDIANS OLD AND YOUNG ON RESERVATIONS MUST BE GIVEN BEST CARE AND PROTECTION POSSIBLE. IMPORTANT THAT INHABITED SCHOOL BUILDINGS BE KEPT AT UNIFORM TEMPERATURE FROM SIXTY-EIGHT TO SEVENTY DEGREES GOOD VENTILATION MAINTAINED AND ALL FORMS OF DETRIMENTAL EXPOSURE OF PUPILS VERY CAREFULLY AVOIDED PARTICULARLY DURING ILLNESS AND CONVALESCENT PERIOD DISCONTINUE CLASSROOM AND OTHER ASSEMBLAGE WHEN CONDITIONS WARRANT ALLOWING NO INTERMINGLING OF PUPILS OR EMPLOYEES UNDER CONDITIONS OF OVERCROWDING, AND TO THE EXTENT YOU FIND IT DESIREABLE ENFORCE ISOLATION QUARANTINE FOR PREMISES CONSULT AND COOPERATE WITH LOCAL HEALTH OFFICERS AND SERVICE PHYSICIAN WHEN CONDITIONS JUSTIFY YOU ARE AUTHORIZED TO CEASE ALL ACTIVITIES NOT URGENTLY REQUIRED SO EMPLOYEES MAY BE AVAILABLE FOR NURSING AND OTHER INFLUENZA WORK

EMPLOYING EXTRA HELP WHEN STRICTLY NECESSARY KEEP OFFICE ADVISED.

SELLS
COMMISSIONER
530 PM

STATE COLLEGE IS QUARANTINED
ENTIRE FOURTH WARD AT AMES IS SHUT OFF FROM OUTSIDE WORLD.
GENERAL LINCOLN SAYS CONDITIONS ARE IMPROVED

Fewer New Cases of Influenza Developing in Recent Days—Some of the Students Seriously Ill—Four Deaths Reported on Thursday But Demise of Only Two Is Confirmed.

EVENING TIMES REPUBLICAN

Ames, Iowa (Oct. 11, 1918) – Following their adopted plan of doing everything in their power to prevent the spread of Spanish influenza in the city, at Iowa State College and among the soldiers and members of the students' army training corps, the local b6ard of health, acting in conjunction with the military authorities, cooperating with college officials, decided to quarantine the Fourth ward from the rest of the city beginning at 6 o'clock last night, while a stronger forbidden circle will be placed around the campus. All efforts will be made to stamp out the disease which has found root here.

According to the statement of General Lincoln, the condition at the training detachment and with the S. A. T. O. is showing signs of a big improvement. Enough cases had been removed from the different hospitals to make it possible for certain buildings to be fumigated, and the number of new cases is decreasing while those being dismissed from confinement are increasing.

"Conditions are bright, better, and improving, the hospital nurse reported to me," said General Lincoln, commandant of the Iowa State College training department and the students' army training corps. "Of course, we have many sick boys, but the number of sick boys, but the number of sick is less, by half, than the number reported Wednesday and the number reported yesterday is less than the number reported Tuesday."

It was first reported that the streetcars would discontinue service between the college and the city proper, but this is denied by General Lincoln, who declares they will be permitted to operate as long as they conform to the rules which are to be laid down by the commandant.

Must Have Passes.

"There is to be no unnecessary travel between the Fourth Ward and the city," the general said. "Every person must show some reason for his or her going back and forth." A guard will be stationed at the first bridge on the highway as well on the bridge at Russell Avenue, and passes will be issued.

"Those who are connected with the college and who are forced to travel the distance between the city and their place of employment will be furnished passes by the commandant's office when requested by the head of their four days or more, according to the severity of the attack. Those who are employed

in the city and who live in the Fourth Ward, will be furnished passes when they have established their identity to the satisfaction of the guards," the general said.

Delivery of foodstuffs and other articles will be permitted as in the past, excepting the delivery men cannot enter the house, placing the goods within the yard.

General order number five, issued by Captain Lane, adjutant, by order of General Lincoln, says:

"A close quarantine will be enforced including the entire campus and buildings of the Iowa State College or agricultural and mechanic arts, and no admittance unless by having a pass from headquarters S. A. T.C.

"A limited quarantine will be enforced, including the entire Fourth ward, excepting territory covered by paragraph one, which will prevent intercourse between Ames and the Fourth ward, except travel on public highways.

"This quarantine will go into effect at 6 o'clock p. m. Oct. 10, 1918.

"It is hoped that the same spirit of helpfulness that has prevailed, with such good results, will continue until we can be freed from all sickness and the need for the sacrifice of comforts and conveniences shall have passed. The Fourth ward will always be held in the highest esteem which their work for the general welfare has gained them."

The quarantine will be lifted; it is declared just as soon as it is possible to do so with safety. While the situation here is serious, it is declared there is no need for panic. The patients are well cared for, and everything possible to do for them is being done.

Four Deaths Thursday.

There are several serious cases, but the total number under observation and which has developed into Spanish influenza was not made known, either at the college or downtown. Several new cases, however, have been reported together with four deaths. Henry M. Larson. of Graettinger, Iowa, a member of the students' army training corps, passed away yesterday in the college hospital from the effects of pneumonia. Walter F. Riess, of North English, who was a member of the S. A. T. C., but who reported to the physicians downtown, died while under treatment for pneumonia at the Mary Greeley Hospital.

The names of the other two men could not be learned at this time.

Double Funeral for Dr. and Mrs. Arnold R. Moon at Williamsburg.

Special to Times-Republican.

Iowa City (Oct. 11, 1918)—A double funeral marked the laying to rest of Dr. and Mrs. Arnold R. Moon, of Williamsburg. The young physician and surgeon, a graduate of the colleges of liberal arts and medicine, S. U. I., was a victim of pneumonia, superinduced by Spanish influenza, during the epidemic of which he had refused to rest while patients needed his services. His wife was stricken at the same time and died twenty-four hours after her husband. Dr. Moon was in partnership with his father, in the Moon hospital, and the home of the latter, Dr. Arnold C. Moon, was the scene of the double funeral.

BAN ON PUBLIC GATHERINGS.
Lid on at Iowa Falls in Effort to
Check Spread of Influenza.
Special to Times-Republican.

Iowa Falls. (Oct 11, 1918)—As a precautionary measure against the spread of the Spanish Influenza, the local board of health put the lid on all assemblages this morning, and as a result, the public schools are closed. All public gatherings, such as audiences at the theaters, congregations at churches and other public places are under the ban. This action was taken on the advice of the physicians of the city and with the hope of preventing the disease from gaining much of a hold. Ellsworth College, being under the direction of the government, is not affected by this order.

Three Story Towns Closed.

Special to Times-Republican.

Nevada, (Oct. 11, 1918)—Several Story County towns were closed because of the prevalence of Spanish influenza. At Roland, there is an estimate that 150 cases prevail in the community. Two deaths have resulted, and the schools, churches, moving picture theaters, and the public gatherings closed.

Story City and McCallsburg also have many cases and are closed in like manner. At Ames, the churches and theaters are closed, but the schools are still open, and it is stated that there are but few cases there other than at the army camp on the campus.

Clarion Woman Dies of Influenza

Clarion, Iowa (Oct 11, 1918)—A message was received here announcing the death of Mrs. Joe Henely at Pensacola, Fla, of Spanish influenza. Mr. Henely is also ill in the same hospital with the same complaint but was improving at the latest report.

He has been employed at the shipyards in that city, and Mrs. Henely had gone south to stay with him. The body will be brought to Bade Grove, where Mrs. Henley's parents reside.

Pneumonia Kills Glidden Girl.

Glidden, (Oct, l0, 1918)—Miss Edna Heaton, the youngest daughter of Mr. A. J. Heaton died as the result of pneumonia complicated with heart trouble. On Monday, Miss Heaton assisted her mother with the housework and was not taken ill until that evening, her condition becoming serious yesterday forenoon.

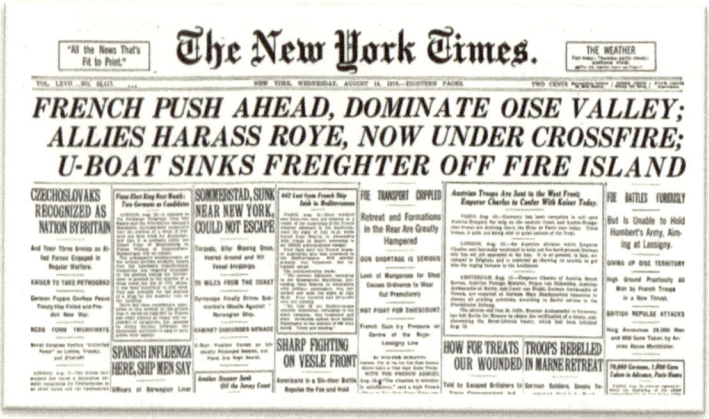

LONG ISLAND WRECK SERIOUSLY INJURES 9

All ambulances, surgeons, and hospitals busy with influenza patients

NEW YORK TIMES

Oct. 12, 1908 – Nine persons were seriously injured last night when a Long Island electric train from Flatbush Avenue, Brooklyn, to Rockaway Beach, ran through an open switch near Lalance & Grosjean agateware factory at Woodhaven and crashed into a freight train on a siding. The injured were without immediate attention because all of the ambulances and surgeons of St. Mary's Hospital, Jamaica, and other hospitals in Brooklyn and Queens were busy caring for influenza patients.

Those taken to St. Mary's Hospital were: Robert Bauer, 576 Atlantic Avenue, Brooklyn, Edward Miller of Glendale, L.I., Emma and Harriet Klotz of 51 Diner Street, Rockaway Beach; Edward Dawson of 607 Kosciusko Street, Brooklyn; Sophie Brady of Edgemere; Catherine Stewart of 24 Beach 104th Street, Rockaway Park, and David E. Jacobs of 404 Boulevard, Rockaway Beach.

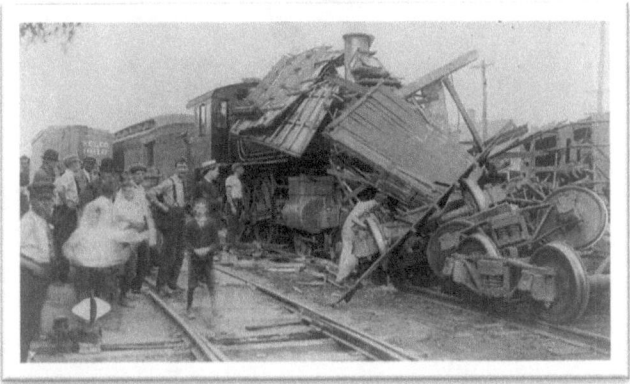

This Long Island Railroad wreck took place in 1909 in a similar fashion to the one in 1918.

5 THEATRES CLOSE TONIGHT
Theatrical Depression Attributed In Large Part to Influence Scare
NEW YORK TIMES

Oct. 12, 1918 – An unprecedented theatrical depression, which managers attribute in large part to the influenza scare, resulted in sudden decisions yesterday to close five playhouses tonight. The attractions departing are "Penrod" at the Punch and Judy; "The Walk-Offs" at the Morosco; "Watch Your

Neighbor" at the Booth; "I.O.U." at the Belmont, and "The Woman on the Index" at the Forty-eighth Street Theatre; "Some Night!" and "The Maid of The Mountains" were previously announced to be closing tonight, making a total of seven.

For the first five of these houses, no incoming attractions have yet been announced. In all, more than a dozen local theatres will be dark next week.

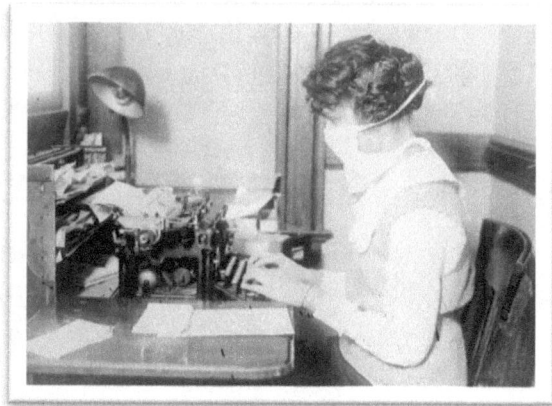

A typist in New York City works with a mask on her face.

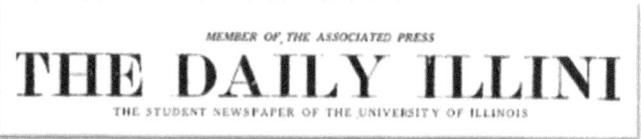

INFLUENZA EPIDEMIC
CLAIMS A SECOND VICTIM
THE DAILY ILLINI Student newspaper at the University of Illinois.

Urbana, Ill. (Oct. 13, 1918) – Authorities Report Total of 300 Cases of Spanish Disease on Campus

Donald J. Miller, 21, of Vincennes, Ind., died yesterday morning at eight o clock at the Phi Kappa Psi house after a short illness with Spanish influenza. The body was taken to Vincennes yesterday afternoon for burial. Miller is the second person to die in the last two days as a result of the epidemic of influenza about the campus. The number of new cases yesterday kept the total at 300, as an equal number were discharged from the hospitals.

 The situation at present is no more serious than it was at this time last week, according to authorities, and there is no reason to believe that the disease will spread much further. The four hospitals are doing their utmost and are caring for the patients with the same facility as a regular hospital system.

Rumors circulating the campus that the situation is much more alarming than it is represented have been branded as false. All persons in the hospitals are well treated, and no causes for complaints have arisen anywhere. Physicians are hoping to have the epidemic on the wane within a few days.

44 DEATHS IN D. C. FROM INFLUENZA REPORTED AT NOON

676 New Cases Were Recorded Today, as Against 1,312 Yesterday.

12,847 CASES WITH 485 DEATHS DURING OCTOBER

Daily Record for First Fourteen Days of the Month—Shortage in Physicians' Report Cards.

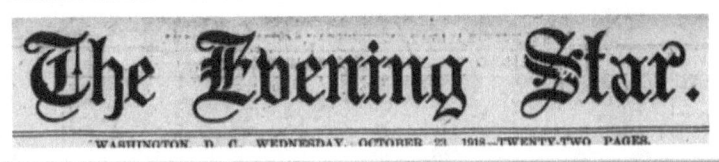

THE EVENING STAR

Washington, D.C. (Oct. 14, 1918) – Influenza continued to reap a heavy death toll in the District today, forty-four deaths being recorded up to noon since 9 o'clock last night.

New cases reported, however, showed a big decline. As compared with 1,312 cases registered yesterday, only 676 were recorded up to noon today.

This may not indicate a slowing up in the progress of the epidemic since there has been a shortage of cards on which the disease is reported by physicians. It is possible that some physicians are out of the cards and have delayed making reports of cases under their care.

12,847 Cases; 485 Deaths.

The influenza record from and including October 1, up to noon today, shows a total of 12,847 cases reported and 485 deaths registered. The record by days is as follows:

	New cases.	Deaths.
October 1	162	10
October 2	39	10
October 3	56	3

October 4	618	23
October 5	276	35
October 6	279	18
October 7	1,150	32
October 8	2,174	43
October 9	1,466	19
October 10	1,701	57
October 11	1,594	73
October 12	1,344	65
October 13	1,312	83
October 14 1/2	676	44
Total	**12,847**	**485**

Public Health Service Is
Rushing the Preliminaries
for Influenza Hospital.

The public health service today rushed plans for equipping an influenza hospital with 500 beds in the building at 19th Street and Virginia Avenue, vacated last week by the quartermaster general's office.

At the same time, the Red Cross was making every effort to obtain nurses for this and other hospitals. Up to noon, the Red Cross branch at 14th and F streets had received an offer of services as nurses from about fifty persons employed in government departments and elsewhere.

This is only about half the number of nurses required now.

The effort to Obtain Nurses.

Commissioner Brownlow yesterday appealed to the heads of government departments and business establishments that they take a! census of their employees this morning to recruit nurses and hospital help. It was expected the appeal would result in services being volunteered by many persons during the afternoon.

Beds have been ordered for the new hospital, and the institution probably will be ready to receive patients in two or three days.

Health Officer Fowler today commandeered Washington's coffin supply. This action was taken to prevent coffins being shipped out of the District. The demand for caskets in Alexandria and other nearby points outside the District is more than the supply, and effort has been made to obtain them in Washington.

Appeal from the outside is being made to Washington for nurses, but the authorities are taking steps to keep in the District all those qualified and willing to render service of this character. Even this does not promise that the local situation will be adequately met.

Gauze Masks for Public Considered

Held in abeyance by the Commissioners today were the proposals looking toward an order for the wearing of gauze masks by the entire population and the closing of poolrooms and other places of business. It appeared probable that the wearing of masks would not be made mandatory, especially if the situation does not become worse. The Commissioners are not disposed to close poolrooms unless such action should appear more required than at present.

To take this step would open the question of closing cigar stores and similar business establishments.

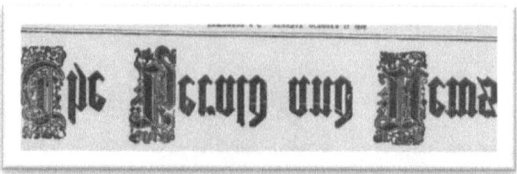

SPANISH INFLUENZA – THREE DAY FEVER – "THE FLU"

The Herald & News Oct. 15, 1918
(Newberry, South Carolina)

By Rupert Blue, Surgeon General j

What is Spanish Influenza? Is it something new? Does it come from Spain?

The disease now occurring in this country and called "Spanish Influenza" resembles a very contagious kind of "cold" accompanied by fever, pains in the head, eyes, ears, back or other parts of the body, and a feeling of severe sickness. In most of the cases, the symptoms disappear after three or four days; the patient then rapidly recovering; some of the patients, however, develop pneumonia, or inflammation of the ear, or meningitis, and many of these complicated cases die.

Whether this so-called "Spanish" influenza is identical to the epidemic of earlier years is not yet known.

Epidemics of influenza have visited this country since 1647. It is interesting to know that this first epidemic was brought here from Valencia, Spain. Since that time, there have been numerous epidemics of the disease. In 1989 and 1890, and epidemic of influenza, starting somewhere in the Orient spread first to Russia, and thence over practically the entire civilized world.

Three years later, there was another flare-up of the disease.

Both times the epidemic spread over the United States.

Although the present epidemic is called "Spanish influenza," there is no reason to believe that it originated in Spain. Some writers who have studied the question believe that the epidemic came from the Orient, and they call attention to the fact that the Germans mention the disease as occurring along the eastern front in the summer and fall of 1917.

How can "Spanish Influenza" be recognized?

There is as yet no certain way in which a single case of "Spanish influenza" can be recognized; on the other hand, recognition is easy where there is a group of cases. In contrast to the outbreaks of ordinary coughs and colds, which usually occur in cold months, epidemics of influenza may occur at any season of the year; thus, the present epidemic raged most intensely in Europe in May, June, and July. Moreover, in the case of ordinary colds, the general symptoms (fever, pain, depression) are by no means as severe or as sudden in their onset as they are in influenza. Finally, ordinary colds do not spread through the community so rapidly or so extensively, as does influenza.

In most cases, a person taken sick with influenza feels sick rather suddenly. He feels weak, has pains in the eyes, ears, head or back, and often is sore all over. Many patients feel dizzy, some vomit. Most of the patients complain of feeling chilly, and with this comes a fever in which the temperature rises to 100 to 104. In most cases, the pulse remains relatively slow.

In appearance, one is struck by the fact that the patient looks sick. His eyes and the inner side of his eyelids may be slightly "blood-shot" or "congested," as

145

the doctors say. There may be running from the nose, or there may be some cough. These signs of a cold may not be marked; nevertheless, the patient looks and feels very sick.

In addition to the appearance and the symptoms as already described examination, the patient's blood may aid the physician in recognizing "Spanish influenza," for it has been found that in this disease, the number of white corpuscles shows little or no increase above the normal. It is possible that the laboratory investigations now being made through the National Research Council, and the United States Hygienic Laboratory will furnish a more certain way in which individual cases of this disease can be recognized.

What Is the course of the disease?
Do people die of It?

Ordinarily, the fever lasts from three to four days, and the patient recovers. But while the proportion of deaths in the present epidemic has generally been low, in some places the outbreak has been severe, and deaths have been numerous. When death occurs, it is usually the result of a complication.

What causes the disease, and how is it spread?

Bacteriologists who have studied influenza epidemics in the past have found in many of the cases a very small rod-shaped germ called, after its discoverer, Pfeiffer's bacillus. In other cases of apparently the same kind of disease, there were found pneumococci, the germs of lobar pneumonia. Still, others have been caused person to person, the germ being carried with the air along with the very; small droplets of mucus, expelled by coughing or sneering, forceful talking and the like by one who already has the germs of the disease. They may also be carried about in the air in the form of dust coming from dried mucus, from coughing and sneezing, or from careless people who spit on the floor and on the sidewalk, as in most other catching diseases, a person who has only a mild attack of the disease himself may give a very severe attack to others.

What should be done by those who catch the disease?

It is very important that every person who becomes sick with influenza should go home at once and go to bed. This will help keep away dangerous complications and will, at the same time, keep the patient from scattering the disease far and wide,

It is highly desirable that no one is allowed to sleep in the same room with the patient. In fact, no one 'but the nurse should be allowed in the room.

If there are cough and sputum or running of the eyes and nose, care should be taken that all such discharges are collected on bits of gauze or rags or paper napkins and burned.

If the patient complains of fever and headache, he should be given water to drink, a cold compress to the forehead, and a light sponge. Only such medicine should be given as is prescribed by the doctor. It is foolish to ask the druggist to prescribe and may be dangerous to take the so-called "safe, sure, and harmless" remedies advertised by patent medicine manufacturers.

If the patient is so situated that he can be attended only by someone who must also look after others in the family, it is advisable that such attendant wear a wrapper, apron, or gown over the ordinary house clothes while in the sick room and slip this off when leaving to look after the others.

Nurses and attendants will do well to guard against breathing in dangerous disease germs by wearing a simple fold of gauze or mask while near the patient.

Will, a person who has had influenza before catching the disease again?

It is well known that an attack of measles or scarlet fever or smallpox usually protects a person against another attack of the same disease. This appears not to be true of '"Spanish influenza."

According to newspaper reports, the King of Spain suffered an attack of influenza during the epidemic thirty years ago and was again stricken during the recent outbreak in Spain.

How can one guard against Influenza!

In guarding against the disease of all kinds, the body must be kept strong and able to fight off disease germs. This can be done by having a proper proportion of work, play, and rest by keeping the body well clothed and by eating sufficient, wholesome, and properly selected food.

In connection with diet, it is well to remember that milk is one of the best all-around foods obtainable for adults as well as children. So far as a disease like influenza is concerned, health authorities everywhere recognize the very close relation between its spread and overcrowded homes. While it Is not always possible, especially in times like the present, to avoid such over-crowding, people should consider the health danger and make every effort to reduce home overcrowding to a minimum. The value of fresh air through open windows cannot be overemphasized.

Where crowding is unavoidable, as, in streetcars, care should be taken to keep the face so turned as not to inhale directly the air 'breathed out by another person.

It is especially important to beware of the person who coughs or sneezes without covering his mouth and nose.

It also follows that one should keep out of crowds and stuffy places as much as possible, keep homes, office, and workshops well aired, spend some time out of doors each day, walk to work if at all practicable. In short, make every effort to breathe as much pure air as possible.

"Cover-up each cough and sneeze; if you don't, you'll spread disease."

Dr. William E. Pelham, Jr.

The State. (Oct. 15, 1918)

Newberry, S.C. – Newberry was one of the first of the cities of South Carolina to suffer seriously from the epidemic and was the peculiar misfortune of the community that one of the victims of the disease was a physician, Dr. William Ellerbe Pelham Jr., of great usefulness and promise of expanding usefulness. He was in his fortieth year, a graduate of the medical department of Tulane University, where he won his degree with honors in the class of 1915. He was a gentleman of irreproachable character, a deacon in the Presbyterian Church, and by his faithful ministrations had endeared himself to a large circle of friends. The harvest of death has been so great in South Carolina and elsewhere in the last fortnight that it is not practicable for newspapers to call attention to the virtues of many of those who have died. The death of a young and beloved physician of talent and attainments is, however, an incident of more than ordinary sadness even in a time when so many homes have been bereaved. Outside of

Newberry as well as in that city, there is felt profound sorrow for the loss to the family and to the people of this talented doctor whose services were so greatly needed and so cheerfully given.

THE INFLUENZA SITUATION SEEMS TO BE IMPROVING

While there are a good many people sick and a good many who are very ill and there have been several sad deaths, the situation in the prevailing epidemic it seems to us is improving in the city.

Three doctors came to our assistance last week, and several nurses and everything possible is being done to care for the sick and to alleviate suffering.

The conditions in the country in rural districts are not so good as the disease seems to be spreading in these sections, and a good many deaths have been reported, especially among the colored people.

It has suspended all business, and especially has it hit hard the newspapers because the merchants are not advertising as the people are requested to stay away from crowds and from town, in fact.

The State Board of Health does not order the country gins to close but requests those in authority to see to it that there Is no crowding of the people and that those who come to the gin stay out in the open. That is the order sent to Sheriff Blease.

****

(Oct. 15, 1918, Newberry, S.C.) – The influenza is prevailing in Greenville, and there have been a great many deaths among the civilians and at Camp Sevier. The hearses and ambulances wore going all day, and there were dead at the morgues at all of the undertaking establishments. There was a military funeral in the afternoon, and it was sad and impressive. Among the civilians, two prominent preachers had died during the last few days, Dr. Turnipseed of the Methodist church and Dr. Griffin of the Presbyterian church.

Two Funerals at the Same Time
Held at St. Paul's Church.

NEWBERRY, S.C. – (Oct. 15, 1918) – On Tuesday, Oct. 8, there were two funerals at the same time at St. Paul's church near Pomaria, and both from the same house in Newberry.

Anna Elizabeth Beggs died first. Her age was 24 years, five months, and 22 days. Frank S. Summer, her stepfather, died a little later. His age was 57 years, four months, and 21 days.

Both died of Spanish influenza. The funeral was conducted by the Rev. S. P. Koon assisted by the Rev. Driggers of the Baptist church. Their bodies were laid to rest in St. Paul's cemetery to await the resurrection. May the Holy Spirit comfort the bereaved family.

The Sheriff Enforcing the Order.

Sheriff Cannon G. Blease is seeing to it that the order of the State Board of Health is being carried out in this county. He has notified the mayor and magistrate and other officials throughout the county that they have the order obeyed. To that end, Sheriff Blease went to work immediately upon receipt of the following: "Under the authority of paragraph 1614 South Carolina code you are directed to close all schools and other institutions of learning, churches, picture shows and all other places of public gathering in your county. See that there is no crowding in stores and public conveyance.

James A. Hayne, Secretary and State Health Officer.

So far, however, as the City of Newberry is concerned, the board of health had already ordered closed the places above mentioned, which order went promptly into effect and is still of force.

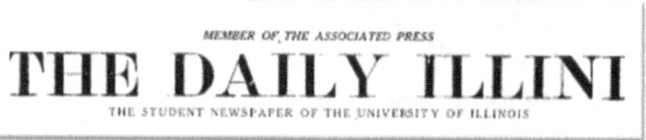

INFLUENZA EPIDEMIC CLAIMS
THREE MORE FROM UNIVERSITY

Carl E. Pike, Instructor, and Two Students Yesterdays Toll—

Death Total Reaches Seven.

THE DAILY ILLINI

(Oct. 16, 1918) – Carl E. Pike, an instructor in the department of physics, died this morning at 3:45 o'clock in the emergency hospital at College Hall.

He had been ill about a week with influenza which developed into pneumonia, Pike was 27 years old and had been a member of the faculty of the University for two years. His body was taken to Central City, Iowa, by his parents, who were with him when he died. Albeno Rodighiero, 22 of Chicago, was the second victim of influenza yesterday. He died at four a. m at the Beta Theta Pi house. His parents, brother, and sister were at his bedside. The body has been taken to Chicago for burial. Byron. Daugherty, 22, of Streator, died at 6:30 o 'clock yesterday morning in the isolation hospital on the south campus. Daugherty was twenty years old and had been sick since last Thursday night. His father and mother have taken the body to their home in Streator.

The toll of Spanish influenza now totals seven victims, all having died since last Friday afternoon. All of the five emergency hospitals are full at present, with more than 300 patients being cared for. Except for those cases which have resulted fatally, most of the patients are in no serious condition, many of the cases being not much more than heavy colds and attacks of grip.

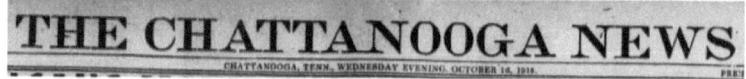

NEED FOR MORE NURSES

THE CHATTANOOGA NEWS

Oct. 16, 1909

CHATTANOOGA, TENN. – Dr. T. S. McCallie has gone to Ringgold, Ga., today to attend the funeral of Miss Jamie Edwards.

Things are a little quiet at the Red Cross office. The rush for the little white masks has subsided, and R. F. Hudson of the nurses' department, says that conditions have evidently improved over Tuesday.

More nurses can be used In the city, said Mr. Hudson, and there is a demand for the Good Samaritan spirit.

Many homes need sonic one to go and prepare the food for the sick. In some households, the mother of little children is ill and no servant to attend the children or nurse to care for the patient's wants. In some families, there are several cases and the overworked mother badly in need of assistance. It is next to Impossible to obtain servants, even where the families can pay them. Unless there are volunteers for those families, unnecessary Buffering will undoubtedly be the result

SOCIETY PERSONALS

Mrs. Uri Bachtel, of Montgomery, Alabama, was here by the death of Carl MacIntosh.

Burton Jones, of the St. James Drug Company, and his son, Carroll Jones, recovering from an attack of influenza.

News has been received here by friends of the safe arrival overseas of Corp. J. Walter Childress of the Fifty-Seventh pioneer infantry.

Mrs. John C. Beeson has been removed to her home on Vine Street, from the Newell infirmary, where she underwent an operation.

INFLUENZA

Mrs. Douglas McMillin, who has been very ill of influenza at West-Ellis Infirmary, is reported as much improved.

Miss Clara Pindell is recovering from an Illness of Influenza.

Miss Willie Mae Sutton, of McCallie Avenue, who has been ill of Influenza, is convalescing.

Miss Stella Alexander has gone to Reeves, Ga., where she will undergo treatment at the Battle Creek Sanitarium.

Mrs. William Bryan is improving from her recent illness at the home of Mrs. E. P. Sisson in St. Elmo.

Miss Emma Sue Smartt, who has been ill, is now able to be out.

Mrs. Ben Allison is ill of Influenza at her home in St. Elmo. Masters Joe and Ben Allison Jr. have recovered from their recent illness.

Misses Emma and Nellie Greenwood have returned from Martha Washington College. Owing to the epidemic of influenza, the college will be remained closed until Nov. 1.

HEAVY TOLL OF INFLUENZA

Washington, D.C. (Oct. 16, 1918). There were 6,122 deaths from Spanish Influenza in thirty cities during the week ending Oct. 12, as compared with 19 for the week ending Sept. 14, when the disease got its first foothold In Boston. In the same period, there were 4,409 deaths from pneumonia.

These figures, announced today by the Bureau of the census, do not Include figures from army camps, and, with reports missing from all other cities and towns and country districts, there was no way of estimating the total number of deaths.

The heaviest toll from influenza was 1,697 in Philadelphia. The New York total was 969, Boston 850, and Chicago 871.

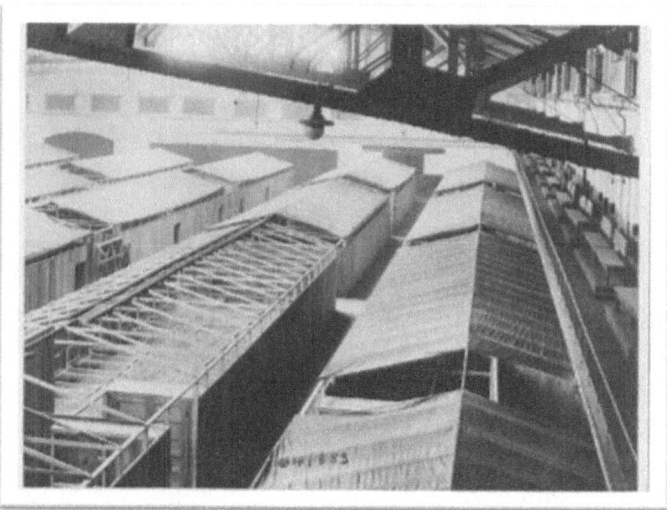

The Medical Department of the Army set up a Military hospital in the Boston Armory to treat those inflicted by the Spanish Influenza during the critical months of September, October, and November of 1918. *Photo from Boston Transcript.*

STATE FAIR NOT TO OPEN
Health Authorities Refuse to Allow the Mississippi Fair to Proceed.

Jackson, Miss., Oct. 16. Dr. W. S. Leathers, executive officer of the state board of health, has ordered the Mississippi State Fair, which was to have opened In this city Oct. 21, not to be held on account of the Influenza epidemic.

The situation generally Is Improving rapidly. Dr. Leathers says.

HAROLD CROUCH RECOVERS
Influenza Has Kept Him in Naval Hospital Several Days.

Mr. and Mrs. G. O. Crouch received a letter Tuesday from their son, Harold, who is in the navy at New Orleans, in which he stated that he was just recovering from two weeks' illness of Influenza. He has been in the hospital.

The young man's message relieved the anxiety of his parents, as they had not heard from him for several days.

Harold Crouch offered his services to his country and flag last winter and began active duty in January. For a while, he was on a patrol boat. Lately, he has been stationed at New Orleans. He Is one of Chattanooga's best-known young men.

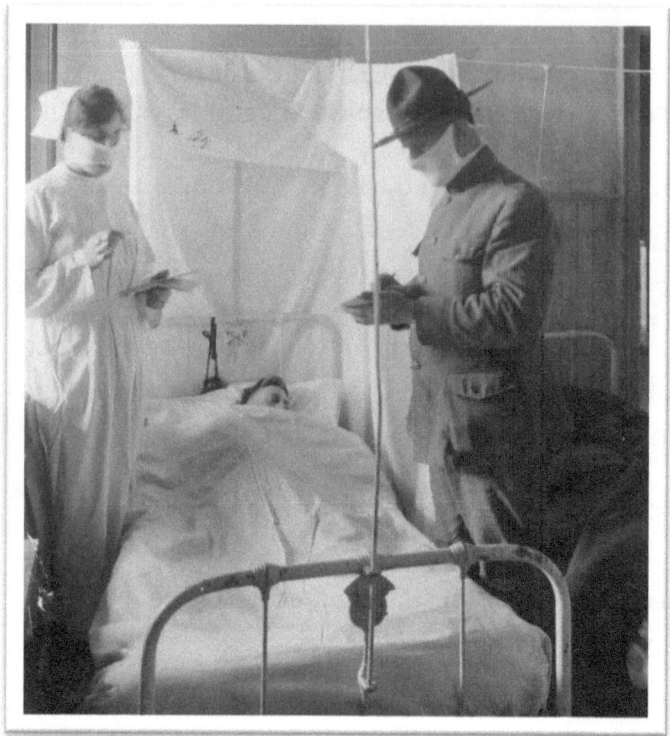

Medical Department - Influenza Epidemic 1918 - Spanish Influenza in army hospitals. Masks and cubicles used in United States of America General Hospital Number 4, Fort Porter, New York. Patients' beds are reversed, alternately so breath of one patient will not be directed toward the face of another.

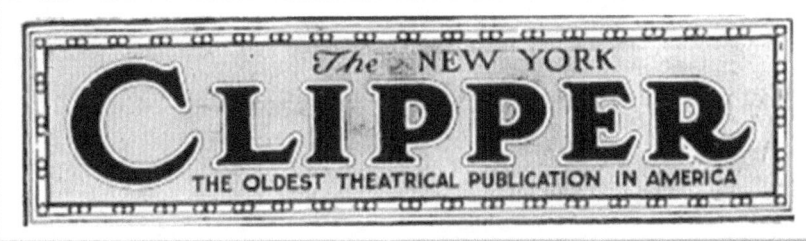

VAUDEVILLE CIRCUITS STOP
ROUTING FOR TIME BEING

Closing of Houses in Practically Every State in the Middle West
and South Throws Booking Men Into a Tangle
Never Before Experienced

THE NEW YORK CLIPPER

The Spanish influenza epidemic completely tied up all of the western and southern vaudeville circuits this week, routing being discontinued for the time being by the Interstate, Western Vaudeville Association, Finn, and Heiman, Jones, Linick and Schaeffer and other organizations operating theatres in the middle west and southern states. Thousands of vaudeville actors are now laying off in Chicago, and more are arriving every day. The vaudeville booking men have no means of telling exactly when the ban will be lifted in the various sections affected by the Spanish pest, but are hopeful that before another week has passed, the situation will have at least improved in spots.

The "Flu" is very bad at present in the Middle West and South. Detroit and Grand Rapids were the only cities open in the State of Michigan on Saturday, and their closing this week means that there is not a vaudeville theatre operating in the states of Illinois, Wisconsin, Indiana, Ohio, Iowa, Missouri, Mississippi, Texas, Louisiana, Alabama, and Kentucky. Conditions are decidedly unfavorable for an early opening in Chicago. Meanwhile, all concerned are holding a pat hand and hoping for the best.

FLU HALTS MINTURN STOCK

NEW YORK CLIPPER

MILWAUKEE, Wis., Oct. 10, 1918. —The Harry Minturn stock at the Shubert Theatre, in common with all the other shows in the city, was ordered closed today by the local authorities.

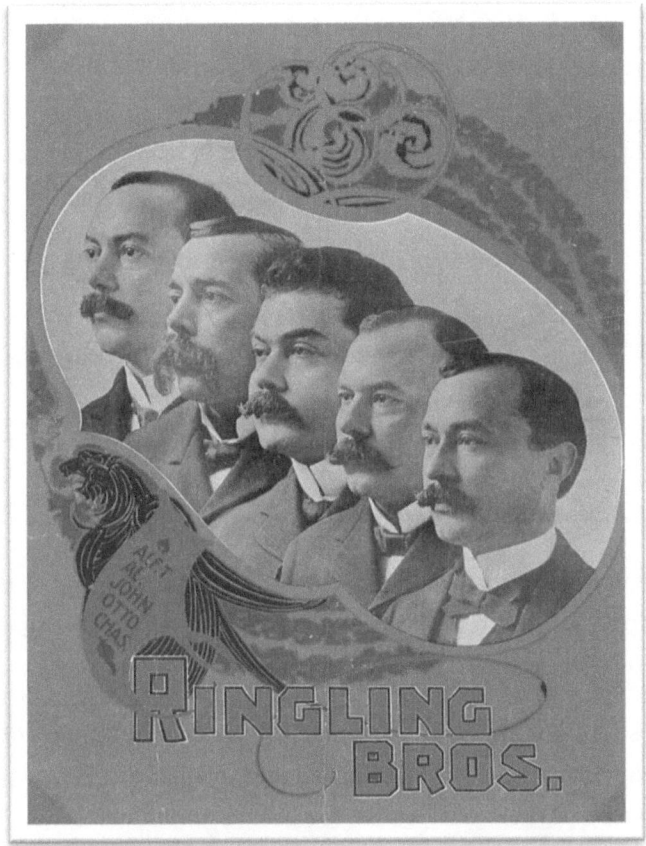

Ringling Brothers, 1900, Library of Congress

RINGLING BROS. CHANGE WINTER TOWN

NEW YORK CLIPPER

For the first time in the history of the Ringling Brothers Circus, the big show will not be wintered at Baraboo, Wis., as formerly. The aggregation will move into the Barnum and Bailey headquarters at Bridgeport, Conn.

The show was forced to close two weeks before the scheduled end while playing in Waycross, Ga., due to Spanish influenza. The Barnum and Bailey Circus was also ordered closed while it was playing at Houston, Texas. Both will winter at Bridgeport, Conn.

The North Mississippi Herald

INFLUENZA RAGING IN WATER VALLEY

Over 1200 Cases Reported; Doctors Unable to Care for Patients – Only Two Deaths Resulted

THE NORTH MISSISSIPPI HERALD

Water Valley, Miss. (Oct. 11, 1918) – Spanish influenza, or the common old grippe as Health Doctor Cox diagnosis it, is raging in epidemic form in Water Valley.

The disease struck the city last week and spread rapidly until practically every section of the city is affected and in all over 1200 cases have been reported.

The fatalities from the disease have been remarkably low, only two, so far, which goes to show that there is no cause for the people to be unduly excited as there is very little danger if the patient will receive immediate attention and take proper care of himself.

The four physicians of the city have worked night and day heroically in their efforts to serve the people, and then it was impossible for them to see all the patients, especially as often or at times when needed.

The big Yocona Mills were compelled to close down Tuesday on account of fully three-fourths of the working force being stricken with the disease.

Thursday morning, over 300 employees of the Illinois Central railroad shops failed to report for duty while the train crews have been hit hard. The company has so far managed to keep the trains running while the shops continue operation but in a very limited and disorganized manner.

The Mayor and City Aldermen met Monday night and passed a "closing up" ordinance prohibiting all public gatherings of any kind as well as unnecessary traveling on the streets.

The picture shows schools, churches, etc. were included in the order of closing until the endemic shall have passed.

THE HERALD HIT BY THE SPANISH "FLU"

The Herald comes out several days late this issue on account of the force suffering from attacks of the Spanish Influenza.

Miss Christina Mae Allen, our Linotype operator, was stricken Tuesday and confined to her bed until Saturday, three other members of the family being down at the same time.

Several members of the editor's family are down, and the editor himself has been sick for over a week but somehow manages to keep going.

It is utterly impossible to secure additional help, and all we can do is to do the very best under the circumstances.

We ask our subscribers to be as considerate as possible in our shortcomings while in the throes of the epidemic now raging in the city.

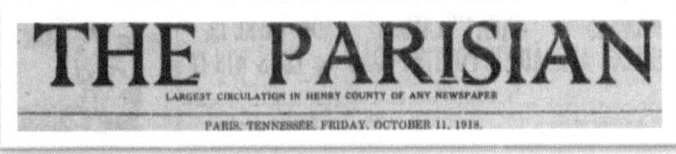

LARGEST CIRCULATION IN

HENRY COUNTY OF ANY NEWSPAPER

REAPER WHOSE NAME IS DEATH
His Sickle Keen Reaps The Beaded Grain and Flowers Between

PARIS, TENNESSEE, (OCTOBER 11, 1918) – The opening verse of Longfellow's poem "The Reaper and the Flowers" seem appropriate in Henry County this week, as the number of deaths has been unusually large and comprise the childhood and womanhood referred to as flowers and manhood as the bearded grain.

The ages have ranged from infancy to old age of those who have passed away, leaving sorrowing relatives to cherish their memory.

The following are the deaths which have occurred since our last issue:

WALTER B. GRIZZARD.

On Monday night, Walter B. Grizzard, who has been in feeble health for several months, passed away in Huntingdon at a ripe old age. He was 84 years of age and was the father of Mrs. W. J. Holman of West Wood Street, with whom he spent a part of his time.

His death was possibly due to heart failure, as he was found dead in bed. The interment was in Huntingdon. He was a splendid citizen and was well known to the citizens of Paris of half a century ago, where he visited. He was the father of six children.

HARLEY ADAMS.

At an early hour Tuesday morning, at his home near India, Harley Adams passed away from pneumonia following an attack of influenza.

He appeared to be getting along as well as could be expected when his brother, W. G. Adams, left his bedside about midnight, but later, he grew worse and passed away.

He was 24 years of age and is survived by his wife and child, both of whom are reported critically ill. His father and several brothers also survive him.

Thursday morning, the funeral services were conducted at the residence by Rev. D. T. Spaulding, and the remains were taken to Sedalia, Ky., his old home for interment.

MRS. WHEATLEY.

A death of unusual sadness occurred here Monday when Mrs. Arthur Wheatley passed away, and about an hour later, death claimed her baby.

Mr. and Mrs. Wheatley both have been suffering from influenza, and after their baby came, she grew worse, and death resulted; her infant also passing away.

Mr. Wheatley was so ill that he could not accompany the remains to Faxon, their old home, where the interment took place. Mrs. Wheatley was twenty-eight years old.

R. H. WISEHEART.

On Sunday, at the Western Hospital at Bolivar, Robert H. Wiseheart passed away at the age of 45 years years.

The body was brought to Paris, and after funeral services at the family residence near Paris on Tuesday, the remains were laid to rest in Maple wood cemetery. The funeral services were conducted by Rev. D. T. Spaulding. He was highly esteemed by a large circle of friends who extend their sympathy to his wife and relatives. He was a member of the First Baptist church.

V J. HORACE DORAN

At an early hour Monday morning, at the home of his father, M. E. Doran, in the Whitlock section, J. Horace Doran, the youngest son, died of pneumonia following an attack of influenza.

He was a splendid young man, 28 years of age, a member of the local company of National Guards, and a prominent member of the Woodman of the World organization.

The remains were interred at Maplewood cemetery on Tuesday after services by Revs. D. C. Gray of Whitlock, C. B. Clayton, and Davis, of Paris.

FRED COLLINS.

A telegram from Camp Mills, New York, announced the fact that Fred Collins died on Sunday at that place. Mr. Collins was 23 years six months and three days old and was the son of John T. Collins of the India neighborhood. The young man will be remembered by the businessmen as having been connected with the Southern Express Company here for some time.

He volunteered in Battery D., of the 114th Field Artillery here, but was rejected. Later he was sent to Camp Gordon as a selective draftsman, and having qualified for The mail service in France was en route when his death occurred.

The remains arrived Wednesday, and the interment took place at Edgar burying ground in the old Fourth district.

MRS. MARTHA JONES.

On Monday, Mrs. Martha Jones, wife of Burrel Jones, passed away at her home near the Louisville & Nashville depot. Her death was due to pneumonia. She was 73 years of age. She leaves several children. The body was taken to Calloway County, Ky., her old home, for interment. Rev. C. B. Clayton, of Paris, conducted the funeral services.

COUNTY BOARD
OF HEALTH ORDERS CLOSINGS
Vaccine Now Available

Paris, Tennessee (Oct. 11, 1918) – On Wednesday afternoon, the County Board of Health met in the office of the County Court Clerk and decided that there should be no more public gatherings in Henry County until further orders.

This action was in line with that taken earlier in the week by the City Board of Health and is a movement by which it is hoped to speedily stamp out the epidemic of the so-called Spanish influenza.

This means that all the school of Henry County will be closed and that churches and lodges will not be held until further notice.

Prompt action is deemed necessary all over the country in order that the malady may be reduced to the minimum.

Owing to the prevalence of Influenza, the Board of Health of Paris and Henry County, have issued the

following order:

First: That all public assemblies, schools, playhouses, shows, churches, and public gatherings be closed temporarily and until the subsidence of the epidemic.

Second: That all persons who may be suffering from the disease, or who have severe colds, headaches, fever and other symptoms of la grippe or influenza, are hereby requested and urged to remain indoors, as this course will be best both for those who are sick and for the public.

Third: That persons known to have the disease should not return to their respective avocations or work until the attending physician shall give permission for them to do so.

Fourth: It is requested that visitors to those who are sick with the disease, will exercise proper care to protect themselves as far as possible against the infection.

Fifth: In conformity to the laws of the state and the rulings of the State Board of Health, all soda water and soft drink stands are required to furnish other paper cups or sterilized cups or glasses for all customers, and customers should see that such articles are provided.

We have been asked if there is any preventive of the disease known as Influenza which is the same as Lagrippe and would state that there is now a vaccine that is said to prevent it, and which is being used in the Army Camps, and also by our local physicians. We suggest that more extensive use of the Vaccine be resorted to with a probability that it will prevent the disease and, if not shorten it, and prevent complications.

Signed:

Board of Health of Paris.

Board of Health of Henry Co.

BAN ON PUBLIC GATHERINGS
In Many Other Towns and Cities Schools and Gatherings Close

THE PARISIAN

Paris, Tennessee (Oct. 11, 1918) – For an indefinite period, the schools of Paris will be closed. The order affecting the closing also obtains as to churches and theatres, and all other public gatherings.

This was determined on Monday afternoon at a meeting of the County Board of Health upon advice from the State Board of Health and following certain instructions received by Mayor Joel M. Porter.

This is a precautionary measure that is being adopted in many of the larger cities and other towns of a similar or smaller size as compared to Paris.

By this, it is hoped to prevent the spread of any contagion which may be communicated from one person to another in crowds. The measure is especially aimed at the so-called Spanish influenza.

There are numerous cases of the malady in Paris and Henry County, but fortunately, it is believed that a majority have been in a mild form.

The disease in itself is not so much dreaded but for the complications which often attend it, and the fact that it may be easily communicated.

A telegram from Washington says that the surgeon general of the army issues the following rules to the public to safeguard against the spread of respiratory diseases:

How to strengthen our personal defense against Spanish influenza:

First: Avoid needless crowding. Influenza is a crowd disease.

Second: Smother your coughs and sneezes. Others do not want the germs which you would throw away.

Third: Your nose, not your mouth, was made to breathe through. Get the habit.

Fourth: Remember the three C's: a clean mouth, clean skin, and clean clothes.

Fifth: Try to keep cool when you walk and warm when you ride and sleep.

Sixth: Open the windows always at home at night, at the office. When practicable. '

Seventh: Food will win the war if you give it a chance. Help by choosing and chewing your food well.

Eighth: Your fate may be in your own hands. Wash your hands before eating.

Ninth: Don't let the waste products of digestion accumulate. Drink a glass or two of water on getting up.

Tenth: Don't use a napkin, towel, spoon, fork, glass, or cup, which has been used by another person and not washed.

 Eleventh: Avoid tight clothes, tight shoes, tight gloves, seek to make nature your ally, not your prisoner.

Twelfth: When the air is pure, breathe all of it you can; breathe deeply.

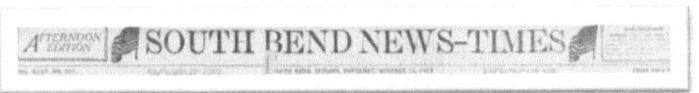

HENRY RINGLING DIES

BARABOO, WIS. (Oct. 12, 1918) – Henry Ringling, youngest of the six brothers who during the last 25 years have been prominent in the circus world, died yesterday of heart and other internal disorders, it was learned today. He is survived by his wife and a son.

HOME GUARDS TO OBSERVE RULING

SOUTH BEND NEWS-TIMES

South Bend, Indiana (Oct. 12, 1918) – The closing order issued by the board of health affects the home guards as well as other organizations. Consequently, work on the target range will be abandoned for the present, or until such time as the health order is rescinded. There will be no drills or other gatherings of the guards unless in a case of emergency.

LIBRARY TO CLOSE READING ROOMS

Both the adult and children's reading rooms at the public library will be closed to the public, beginning Saturday, Oct. 12, until further notice is given. No meetings will be held in the social room at this time.

Books may be returned, and they will be loaned as usual, but the privileges of the social and reading rooms will be withdrawn for a short time because of the influenza epidemic. Hence, the library will close at 8 p. m. instead of 9 as the last hour of the day was for reading room purposes only.

KNIGHTS OF COLUMBUS

The meeting scheduled for Monday evening, Oct. 14, postponed indefinitely in accordance with the health board's closing order.

W. E. Konzen, Grand Knight.

L. H. Weber. Recorder. Advt.

COUNTRY SCHOOLS CLOSED FOR WEEK

South Bend, Indiana (Oct. 12, 1918) – All of the township schools were ordered closed for one week by Trustee James L. Kennedy last night. A number of Spanish Influenza cases are reported among the pupils and teachers of these institutions, one school being almost depleted of scholars. Should the disease show no abatement by Monday week, the embargo will be continued.

PUBLIC DANCING BARRED
BY CHICAGO AUTHORITIES

International News Service

CHICAGO, ILL. (Oct. 12, 1918) – With deaths from influenza and pneumonia yesterday totaling 212, Chicago took drastic steps today toward checking the epidemic. Public dancing is to be no more in this city until further notice, and public attendance at funerals are forbidden.

These rules apply to the entire state. In order to relieve traffic congestion, shoppers are urged to do their buying early after the morning rush.

WILLIAM MCMAHON IS FLU VICTIM IN CAMP

South Bend, Ind. (Oct. 12, 1918) – William McMahon, 224 N. St. Peter St., formerly a member of the South Bend Police Department, but now in the Army and stationed at Camp Zachary Tayler is very ill with Spanish Influenza, according to a report received here. Pvt. McMahon left for Camp Taylor July 22. He was a member of the police department for five years.

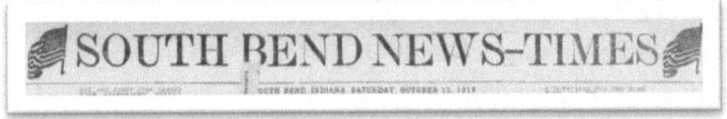

Modern Methods of Quarantine

SOUTH BEND NEWS-TIMES

SOUTH BEND, IND. (Oct. 12, 1918) – The world is growing smaller every day. Not only, as the geologists assure us, by the wrinkling of its crust as its red hot molten interior cools and shrinks, but also by the genii of Aladdin's lamp of science, steam and gas and "Juice" bring us closer to every other habitable part of it. For all practical purposes, the Atlantic

Ocean is only a tenth as wide as it was in the days of the Mayflower, and 20th of its vast and howling stretch in the time of Columbus.

Nowhere is this better illustrated than in the sweep of pestilences and the spread of epidemics. Contrary to traditional belief, these visitations of the wrath of God do not fall from the skies or travel upon the wings of the wind. They have to be laboriously carried from place to place by messenger, and the couriers who deliver these dispatches of death, are nine times out of ten either human beings or insects.

It may be an open question of whether trade follows the flag or not, but there can be no manner of doubt that epidemics spread along the trade routes. When the traveling merchant packs his grip and sets forth to cover his territory, he carries with him, unwittingly, a sideline of samples, which display themselves without any effort on his part.

As cars travel far faster than caravans, and steamships than schooners, epidemics spread at something like ten times the rate that they used to. An outbreak of cholera or influenza in Russia or Egypt interests us more keenly and reaches than one just on the other side of the Alleghanies did a hundred and fifty years ago.

Consequently, when last June the cables flashed the reports of a nation-wide outburst of influenza in Spain, and in July of an outbreak of cholera in Petrograd and Moscow, health officers in the ports all up and down our Atlantic coasts began to prick up their ears and sniff the air figuratively speaking. In peaceful times cases of both diseases would have reached us long ago in the emigrant-crowded steerages of our great Atlantic liners, but the war by its almost complete wiping out of emigration has done us this one small favor at least of delaying their arrival and diminishing our risks.

Strange as it may seem, the "flu" gives us far more uneasiness than cholera, because after we have boiled the drinking water and sterilized the food and isolated the sick and vaccinated those who have come in contact with them, all we have to do is to deal with the carriers, and the pestilence is down and out.

These carriers are human hosts of the disease germs, who thought themselves in fairly good health, carry the "bugs" about with them, and may spread them broadcast.

They are probably the means by which the disease survives over from one season to another. Wherever there has been an epidemic of cholera in a given season, no matter how thoroughly it has been apparently stamped out, health officers are now always sharply on the alert the next summer to detect and head off small scattered outbreaks which will start from these human incubators of the germ.

We can head off, and short circuit this quite quickly this method of spread and reappearance of the diseases. This is by the systematic microscopic, and bacteriological examination of the discharges from the bowels of those who have either recovered from the disease or have come in close contact with it, to see whether the germs of cholera serum and with intestinal antiseptics and kept in an isolation hospital or camp until all traces of the spirilla have disappeared.

This gives us quite effective and reliable practical control of the disease, as illustrated by the admirable fight against it made by the Italian army medical corps. In the first year of the war, cholera was brought into the Italian lines by some Austrian prisoners, and the infection had been widely spread before it was discovered, reaching a total of 10,000 cases among the prisoners and Italian troops brought into contact with them within a few weeks. Then the situation was promptly attacked, the drinking water sterilized, the patients and contacts isolated, the infected barracks burned and flooded with corrosive sublimate solution, with such success that barely a thousand more cases appeared. The deaths were kept down to about two thousand. The following spring, several small epidemics started from carriers that had escaped detection, but these were promptly snuffed out before they had reached two thousand cases, all told, with only a few hundred deaths. This was practically the end of an epidemic, which under the sanitary conditions which have obtained in previous wars, would certainly have mounted up into the hundreds of thousands of deaths.

We also have a cholera vaccine, which, if given in advance, very considerably diminishes the risks of catching the disease, although it is not complete protection. And a serum which seems to diminish the deadliness of the disease when it does occur, so that by the aid of this and modern methods of medical treatment, particularly the injection of large amounts of salt solution into a vein to make good the terrific flooding of the body fluids out in the profuse discharges have reduced the death rate from 30, 40 and even 50 percent down to about 15 or 20.

FLU CLOSES KEITH PLAYERS
THE NEW YORK CLIPPER

UNION HILL, N. J., Oct. 17, 1918 —Manager William Wood, of Keith s Players at the Hudson Theatre, was notified by the local authorities to close his company because of Spanish influenza. This city was the last in the State to be ordered closed, and for a time it was thought it would not be closed at all. However, the increase this week of influenza cases caused the city fathers to follow the action taken by other cities in New Jersey and close all places of amusement.

MARION HAFF IN NEW YORK

Marion Haff arrived in New York last week from South Royalton, Vt., where she was ill for nearly two weeks with Spanish influenza. Miss Haff went to South Royalton about three weeks ago and was taken ill a few days after her arrival. She is still very weak from the effects of the disease and will rest in this city for several weeks.

FLU HALTS K. C. OPENING

KANSAS CITY, MO., Oct. 14. —The Oliver Players (Western) were to have opened here at the Auditorium next week, but the city amusement resorts are closed up tight owing to the flu. The epidemic closed the company last week at Wichita, Kansas. Manager Oliver will reorganize the company and reopen early in November.

MANY HIT BY INFLUENZA

Many performers are reported ill from Spanish influenza here this week. Jack Rose, in vaudeville with Mike Bernard, was removed to the American Hospital, suffering from the ailment. Physicians there state that he has but a slight touch of the disease.

Oscar White, of the Clifton Kelly Shows, was brought into Chicago and placed in the American Hospital suffering from a serious touch of influenza-pneumonia. When brought to town, White was in a very serious condition. Hospital officials believe that he will be able to pull through.

Rose Morrisey, formerly with stock burlesque aggregations, is at the American Hospital with a serious touch of influenza-pneumonia.

Mrs. Amelia Newman, the wife of the president of the United States Tent and Awning Company, died at the American Hospital with influenza-pneumonia. She was buried last Saturday.

MASSACHUSETTS STOCK COMPANYS REOPEN

STATE NEARLY NORMAL AGAIN

(Oct. 14, 1918) – As a result of the removal of the ban on amusements, twelve permanent stock companies in the State of Massachusetts are reopening this week. The companies thus affected are located in the eastern part of the State, where the epidemic has shown a decline to warrant the authorities issuing orders permitting the return to normal business conditions.

Heading the list of cities is Boston, where the players at the Copley

Square Theatre resume their engagement under the direction of Henry Jewett.

Other stocks opening are The Warren O'Hara Stock at Hathaway's, Brockton, with Lilac Time; Emerson Players, at the Academy, Haverhill, with As Ye Sow; Shea Players, at the Holyoke Theatre, Holyoke, with Lilac Time; Auditorium Players, Auditorium, Lynn, with Daddy Long Legs; Goodhue Players, Central Square, with Mary's Ankle; Emerson Players, Colonial, Lawrence, with Lilac Time; All-Star Players, Opera House, Lowell, with The Man They Left Behind, and the Players, New Bedford Theatre, New Bedford, with The Only Girl. The Auditorium Players, at Maiden, Harry Katz's Stock at the Empire, Salem, and the Somerville Players, Somerville, are also slated among those opening.

Of the companies mentioned earlier, Manager Ohara, at New Bedford, was closed for the longest time, it is nearly three weeks since the organization was ordered to close. New Bedford, next to Fall River, was the hardest hit by the epidemic of any of the Massachusetts towns near Boston and was closed several days before the big towns of the Bay State.

Except for the two towns above mentioned, the majority of the towns in Massachusetts closed with Boston and have been darkened, so far as amusements were concerned, for- two weeks. The Shea-Kinsella Stock, at the Warburton Theatre, Yonkers, N. Y., which was closed on Tuesday, October 8, is another company joining the active ranks this week; It will resume with The Brat. While the majority of the companies reopen with the same roster they closed with, several have lost members either through the draft or because players have taken other engagements.

Warren O'Hara's Brockton company was the worst hit in this particular and reopened with four new members.

LINCOLN STOCK CLOSED BY FLU

NEW YORK CLIPPER

LINCOLN, Neb., Oct. 16, 1918 —The Otis Oliver Players at the Lyric Theatre were closed last Saturday, the order of closing taking effect at noon. Last week was the forty-sixth for the company in this city, and it will lay off until the ban caused by the epidemic is lifted and then resume with Freckles as the bill and Playthings to follow.

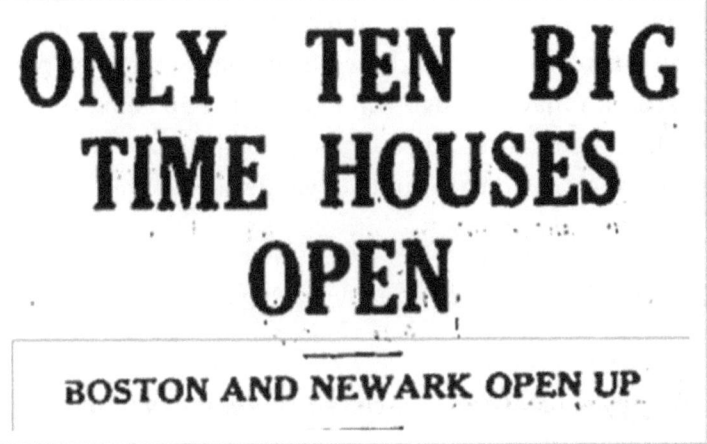

ONLY TEN BIG TIME HOUSES OPEN

BOSTON AND NEWARK OPEN UP

The United Booking Offices early this week reported that all but nine of the big-time houses on its route sheets were closed as a result of the Flu epidemic.

Seven of the big time-vaudeville houses remaining open are in Greater New York.

These are the Palace, Riverside, Colonial, Alhambra, and Royal in Manhattan and the Orpheum and Bushwick in Brooklyn. Keith's Boston was added to the handful of big-time houses doing business at present, reopening on Sunday night with the following bill: Lew Dockstader, Chas. Grapewin, Kaufman Bros., Sylvia Clark, Harold Dukane Trio, Kerr and Weston, Darras Bros., Herbert Clifton, Elinore and William, and "Somewhere with Pershing."

The health officials of Newark also permitted the theatres to re-open on Monday night. Proctor's announcing a well-balanced bill for the current week. In addition to the big-time houses, all of the smaller theatres in Boston and Newark, booking attractions through the United offices, also resumed operations Monday.

The Family Department of the U.B.O. reported that the following cities holding small-time franchises permitted the theatres to reopen on Monday: Norwich, Conn.; Lynn, Mass.; Dorchester, Mass.; Manchester, Vt., and Quincy, Mass., New London, New Haven, Hartford, Bridgeport, Conn., and Ithaca, N. Y. have not been affected by the epidemic sufficiently to close the theatres and are going along in their usual manner, receiving their customary quota of vaudeville bills biweekly.

With a very few scattered instances, the cities mentioned above constitute the entire list of towns regularly playing the small bills that remain open.

Every house on the Pantages Circuit is closed at present, with the date of reopening unknown.

St. Paul is the only city on the Orpheum Circuit that remains open. At the Orpheum offices, it was stated that it is impossible to say when the affected cities would resume reopening being entirely dependent on circumstances.

CHANGES ON BILLS

Harry Holman and Company replaced Daisy Jean at the Royal Monday.

Van and Schenck were replaced on the Palace bill Friday night by Harris and Manion owing to the illness of Van, who is in serious condition from influenza. On Saturday, Blanche Ring was put into the bill in their place.

Gardner and Hartman replaced the Van and Schenck act at the Proctor's Twenty-third street where the latter was booked for the first half.

Edith Clifford, although booked for the Palace bill, this week, did not appear.

LURA LAWRENCE BACK

Lura Lawrence, a member of the Harry Sauber act, called "The New Model," returned to New York, last week, after having been attacked with influenza in Richmond, where she was ill for eight days.

GEORGIE O'BRIEN IMPROVED

Georgie O'Brien, of the Max Hart office, who has been ill with influenza, is improved and will be about in a few days.

PAN TAKES NEW QUARTERS

The Pantages Circuit moved into its newly acquired New York City offices in the Fitzgerald Building last Thursday. The Western circuit will occupy a suite of three rooms on the fourth floor. Walter Keefe, the Eastern representative of Pantages, stated this week that the circuit would continue to book attractions independently as heretofore, as soon as normal conditions obtained again. No booking affiliation with any Eastern circuit was contemplated, Mr. Keefe asserted.

CALLS IT "QUARANTINE CIRCUIT"

Chief Tenderhoa, who was to fill several engagements over what he has named, the "Quarantine Circuit," has not been able to finish one. He was to open for a week in Lawrence on Oct. 7 but played only three days. In New Bedford, he played, one-half day, Portland had closed when he reached there, and Sanford kept open for only one day after his arrival so that he was forced to return to New York.

PAY LAST HONOR TO AVELING

Many prominent vaudeville performers attended the services held over the body of Edward V. Aveling last Thursday at the Campbell Funeral Church. Among those present were Blanche Ring, Sophie Tucker, Jack Lewis, Irene Franklin, James McIntyre, Nan Halperin, Fanny Brice, Walter Kingsly, Edward Keller, Van and Schenck, Mollie King, LeRoy Barnes, Florence Tempest, W. H. Pollock, and Florence White.

ACTOR TAKEN ILL ON STAGE

Mickey Moran, of Moran and Wheeler, became suddenly ill while performing at the Lincoln Square Theatre, this city, last Thursday afternoon, and fell over the footlights into the orchestra pit. He was removed to his rooms at the Bartholdi Inn. The attending physician announced that Moran's complaint is not Spanish influenza.

CLOSE MUTT AND JEFF

Kissimmee, Fla., October 19, 1918 —The state health department here has closed Mutt and Jeff. The men are laying off in Jacksonville, Florida.

SPANISH INFLUENZA VACCINE IS PROVIDED
THE DAILY CAPITAL JOURNAL, SALEM, OREGON

CHICAGO, (Oct. 17, 1918) – Vaccine originated by Dr. E. C. Rosenow of the Mayo Clinic, Rochester, Minn., will be used in a vigorous campaign against Spanish Influenza.

Dr. Rosenow told the Chicago Influenza emergency commission of his experiments with the vaccine, which has treated 20,000 persons. The commission at once named a committee of physicians to take charge of the manufacture and use of all vaccines and serum in Chicago, including the Rosenow vaccine. Another committee was named to raise funds for

its manufacture and distribution.

Five days will be required to begin the manufacture of the vaccine here; it was stated.

Meantime, Dr. Rosenow will provide a supply sufficient for 100,000 doses from his laboratories at Rochester. The vaccine is designed to provide immunity from the disease, though Dr. Rosenow is unwilling to make specific claims as to its value. He believes it aided greatly to suppress the spread of influenza at Rochester.

THE CATOCTIN CLARION.

A Family Newspaper—Independent in Politics—Devoted to Literature, Local and General News.

VOLUME XLVIII.   THURMONT. FREDERICK COUNTY, MD., THURSDAY, OCTOBER 17, 1918.   NO. 32

Fourteen Dead.
Nine from Maryland State Sanatorium

THE CATOCTIN CLARION

Thurmont, Md. (Oct. 17, 1918) – Monday morning, our undertakers had on hand fourteen dead bodies to prepare for burial, M. C. Creager & Son having nine, several of these coming from the State Sanatorium at Sabillasville, and Wilhide & Creeger had five, all of which were local people.

No County Fairs.

Through the Frederick city papers, it has been announced that the Frederick and Hagerstown Fairs have been called off because of the Flu and pneumonia grip on the country. Quite a disappointment and loss to thousands of people, but a very wise proceeding under present conditions.

Card of Thanks.

Mr. and Mrs. Thomas Buchanan McPherson and Miss Louise McPherson desire publicly to thank their neighbors from Catoctin and Thurmont by whose efforts their home was saved from destruction by fire last Wednesday.

In the face of all the illness and sorrow in the community, the prompt assistance of their friends will never be forgotten but will be constantly recalled with deep gratitude.

Personal.

Mrs. Ed. Baxter has been very ill with pneumonia.
Mr. Russell Baxter, merchant, is ill with pneumonia.
Mrs. Mary Tenney has been ill the past week.
Mr. Roy English, who had a severe attack of Flu at the Norfolk Navy

Hospital, writes that he is much improved and able to walk out.

Private Paul Fleagle was home this week from Camp Humphrey, Va. He is recovering from an attack of Flu.

Mr. Latimore Schildt and his family, who were ill last week, have all recovered.

Mrs. Geo. E. Wilhide has been very ill with pneumonia the past week.

Mr. Wm. Harman is yet very ill with pneumonia, the members of his family now being on the mend.

Death Rate Still High.

Imports from All Sections
Indicate That Flu Is Not Checked

Reports in Baltimore papers would indicate that the number of new cases of Spanish Flu and pneumonia and the number of death from there are not diminishing. In some sections of the State, the disease has abated somewhat, while in other places, it is increasing.

Locally it would seem that perhaps the worst has been faced. There are at this time several persons seriously ill, but the new cases are not so numerous. The demand for nurses to care for the sick has been great, but few are to be had. Whole families have been afflicted, and many times, neighbors have not been altogether willing to enter the home and do nursing.

Of those who have passed away in this community the past week, we report the following.

Flohr.

Mr. William Flohr, a highly respected citizen, residing near Thurmont, died at the home of his daughter, Mrs. Harry Flohr, Sunday morning, October 13th, after an illness of several months and an attack of paralysis, aged 78 years, eight months and seven days. Funeral services were held Wednesday morning at 9.30 o'clock at the home of Mr. and Mrs. Harry Flohr and interment made in the United Brethren cemetery. Elders Fike and Weybright officiating. Wilhide & Creeger funeral directors.

Crouse.

George Sefton Crouse, the oldest son of Mrs. M. M. Crouse of Thurmont, died at his home in Great Falls, Montana, of influenza. October 12th, aged 26 years and seven months. He is survived by his wife and three daughters. At the age of 17 years, Mr. Crouse left Thurmont, went west, later marrying and taking up a homestead in Montana. For the past 27 years, he has been a superintendent at the Boston Montana Smelter Works. Interment will be made at Great Falls. Mrs. Margaret Crouse, his mother, Mrs. G. F. Rogers, and Miss Ada Crouse of Thurmont, sisters, and Mr. Warren Crouse of California, a brother, also survive.

Fleagle

Maude Margaret and Sophia Beatrice Fleagle, twin daughters of Mr. and Mrs. Parker Fleagle, of Thurmont, succumbed to the epidemic prevalent at this time, Margaret passing away Friday, October 11th at the home of her parents, and Beatrice, Sunday, October 13, 1918, at the home of her grandparents, Mr. and Mrs. David Wireman, near this place. These sisters were more or less afflicted from infancy both in the same manner, and while funeral services were being held for Margaret, Beatrice died. Margaret was aged 16 years, eight months, and 28 days. Beatrice is surviving her two days. Funeral services for Margaret were conducted Sunday at her home by her pastor, Dr. P. E. Heimer, and Tuesday afternoon at the home of the grandparents by Dr. Wentz. Interment in the United Brethren cemetery. Wilhide & Creeger directors.

Miller

John Henry Miller, son of Joseph Miller, died of pneumonia at his home at Catoctin Furnace, Saturday, October 12th, aged 30 years, nine months, and ten days. Funeral Services and interment at Lewistown Monday of this week. Wilhide &Creeger directors.

Poole.

Harry W. Poole, son of Charles W. Poole, died at the home of his-parents at Thurmont, Sunday, October 13th of pneumonia, aged 18 years, three months, and 25 days. Funeral services and interment at Lewistown Tuesday. Wilhide & Creeger directors.

Dewees

Samuel Howard Dewees died at his home about two miles east of Thurmont Tuesday morning at 1 o'clock, October 15th, after a brief illness of influenza and pneumonia, aged 38 years, 0 months, and 28 days. Funeral services today at 2 o'clock at home. Interment in the U. H. cemetery at Thurmont, Rev. E. O. Pritchett is officiating. The deceased is survived by his wife and seven children, also by his mother, Mrs. William Dewees, one sister, Mrs. Aaron Stull, and brother, Edw. Deweese. The deceased was a member of Good Samaritan Lodge of Odd Fellows, Wilhide & Creeger directors.

Fraley

Herbert Fraley, aged 25 years and a son of Mr. and Mrs. Harry W. Fraley, died Monday morning, October 14th. At the home of his parents near Catoctin, I Furnace, of pneumonia and influenza. His brother, William Thomas Fraley, who died last week at Camp Colt, Gettysburg, of pneumonia, was buried Sunday at Lewistown. Funeral services for Herbert were held Wednesday at his home, Rev. C. E. Wolfe had charge of the funeral services. The deceased was a member of Chancellor Lodge K. of P., of Thurmont. M. L. Creager & Son funeral directors.

Stocksdale

George Frederick Stocksdale, aged 39 years, eight months and 26 days, son of Mrs. T. C. Stocksdale formerly of Thurmont, died at York, Pa., Monday, October 14, 1918, of bronchial pneumonia. His body was brought to Thurmont and taken to the home of his grandfather, Mr. George W. Stocksdale. Burial services were held Wednesday, and interment made in the United Brethren cemetery at Thurmont, Rev. E. O. Pritchett officiating. The deceased is survived by his mother, two brothers, and three sisters—Wilhide & Creeger's funeral directors.

Sweeney

Melvin Sweeney, aged 37 years, died at his home at Catoctin Furnace Monday morning, October 14, 1918, of pneumonia, The funeral Look place Wednesday afternoon at his home, interment at Lewistown. The deceased was a member of Good Samaritan Lodge of Odd Fellows. M. L. Creager t Son directors.

Deweese

Lulu Gertrude Deweese died at the home of her mother, Mrs. William Deweese, at Franklinville one mile north of Thurmont, Thursday, October 10, 1918, of pneumonia, aged 36 years, seven months, and 28 days. Funeral services were held on Saturday at the house and interment made in the U. B. cemetery, Rev. E. O. Pritchett officiating. M. L. Creager & Son funeral directors.

Ohler

Vernon Ohler, son of Mr. and Mrs. Beecher Ohler of near Emmitsburg, died October 10, 1918, at Camp Meade.

Gingell

Thomas Gingell, aged about 25 years, and residing near Emmitsburg, died at his home Friday night last of pneumonia. He is survived by his wife, who before marriage was Miss Mary Weller of Thurmont and two children.

Shaffer.

Mrs. Mary Fraley Shaffer, the wife of Frank Shaffer, residing near Catoctin Furnace and daughter of Mr. and Mrs. Henry Fraley, died Tuesday, Oct. 15, 1918, of influenza. Funeral services will be held Friday and interment made at Lewistown. The deceased is survived by her husband and five children, the oldest boy, Wallace being ill at this time.

Wetzel.

Charles Luther Wetzel, aged eight months, died at the home of his grandmother, Mrs. Lee Dubel, at Lewistown Wednesday morning, October 16th, of pneumonia. Funeral service and burial at Utica Friday.

Wilhide and Creeger directors.

James S. Waters.

Mr. James S Waters, aged about 19, died of pneumonia at St. John's Naval Hospital, Annapolis, Wednesday, October 16, 1918, after a brief illness due to pneumonia. The deceased is the only son of Mr. and Mrs. Charles Waters of Thurmont. The body will be brought to their home in Thurmont today by Wilhide Creeger's funeral directors. Arrangements for the funeral have not been announced.

Not Yet.
(Newspaper manager fills all posts, has yet to write his own obituary)

The Flu has not struck The Clarion Office directly, but due to illness at home, our help has been home since Monday of last week. The manager is serving in all branches in newspaper and job work and is giving the readers the best he can under present conditions. Help in a print shop is very hard to secure. ,

Carson City Daily Appeal

Whole Town Is Influenza Victim

San Francisco Churches Will Hold Sidewalk Services

By United Press

SACRAMENTO. Oct. 18, 1918 – Four hundred, nearly the entire population of Needles, Calif., are influenza victims.

There have been thirteen deaths. An appeal has been sent to Governor Stephens for nurses and doctors, as the only two resident doctors have worked night and day, and entire families are dying for lack of care. Depopulation is threatened.

Not to Be Outdone

By United Press

SAN FRANCISCO. (Oct. 18, 1918) – Churches here will hold sidewalk services Sunday, the Board of Health has granted the necessary permission.

Close Public Libraries in Frisco

SAN FRANCISCO. (Oct. 18, 1918) – The public library and all of its branches have been closed to prevent the spread of influenza. At noon today, the total number of cases in the city had reached 3,275.

Camp Lewis to be Quarantined

TACOMA. Oct. 18. Camp Lewis is to be quarantined to the limits of the military reservation, beginning tomorrow, the authorities announced today. This action has been taken on account of influenza.

SINKS IN COLLISION

British Freighter Sinks When She Collides With War Vessel.

New York, Oct. 18. The British freight steamship Port Philip, outbound, was sunk in a collision with a United States war vessel off Swinburne island In the lower bay this forenoon. The Port Philip's crew of forty men was saved.

Steamer Sinking.

New York, Oct. 16. A large steamship was reported to lie sinking in the lower harbor today. The vessel was bound outbound when it signaled for help.

VICTIM OF AIRPLANE

Lieut. Edward Little Killed and Instructor Seriously Injured.

FULTON, KY. Oct. 16. Lieut. Edward Little was killed here today, and Instructor K. C. Smith received serious injuries when their airplane fell out of control from a considerable height. The accident is the sixth of its kind to occur at Fulton in the past year.

CONVENTION CALLED OFF

Educators of Tennessee Postpone Meeting on Account of Influenza.

The executive committee of the East Tennessee Educational Association has canceled the coming meeting, which was to have been held in Knoxville Oct. 31 to Nov. 2. This action was taken by the executive committee because of the very rapid spread of Influenza, rendering it very improbable that public meetings could be held in Knoxville at the time set for the meeting. The spread of influenza has also greatly interfered with the program, as a large number of persons to take part would not be able to fill their engagements. Owing to the unsettled state of affairs the association has deemed it wise to not attempted to hold the meeting until next year when every effort will be put forth to reach the goal of attendance set for this year – 2,500 – and to have the greatest meeting in all respects in the history of the association. Last year 2.072 teachers, or 60 percent of the public teachers of East Tennessee, were registered and were in attendance upon the meeting at Knoxville.

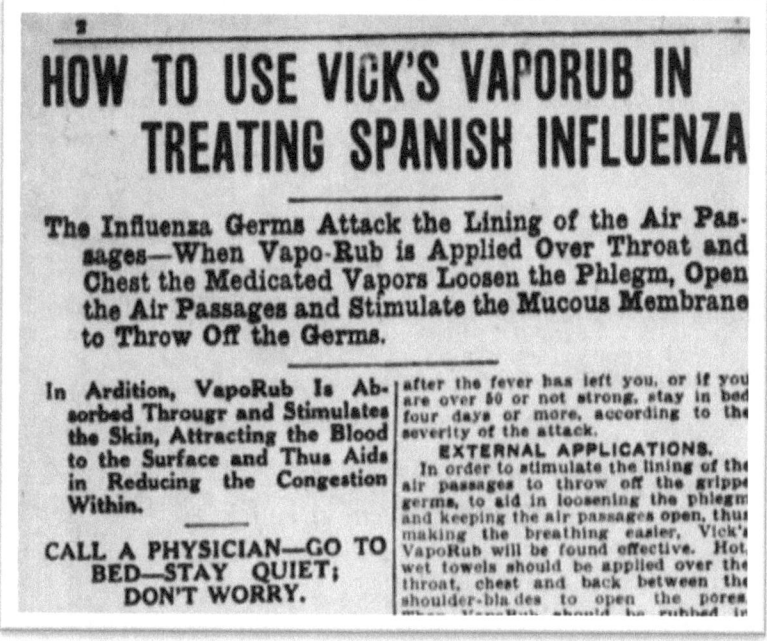

HOW TO USE VICK'S VAPORUB IN TREATING SPANISH INFLUENZA

The Influenza Germs Attack the Lining of the Air Passages—When Vapo-Rub is Applied Over Throat and Chest the Medicated Vapors Loosen the Phlegm, Open the Air Passages and Stimulate the Mucous Membrane to Throw Off the Germs.

In Ardition, VapoRub Is Absorbed Througr and Stimulates the Skin, Attracting the Blood to the Surface and Thus Aids in Reducing the Congestion Within.

CALL A PHYSICIAN—GO TO BED—STAY QUIET; DON'T WORRY.

after the fever has left you, or if you are over 50 or not strong, stay in bed four days or more, according to the severity of the attack.

EXTERNAL APPLICATIONS.

In order to stimulate the lining of the air passages to throw off the grippe germs, to aid in loosening the phlegm and keeping the air passages open, thus making the breathing easier, Vick's VapoRub will be found effective. Hot, wet towels should be applied over the throat, chest and back between the shoulder-blades to open the pores.

SOLDIER CAN KISS GIRL
Recorder of Atlanta So Rule and
Warn Police Not to Interfere.

Atlanta, Ga., Oct. 16. Soldiers departing for overseas may publicly kiss their sweethearts good-by without fear of police interference, according to a ruling made today by Recorder George E. Johnson, of this city.

The momentous opinion was the case of Miss Ruby Young, of 168 Marietta Street, who was arrested by a local patrolman for publicly receiving the silent salute provided for in the manual of arms of Col. Daniel Cupid. The patrolman declared that he was guided by the impropriety of the publicly administered salute and by the fear that the osculation might increase the spread of Spanish Influenza.

Neither consideration weighed with Recorder Johnson.

"If this young lady wanted to kiss her soldier farewell,"

the recorder declared, "far be it from this court to interfere. The case is dismissed."

"FLU" EPIDEMIC ALARMING
Business Houses Closed and Other Restrictions Taken to
Combat Disease

Huntsville, Ala., Oct. 16. – (Special) – From 2 o'clock Monday afternoon up to Tuesday morning, nine people have died of Spanish Influenza. Madison County seems a nest hole for the epidemic, as hundreds of cases are reported from the country. County and city health officer Dr. Grote have issued orders that business hours be only from 9 to 5.

Every known means is being used to stamp out the disease. Several cases have developed into pneumonia, and the stage seems fatal. Albert Vaughan, a well-known restaurant man, died today. Miss Cecil Cochran, a trained nurse from New York, who came a few days ago to help out the situation, was taken ill immediately and died today. Doctors, pharmacists, and nurses are coming in daily. Never has there been a time when the people are doing such noble work.

The Red Cross has served the best to the people. The women and girls going out masked and actually working in the sick rooms with hundreds of cases at Abingdon mills, the hotbed of Illness in Huntsville.

Many prominent men have died and eight in the mill district yesterday.

CHICAGO CLOSED TIGHT
More Than 10,000 New Cases
Of Influenza Reported in Illinois.

Chicago, Oct. 16, 1918 – With more than 10,000 new cases of Influenza reported in Illinois today, public health officials prepared to extend the order closing all night schools, theaters, motion picture houses, lodge meetings, skating rinks and other places of public amusement.

An extension of the order to include all saloons in the vicinity of big industrial plants and a possible ban on political meetings was forecast by Dr. St. Clair Drake, director of the State Public Health Department. All public dances have already been suppressed. Many day schools where there is not adequate medical and nursing supervision, also have been closed. An order closing all churches is expected before Sunday.

Reports from 170 Illinois cities of over 1,000 population show a total of 31,800 cases. Of these more than 10,000 were said to be In Chicago. There were 183 deaths from influenza and 134 from pneumonia in Chicago today, while more than 2,000 new cases were reported.

THE CHATTANOOGA NEWS
Published by Chattanooga News Co.
George F. Milton, Editor.
Walter C. Johnson, Business Manager.
Entered Post Office as Second-Class Mail.

INFLUENZA AND THE LOAN.

In considering the influenza epidemic, it is natural for the old-timers to recall former visitations to which the south has been subjected. And there have been several of them. Of course, the yellow fever was formerly the most frequent, but there were others no less dreaded. Speaking of the great yellow fever epidemic of 1878, Col. T. C. Looney, of Memphis, who was in Washington a day or two ago, said: "There is a striking difference in the manner in which this influenza epidemic is being handled and the conditions which prevailed In the south in 1878 when I came to Washington as a student to escape the yellow fever plague. At that time, thousands of persons along the Mississippi River died because medical science then knew little about treating the disease."

"The mortality reached an appalling height of 80 percent. Sanitary measures largely instituted by Gen. Gorgas have triumphed in all modern outbreaks of this scourge. Today the local and federal authorities have been quick to act and to take every precaution to protect the public in the Mississippi valley, as well as elsewhere, and prevent the spread of the flu."

"Warnings are posted everywhere, public gatherings of every kind have been discontinued, columns of advice by the best medical authorities in the land have been published in the newspapers, and I believe a frightful situation has been averted, due to these measures. Too much praise cannot be given that great humanitarian organization, the Red Cross, and other volunteer organizations, whose heroic work has saved thousands of lives."

"While this epidemic has done much to hinder the floating of the liberty loan, I am confident that Memphis and the South, in fact, the whole country, will ever 'go over the top.' The temper of the American people will not be affected by the recent German note, in my opinion. They will keep on buying bonds and fighting until the commander-in-chief gives the command to 'cease firing.'"

The practical banishment of yellow fever, the former southern terror, Illustrates quite forcibly the world's advances in medical knowledge and sanitary science. One shudders to think of the cruel quarantines which the self-preservation instinct once suggested and especially to think that they were entirely unnecessary. The breaking out of yellow fever in one town of the south was the signal for a panic throughout its borders. We know better now.

Col. Looney, however, illustrates a southern trait when he suggests that we are not going to let our distress and uneasiness over the Influenza to distract our attention from the great task in hand – the raising of the liberty loan.

It has been stated that great earthquakes have passed unnoticed by armies furiously engaged in battle. And America is keyed up and concentrated upon the war almost to that extent.

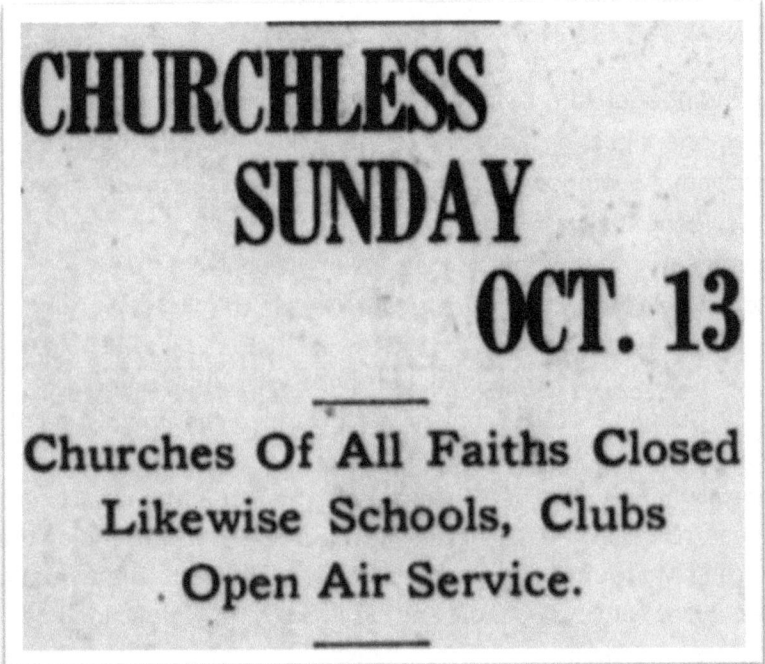

THE BRECKENRIDGE NEWS.

$1.50 a Year; 50c for 4 Months; 75c for 6 Months.   ALL THE NEWS THAT'S FIT TO PRINT. $1.50 a Year; 90c for 4 Months; 75c for 6 Months.

VOL. XLIII.   CLOVERPORT. KENTUCKY, WEDNESDAY, OCTOBER, 16, 1918   6 Pages   No. 16

CHURCHLESS SUNDAY OCT. 13

Churches Of All Faiths Closed Likewise Schools, Clubs . Open Air Service.

THE BRECKENRIDGE NEWS

BRECKENRIDGE, KENTUCKY – Sunday, Oct. 13, 1918, will be remembered as a churchless Sunday not only in Cloverport but all through the State and in many other states as well. Owing to Spanish influenza, the churches of all faiths were closed by order of the State Board of Health. Consequently, there was no public worshiping inside the churches, but an open-air prayer meeting lasting thirty minutes was conducted by Rev. A. N. Couch and Rev. W. O. Rickard at 10:30 o'clock. Only a few attended it as it was not generally known. In all probability, there were many homes where family devotion was observed at the church hour. The day had little social visiting either as this is disapproved by the Board of Health.

Until further notices from the Board the Cloverport Public school will remain closed, likewise the churches, and the women's clubs. The crowds at the post-office during the evening mail have not been allowed to congregate in the lobby of the office as they have done heretofore.

The exact number of "flu" cases is difficult to obtain, but every now and then, when one is passing along the residential streets, they are liable to see more than one window with "Influenza" cards in them, and these were not evident at all last week. While the cases have been genuine, none have been fatal thus far, and it is generally believed that the epidemic can be checked to a very great extent in this vicinity.

REV. DR. SAM MILLER DIES OF INFLUENZA.

The Rev. Dr. Samuel M. Miller, one of the most prominent ministers of the Louisville Conference, died Monday of pneumonia at his home in Owensboro, where he had been in charge of the Settle Memorial church for two years. Dr. Miller was stricken with influenza while attending the Conference in Madisonville, and after coming home, double pneumonia developed. He was forty years old and survived by his widow and one daughter.

SOLDIER BURIED HERE SATURDAY
William Ahl Died in Camp Custer of Influenza. 23 Years Old.

The funeral of William Ahl, the twenty-three-year-old son of Mr. Sam Ahl of this city, was held from the residence, Saturday afternoon, and the burial took place in the Cloverport cemetery, he is the first soldier to be buried there during this war. Services were in charge of Rev. J. S. Henry. Pvt. Ahl left this city some time ago. He had been in the army for several months and was stationed at Camp Custer, Mich. His death was caused from Spanish influenza. Besides his father, he leaves one sister, Mrs. John Kelly of Rockport, Ind.

Mr. John Black Follows Wife in Death.

In a very short while after the remains of Mrs. John Black had been interred in the Cloverport Cemetery, Saturday afternoon a message came here to Mr. and Mrs. S. R. Berry, Sr., bearing the news that their son-in-law, Mr. John Black had succumbed to Spanish influenza at the City Hospital, Louisville. His body was brought here Sunday, and Monday afternoon, the funeral service was held from the home of Mr. and Mrs. Berry. Services conducted by Rev. W. O. Rickard. He was buried beside his wife In the Cloverport Cemetery.

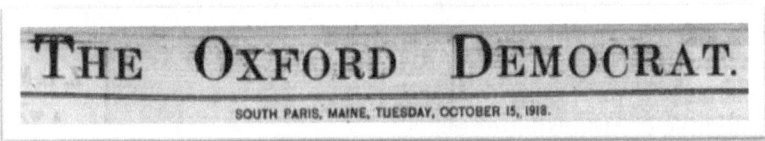

SOUTH PARIS, MAINE, TUESDAY, OCTOBER 15, 1918.

BOSTON TO REMAIN CLOSED

OXFORD DEMOCRAT
South Paris, Maine (Oct. 15, 1918)

The granite cutting industry of Vermont is virtually at a standstill as a result of the spread of Spanish influenza among the quarry and shed workers n Montpellier and Barre.

****

Theatres, motion picture houses, dance halls, and other amusement resorts in Boston, which have been closed for the past week because of the influenza epidemic, were ordered to remain closed until Oct. 14 by the city emergency health committee.
Under the original order, they were to have been permitted to reopen last Monday. So that their employees might not be obliged to travel during "rush" hours, several business houses have put new working hours into effect.

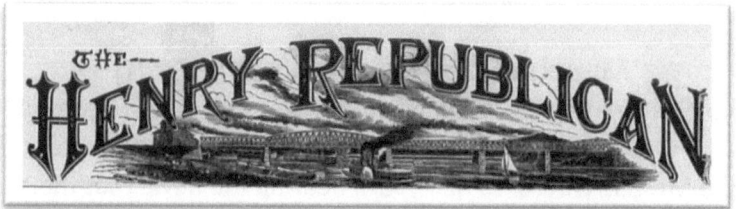

THE INFLUENZA EPIDEMIC.

Special to Henry Republican.

Chicago, Oct. 15, 1918—The results of a statewide survey by telegraph of every Illinois community of 1,000 population or over, given out here tonight by Dr. C. St. Clair Drake, director of the state department of public health, shows that 227 cities and towns in Illinois have been hit by the epidemic of Spanish influenza.

The number of cases reported in these 227 communities is 55,7215, of which 17,943 are in Chicago, and 37,782 downstate.

There have been 2,264 deaths from influenza and pneumonia in Chicago and 491 in the downstate communities, which have been reported.

Convinced that the epidemic had reached proportions that required prompt and vigorous measures, the state department of health has ordered that all theaters, including moving picture shows, all night schools, all lodges, and all places of public amusement, -closed until the epidemic subsides. All public schools which are lacking adequate medical and nursing supervision were Included in the order.

"From the Information we now have," said Dr. Drake, "we believe that every community in Illinois will be affected by Influenza before the epidemic subsides. Based on the reports which reached us today, we estimate that there are now more than 170,000 cases in the state outside of Chicago."

An analysis of the influenza situation in Chicago today shows that the epidemic has not reached its crest here. For the week ending September 28, there were 598 cases reported in Chicago, with 176 deaths. During the week ending October 7, there were 6,106 cases reported with 627 deaths. The week which ended October 14, produced 11,239 cases and 1,461 deaths. The total number of deaths from influenza and pneumonia In Chicago during the past three weeks of 156 for the same period during the past five years.

 Although the situation is bad in many down-state communities, it will get worse before it gets better, according to members of the state influenza commission, which meets daily.

 The town of Assumption in Christian County, with a population of 1,918, has reported 500 cases and has called for help. There are only four doctors and one registered nurse in the town.
Greenup, with a population of 1,224, reported 400 cases. Two doctors live in Greenup, and both are ill with influenza. Peoria reports 10,000 cases and Rockford 6,000. In Peoria, two emergency hospitals have been equipped, and in Rockford, medical help has been loaned from Camp Grant, where the epidemic is rapidly being brought under control.

More than 1,200 cases have been reported in Kankakee. Cairo reports 500. Marengo, with a population of 1,872, reported 496 cases and has asked for the help of outside doctors and nurses. Nokomis, which has a population of 1,973, has reported over 600 eases with no hospital facilities available. Bloomington reports 1,200 cases with 11 deaths.

The state health department urges extreme care to prevent, so far as possible, tile needless further spread of the contagion. All persons are warned to keep sway front crowds, to avoid the person who sneezes, coughs and spits without covering the face with a cloth, and to consult a physician immediately upon the first symptoms of what may seem to be an ordinary cold.

Albert Walter Farling.

The funeral of Albert Walter Farling, private in the national army of the United States, was held at the home of his father, Frank Farling, five miles west of Magnolia, on the afternoon of October 15, -918.

On June 14 of this year, he was called from his work with his father on the farm to take his place among the Putnam County boys in the military service of his country.

For six weeks, he attended the Rahe motor school in North Kansas City, Mo., to finish the preparation he needed as a truck driver in the army.

At the end of that time, he was transferred to Camp Holabird, Baltimore, Md., where he was a member of Company F, 302nd water tank train. About six weeks ago, his father visited him at the camp and found him enthusiastic over his work, though not so vigorous as he ordinarily had been.

When the influenza epidemic reached the camp, he was one of those who took it, and though cared for in the Fort McHenry hospital in Baltimore, he could not ward off pneumonia when the influenza was over.

It was in the hospital that he died on October 9, 1918. Albert Walter Farling was born in Putnam, Putnam County, on March 13, 1896, and moved with his parents to Whitefield township, Marshall county, in 1899. There he spent his boyhood days, again moving to Oxbow, Putnam County, residing there until called to the colors June 14, 1918.

There he enjoyed army life until he was stricken with Spanish influenza, later developing into pneumonia and passed away at Fort McHenry hospital, Baltimore, Md., October 9, 1918, at the age of 23 years, six months and 26 days. His mother passed away when he was but six years old, also a sister passing away in infancy. He leaves to mourn his loss his father and stepmother; brother, James H., residing in Chillicothe; Thomas L., serving his country with a machine gun company in France; Blanche Mae Saner of Peoria, and William I., at home. Those who attended the funeral from a distance were Mr. and Mrs. Fred Saner of Peoria, James Farling of Chillicothe and Mrs. Feathering!!! of Chicago, the latter an aunt of the deceased.

Henry Businessmen Pay Tribute.

Tn honor to the memory of Albert W. Farling, the business houses of Henry all closed, and the proprietors, clerks, and citizens gathered in a line, each carrying an American flag, marched to the Henry bridge and with opened ranks. At the same time, the cortege in entering our city passed through the long columns of sympathizing friends, who escorted the funeral train through our city.

It exemplified pure Americanism in action. It showed the spirit that should exist in every American heart—loyalty to the common cause of humanity. The funeral train continued to Putnam, where a beautiful burial service was conducted by Revs. Young of Magnolia, Van Leer, and Dusenberry of Henry.

The remains were in charge of six soldiers from Camp Herring of Peoria, who acted as pallbearers. After taps were sounded by Albert J. Wimer of Henry, each soldier, in turn, gave his farewell salute to his departed comrade before leaving the grave.

A young, pure life has been taken, sacrificed while in training to answer his country's call. He discharged his full duty and soon was to be called for overseas duty when the terrible disease, pneumonia, seized him, and death ensued.

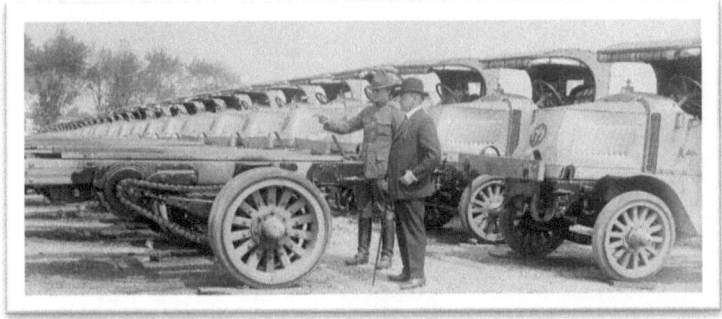

Camp Holabird, Baltimore, Md. 1915 Harris & Ewing

LIEUT. LAVAN TO RETIRE FROM BASEBALL

Great Lakes Manager Will Remain In The Navy

SPANISH INFLUENZA

GREAT LAKES BULLETIN

WEDNESDAY, OCTOBER 16, 1918.

By HENRY W. SHAW
 Lieutenant (j. g.) John Lavan, popular manager of the champion Great Lakes Naval Training Station baseball team, is through professional baseball. Henceforth he will devote his entire time to the Navy.

"I have played my last game," said the Great Lakes manager yesterday. Regardless of what happens in this war, I am through with professional baseball. I like the Navy and intend to stick whether. I do or not will have nothing to do with my future on the diamond. That is settled."

 Lieutenant Lavan intends to return to the practice of medicine in case he should again become a civilian at the expiration of the war.

Had Fine Record

The Great Lakes manager played with the St. Louis Browns for five years. Last winter, he was traded to the Washington Senators in one of the biggest baseball deals of the season. He has always been regarded as one of the best fielding shortstops in the game and as a dangerous man with the bat.

The primary reason for Lieutenant Lavan's decision is that he desires to establish himself permanently. The choice was between the medical profession and baseball, and he chose the former.

 Lieutenant Lavan enlisted in the Navy last December but was not called until late in the summer. He was immediately placed in charge of the baseball team and played a big part in the closing lap of the campaign on the diamond.

Defends George Sisler

Lieutenant Lavan is a personal friend of George Harold Sisler, the Browns' famous first baseman who is now a Lieutenant in the Chemical Warfare Service, U.S.A., and verifies yesterday's dispatches to the effect that Sisler is not a shipbuilder as previously reported.

On leaving St. Louis at the end of the season, Sisler went direct to Washington, where he filed an application for a commission in the Medical Service. He is now in the "offensive" end of the chemical service, one of the most hazardous branches.

When Lieutenant Lavan left Washington to Great Lakes, he was informed by Sisler of his intentions to join the chemical service. "I know that he carried out his plans," Lieutenant Lavan said, "and that he did not play with Hog Island as was reported."

Arthur Henke Is Seriously Ill

GREAT LAKES BULLETIN

Arthur Henke, National sprint champion as a result of his splendid performances in the National A. A. U. championships here last month is seriously ill at his home in Chicago with Spanish influenza. Henke ran for the Illinois A. C. and Lane Tech previous to entering the service.

BLANEY SIGNS MISS HOWELL

NEW YORK CLIPPER

BALTIMORE, Md., Oct. 18. —Virginia Howell has joined the Blaney Stock Company at the Colonial Theatre and will make her debut with the company in "The Girl Who Came Back" when the epidemic permits the house to reopen.

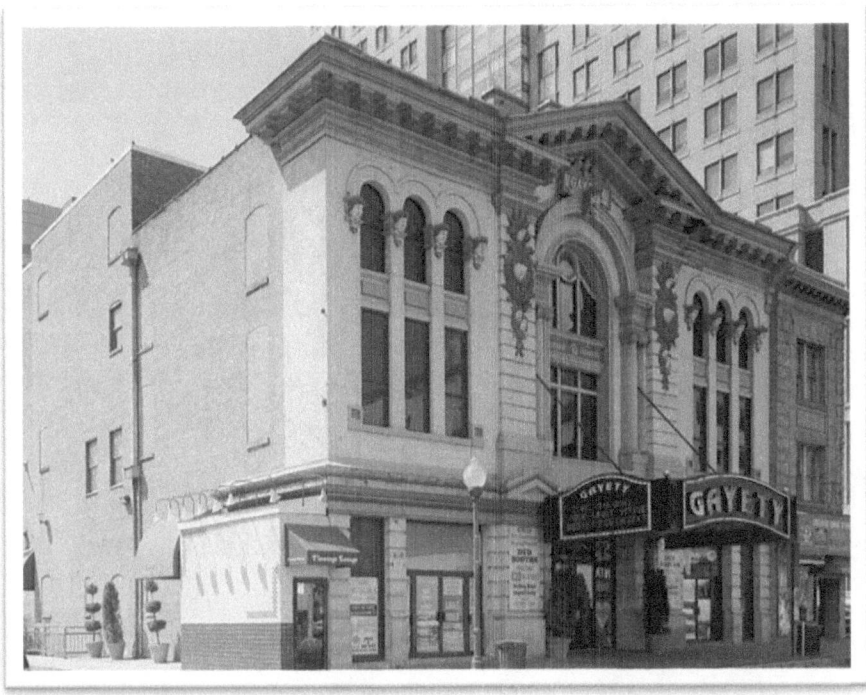

The Gayety Theater in Baltimore was on the circuit, which hosted stars of stage and screen for decades. *Library of Congress.*

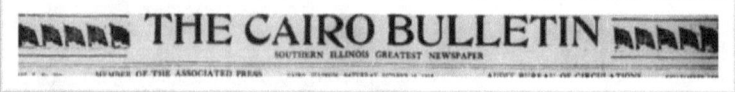

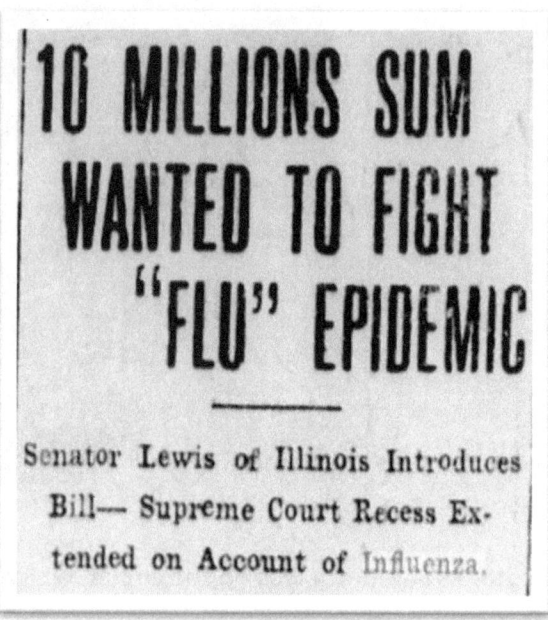

THE CAIRO BULLETIN

Washington, Oct. l8, 1918. (By The Associated Press). The public health service is actively directing the tight against Spanish influenza in thirty states in addition to the whole of New England and the District of Columbia.

Particular attention is being given to providing nurses for the sick, and supplying physicians fur those communities where the doctors are unable to meet all calls made on them.

Despite these and other measures taken by the public health service in co-operation with state and local authorities, the epidemic continues to spread. In parts of New England, it appears to have reached its crest. In

a few states, the num her of new cases is showing decreases.
Continued improvement in conditions in army camps was shown By
reports reaching the office of the surgeon general of the army up noon
today.

New cases of influenza in all camps during the twenty-four-hour period
up to that time totaled 4,454, as against 5,668 the day before.
Pneumonia cases decreased from 1,895 to 1,800, and deaths were 684,
a decrease from yesterday's total.
In discussing the improved conditions in army camps today, Secretary
Baker said no time had been decided upon for resuming the induction
of registrants into the camps.

The military authorities have the matter under consideration, he said,
but they probably will fix no date until the epidemic has further
subsided. Reports on the influenza situation were received by the public
health service today from thirty-three states. Most of the details dealt
with conditions as they existed several days ago and added little new to
dispatches previously sent out from the states affected.

They showed that the disease had reached epidemic proportions in
Nebraska and was spreading in California, New York, Missouri,
Kentucky, Iowa, Illinois, North Dakota, Ohio, Washington, and
Wisconsin. Conditions were described as satisfactory in Oregon,
Minnesota, West Virginia, and Tennessee.
To provide additional funds for fighting the epidemic, Senator Lewis to
Illinois today introduced a bill in the Senate to appropriate $10,000,000
in addition to the $1,000,000 already provided by Congress.

The money would be expended through the health departments of
states and municipalities.
Because of the increased seriousness of the influenzas epidemic in
Washington, the Supreme Court today announced its recess, which was
to have terminated next Monday, will be extended until Oct. 28.
To prevent further overcrowding in Washington while the epidemic

continues, the War Department today joined other government departments in directing that only employees absolutely essential to the conduct of government work be allowed to come to Washington until further notice.

"FLU" SERUM AND VACCINE TO BE TESTED
Preventive and Specific Will Be Used Largely in Combating 'Epidemic in Chicago.

Chicago, (Oct. 18, 1918) – Dr. John Dill Robertson, the health commissioner of Chicago, is going to vaccinate everybody in Chicago against pneumonia following influenza. He made the announcement today in connection with the arrival of the first allotment of 500,000 doses of vaccine from Rochester, Minn. He plans that 100,000 persons shall receive the preventative each day until all are immune. Those who have had the influenza are excepted from the order.

A blood serum used as a curative in the east only in desperate cases of influenza will be tried out in Chicago and Illinois, the State influenza commission agreed tonight.

The commission is faced with a difficult problem to obtain the curative in sufficient quantity, as it was stated that eight ounces of blood must be taken from a patient who has survived the malady to produce three ounces of serum.

The commission received firsthand reports of experiments with this serum from Dr. Herman N. Bundesen of the Chicago Health Department, who returned today from an eastern trip.

The commission laid emphasis on the fact that the serum should not be confused with the vaccine now in use. The vaccine is preventive, and the serum is used as a curative only in very bad cases.

Disease Still on Increase.

Washington, Oct. 18. Reports to the house health service today from 35 states showed that Spanish "flu" still is on the increase in most parts of the country. Conditions in army camps also were less favorable, and the 4,491 new cases reported to noon today showing that the disease apparently was stationary after the marked decline noted for several days.

The epidemic still is more pronounced in the eastern section of the country than it is west of the Mississippi River, due undoubtedly to the more crowded conditions in the large cities.

Although influenza cases in army camps increased slightly, the number of pneumonia cases, 1,599, decreased during the 24 hours ending today at noon. Deaths were 657, against 684 yesterday. Influenza cases reported from all camps since the epidemic began now total 279,945; pneumonia cases 42,576 and deaths 13,681.

California Closes Theaters

San Francisco, (Oct. 18, 1918) – All theaters and motion picture houses in the state were ordered closed today by the State Board of Health as a result of the Spanish influenza epidemic.

200,000 Ill With Flu.

Buenos Aires, (Oct. 18, 1918) – There are 200,000 cases of influenza in Buenos Aires. The medical authorities say that the disease is not Spanish influenza. There have been no deaths from it.

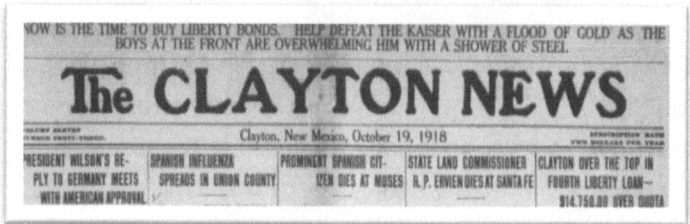

SPANISH INFLUENZA SPREADS IN UNION COUNTY

THE CLAYTON NEWS

Clayton, New Mexico (Oct. 19, 1918) – The dreaded Spanish influenza is with us. It is not only in Clayton, but it is all over the county. Several deaths have been caused by this epidemic. Everyone should be most careful and guard against this disease. Avoid all kinds of public meetings and stay close at home for a few days.

A week ago, we did not think there was a single case in Clayton, and 'today there are perhaps fifty cases of influenza in the city alone. Twelve clerks out of the Otto-Johnson Mercantile Co. failed to report for duty Wednesday morning of this week.

Someone has been missing from every business establishment in Clayton this week with the "flu.".

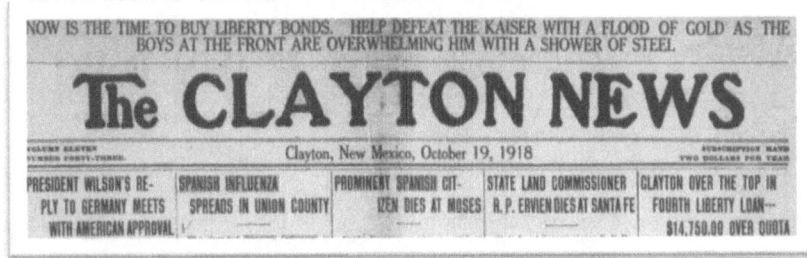

NOW IS THE TIME TO BUY LIBERTY BONDS. HELP DEFEAT THE KAISER WITH A FLOOD OF GOLD AS THE BOYS AT THE FRONT ARE OVERWHELMING HIM WITH A SHOWER OF STEEL.

The CLAYTON NEWS

Clayton, New Mexico, October 19, 1918

PRESIDENT WILSON'S RE-PLY TO GERMANY MEETS WITH AMERICAN APPROVAL | SPANISH INFLUENZA SPREADS IN UNION COUNTY | PROMINENT SPANISH CIT-IZEN DIES AT MOSES | STATE LAND COMMISSIONER R. P. ERVIEN DIES AT SANTA FE | CLAYTON OVER THE TOP IN FOURTH LIBERTY LOAN— $14,750.00 OVER QUOTA

PROMINENT SPANISH CITIZEN DIES AT MOSES

THE CLAYTON NEWS

Clayton, New Mexico (Oct. 19, 1918) – Delfin Espinoza, a pioneer resident of Union County, passed away at his residence at Moses, N. M, on Wednesday of this week.

He was taken ill with Spanish influenza a few days ago, which developed into double pneumonia.

He came to Union County several years ago and has always been active in matters of interest to the community in which he lived.

For the past seven years, he has resided at Moses and has been engaged in the mercantile business.

He was 55 years old and was the very picture of health at the time he was stricken with dreaded influenza.

He leaves a wife and several children to mourn his loss.

Two of the children are at this time sick with the disease that claimed their father.

The remains of Mr. Espinoza will be laid to rest in the Clayton cemetery today.

STATE LAND COMMISSIONER R. P. ERVIEN DIES AT SANTA FE

THE CLAYTON NEWS

Clayton, New Mexico (Oct. 19, 1918) – State Land Commissioner R. P. Ervien died Monday evening October 14th, about 9 o'clock at his home in Santa Fe. Ho was taken sick at Albuquerque, Wednesday evening of last week with Spanish influenza. He hurried home, but the disease grew worse.

Mr. Ervien was born in Pennsylvania, December 8th, 1800, and was 52 years old at the time of his death.

He came to Clayton, N. M., in 1890.

He was in the general mercantile business from 1890 to 1893, Manager of the Clayton Electric light plant from 1893 to 1911. Assessor of Union County from 1901 to 1903; was appointed Territorial Commissioner of Public Lands in 1907. He was elected in 1011 as the first Slat o Land Commissioner and re-elected in 1916 to the same position. He leaves a wife and two sons.

DAUGHTER OF O. A. MURPHY PASSES AWAY

The 16-year-old daughter of O. A. Murphy died Sunday at their home in Clayton. The cause of death was heart failure. The family was under quarantine at the time of her death for scarlet fever. The mother and father were compelled, under the most unfortunate circumstances, to care for their child in the hour death all alone. Two other children of the family are sick, and the attending physician has every hope for their recovery.

PROCLAMATION

Whereas, the Spanish Influenza has made its appearance in Union County. Therefore, it becomes necessary in the interest of the health of our people that all public gatherings, meetings, and schools be discontinued for the present or until further notice. Avoid all crowds and keep your children at home. Keep your homes in a sanitary condition and use every precaution possible. Report all cases promptly to:

Dr. W. A. BRISTOL

County Health Officer

ALL NURSES MUST REGISTER.

According to instructions received by Mrs. M. C. Drake at Red Cross Headquarters this week, all nurses, whether active or inactive, must register. Questionnaires have been received and must be filled out by all nurses. This is not a request but a command. Therefore, all nurses in Union County, who have not already done so, should go at once to Red Cross Headquarters at Clayton and Register or see your branch Chairman. This includes women who have been or are now in one of these classes.

Graduate nurses, pupil nurses, ungraduated nurses, trained attendants, practical nurses, midwives, women who have taken Red Cross courses.

JOHN GUYER PASSES TO THE GREAT BEYOND.

John Guyer, brother of Mrs. Thompson, editor of the *Clayton Citizen*, passed away at Camp Forest, Ga., Tuesday of this week from an attack of influenza. The remains have been shipped to Clayton and will be laid to rest in the Clayton cemetery.

The News force, with her many friends, extends the deepest sympathy to the bereaved family.

Prominent Baptist Minister Dies

The Cairo Bulletin

Oct. 19, 1918 – Rev. W. C. Leonard, pastor of the Tamms Baptist Church, died Tuesday of pneumonia. He was one of the prominent young ministers of the Clear Creek Baptist association. Rev. Leonard is survived by his wife and one child. His home was at Anna.

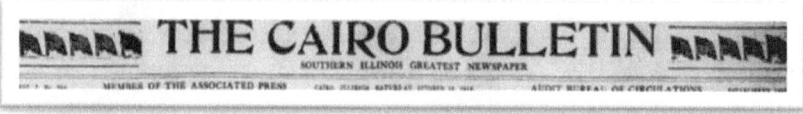

Spanish Influenza Situation Is Not Improving
St. Mary's Hospital Is Crowded.

DEATH RATE CONTINUES TO BE EXTREMELY LOW

Spanish Influenza **Situation is Not Improving—St. Mary's Hospital is Crowded.**

DEATH RATE CONTINUES TO BE EXTREMELY LOW

Only Three Deaths Among Whites of Cairo—May Close All Saloons.

THE CAIRO BULLETIN

CAIRO, ILLINOIS (Oct. 19, 1918) – Influenza conditions In Cairo are not improving to any material extent. Cases are increasing, and St. Mary's Hospital is providing for about as many as the hospital can conveniently accommodate. The death rate, however, remains low, and according to the records of the city, only 16 deaths have occurred in Cairo since Oct 4 from influenza or pneumonia.
Some of these are cases brought to Cairo for hospital treatment from towns in this vicinity.

There have been 31 deaths in Cairo since Oct. 4, a net total of 15 from other causes than influenza. In October 1917, 23 deaths were recorded. This figure is for the entire month. The great majority of the deaths have been among the colored people, there being 11 deaths among just that race from the disease and only five among the white people. Of these, two were brought from out of town.

If it becomes necessary, given the crowded conditions of St. Mary's Hospital, the Marine hospital can very readily be put into use, or the Bondurant Hospital prepared for the accommodation of patients. Both are good buildings, and the convenience necessary for the care of patients is at hand, it is considered to take one of these steps.

Weather like that of the past few days may have its effect on the situation, the misty damp atmosphere offering opportunity for the spreading and rapid contagion of the disease, which means that people must become even more watchful.

Rev. Father James Gillen, pastor of St. Joseph's Catholic Church, accompanied Dr. Clarke in a round of his patients yesterday and expressed himself on what he saw as follows:

"At the invitation and in the company of Dr. Clarke, I visited Thursday noon a few cottages in the Thirty-eighth Street district where the influenza is malignantly prevalent. I should never believe that such scenes here offended the eye, and every other sense were possible this day in an American community."

"In two little rooms, for instance, were five men and women extremely ill with influenza. The bed had no sheets, and the cover was once a quilt. Everywhere was filth and disorder, the air foul, the doors and windows were carefully shut on this balmy day. The faces of the patients gave the expression of despair, springing from a sense of utter forsakenness and helplessness. In short, it was a habitation over which you might write Dante's inscription upon the entrance of another place: 'Let all hope go, ye that enter here.'

"The temptation lies near to seek out the causes of such miserable condition, not of ignorant foreigners, but of true-blood Americans, whose forbears have been such for generations. This, however, is not my present purpose."

"My purpose is to commend our health officer and without exception, our Cairo physicians who have worked so unceasingly and self-sacrificingly to stamp out this insidious disease from our midst."

"Dr. Clark had Thursday afternoon eight of the worst cases removed to the fever ward of St. Mary's Hospital. Another batch will be brought here today. This morning I visited this ward—what a transformation. The patients of yesterday were resting in gowns and sheets as white as snow. Each had received a bath which must have been a luxury inexperienced, perhaps for years."

"They received expert nursing as devoted as though they were millionaires. The Sisters in their charge were radiant with the happiness of those that know the word: *What ye have done to the least of my brethren, ye have done to me.*"

"I should not have dared to draw the picture of Cairo's shame if I could not set it off with Cairo's glory, St. Mary's Hospital, that place of pain with its ministering angels.

B. LESTER BAIN, 21, DIES OF INFLUENZA IN CHICAGO

THE DAILY ILLINI

Urbana, Ill. (Oct. 19, 1918) – B. Lester Bain, 21, died at his home at Morgan Park, Chicago, on Oct.2 following an illness of influenza and pneumonia. Bain, who was a student in the College of Agriculture, was planning to return to school when taken sick. His parents, Rev. and Mrs. A. L. Bain is in Central Africa as Baptist missionaries.

BRIDGEPORT DOING WELL

NEW YORK CLIPPER

BRIDGEPORT, Conn. Oct. 21, 1918 —Polis Players at the Lyric continue to draw good attendance despite Spanish influenza. This week's bill is

Bought and Paid For. Next week we will see a new stock release, The Cabin in the Hills.

HARTFORD BUSINESS POOR

HARTFORD, Conn., Oct. 21, 1918 —The epidemic has had the effect of keeping the public away from the theatres to a very large extent with the result that the attendance at Poli's Palace is far from good. This week s bill is "The Heart of Wetona." Next week, "Pal o Mine."

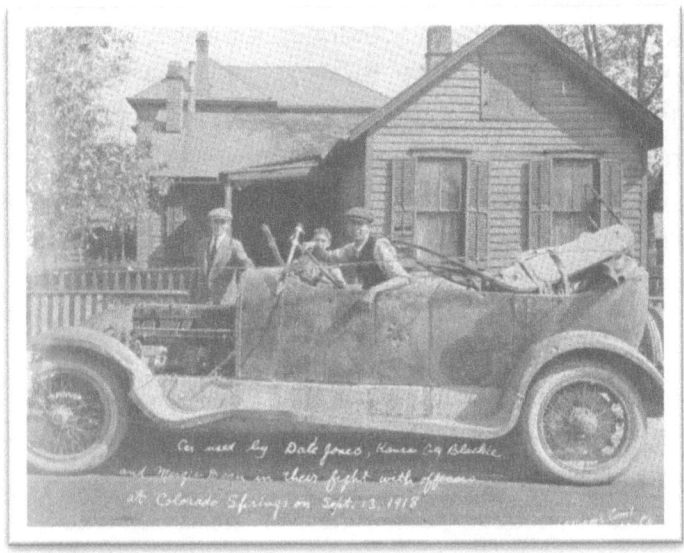

Bloodthirsty bank robber gang of Frank Lewis hacked up a Colorado Springs police officer on Sept. 13, 1918.

BANDIT DIES HERE
Frank Lewis at End of Brazen Criminal Career.
Influenza Fatal to Man With Bullet Wound in His Lung.

Topeka State Journal,
Topeka Kansas (Oct. 17, 1918)

Frank Lewis, alleged gunman, bandit, and train robber died Wednesday afternoon in the Shawnee County Jail, a victim of influenza, which quickly developed into pneumonia. A bullet wound through his lungs inflicted by Colorado Springs police September 13, 1918, made Lewis an easy victim of the disease. It was said that the bandit had been dead about an hour when his body was found in his cell about 4: 30 o'clock by C. W. Hixon, jailer.

Lewis was being held by government authorities in connection with the holding up of a Katy train at Koch, Kan., three and a half miles south of Paola, July 10. 1918. He was brought to Topeka, October 2, 1918, arraigned before C. B. White. United States Commissioner, on the charge of conspiracy to rob a mail train, waived his preliminary meaning and was bound over to the Grand Jury. Since that time, he has been confined in the county jail.

End of a Wild Career.

The career of Lewis was a wild one. Most of his life, it is said, was devoted to crime, and he was engaged in several gunfights to avoid capture by officers of the law. He was alleged to be a member of the famous gang of outlaws headed by Dale Jones, of Kansas City, who is the only member of the gang who has not been captured or killed. Roy D. Sherrill, another member of the gang, was seriously wounded on September 13, 1918, in a pitched battle with Colorado Springs police, at the time Lewis received his wound and is now being held by the government in a Denver hospital. Roscoe Lancaster, better known as "Kansas City Blackie," was mortally wounded by the Kansas City police during a fight that took place on Montgall avenue in that city on September 24, 1918 and died a short time later.

Last July detectives engaged Lewis, Jones, and others in a revolver fight at 3715 Wyandotte street, but the bandits escaped. In the Colorado Springs fight, John D. Rowan, chief of the Colorado Springs detectives, was killed, and John D. Riley, a detective, seriously wounded. It was charged by other members of the gang that Lewis was the one who killed the officer, but Lewis always denied this.

Brothers Were Criminals

Frank Lewis was one of three brothers, all of whom were criminals. Ora and Roy Lewis are serving a term in the Missouri state penitentiary for killing William A. Dillon and John McKenna, St. Louis policemen, April 6,

1916. Dillon tried to arrest the three men for killing McKenna, but the bandits turned on their captor and virtually hacked his body to pieces, it was said. Ora and Roy are serving life terms for the crime.

Lewis's body was taken to Penwell's undertaking establishment Wednesday night. C.C. Jackson, United States Marshal, said this morning that an effort would be made to locate some relatives of Lewis before the funeral was held. The bandit was said to have had a wife and child, but their whereabouts are unknown to the authorities.

Lewis was 25 years old. He was a large, powerfully built man, weighing 225 pounds and in his operations was said to have posed, usually, as a wealthy oilman. While admitting two or three of the many crimes with which he had been charged, he strenuously denied the rest. He told Undersheriff Bob Miller that if he had been guilty of all the misdeeds with which he was attributed that he "wouldn't be able to sleep nights." When reminded that he was still a young man, Lewis's face brightened, and he earnestly expressed the hope that some leniency might be shown him and that after "doing his bit" he could straighten up and live a better life, for the sake of his family. He was said to have begun his life of crime when he was 14 years old.

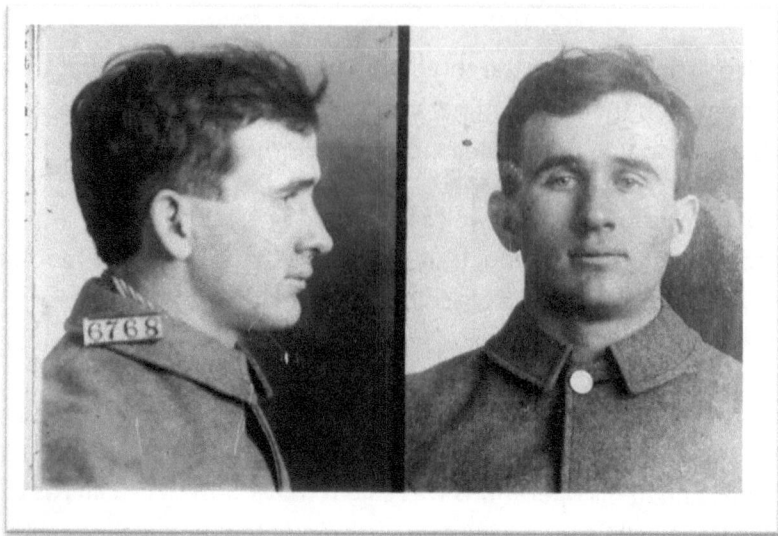

FRANKLY SPEAKING: Surely not the same *Frank the Train Robber* who was shot in the lung and died of influenza, but interesting just the same.

FBI Reward poster for Frank Grigware, who escaped Leavenworth prison in April 1910. He was captured in Canada in 1933 using the name James Fahey, but he was never extradited to the U.S. because many Canadians believed he was innocent of his original mail train robbery charges.

FLU INCREASING HERE; STORES TO CLOSE SAT. NIGHT

Seventy-Six New Cases Reported Up to Noon Today.

High Record Set During Last Thirty-Six Hours.

KEEP CLOSING ORDER IN FORCE

Little Chance for Schools To Open Next Week.

Hospital Is Badly in Need of More Nurses.

CLOSE NEXT WEEK
Kansas May Keep Lid On To
Check Influenza.
Better To Pay for Shows and
Schools Than Funerals.
300 DEATHS A WEEK IN STATE
Two Percent of Number of
Reported Cases In Kansas.
Two Thousand New Cases a
Day Are Developing.

Topeka, Kansas, (Oct. 17, 1918) – Kansas may remain closed during all of next week. Officials of the state board of health will meet tomorrow and determine what action should be taken. Dr. J. J. Sippy, the epidemiologist for the state board of health, said today that he would recommend that the closing order be kept in force another week at least.

"We are getting reports of about the same number of new cases every day," he said. "Wichita, Kansas City, Kan., and Topeka show increases, and there are large increases in southeast Kansas. In the sections where the counties were closed two weeks ago, there is a marked abatement."

"I expect to see the number of cases run along about the same for the next week and then will come the gradual decrease. The matter of closing is a serious proposition. It is serious from an economic standpoint, and then comes the question of whether it is better to pay for amusements and schools than to pay for funerals. Some county health officials have been told that public sales outdoors might be permitted next week if no lunches were served and only grown folks permitted to attend. It is urged that the women keep away from these sales too.

Three Hundred Deaths a Week.

"We figure that the state has around three hundred deaths a week from influenza and pneumonia caused by influenza. This is approximately two percent, and that is the history of the disease in other states. The accurate reports cannot be tabulated until the monthly reports of the vital statistics registrars are available. Only a few deaths are reported to us now. "During the first week the disease was in the state, the new cases ran 190 a day. During the second week, they ran 1,300 a day, an increase of seven hundred percent. During the third week, the present week, they are averaging slightly less than two thousand a day, which indicates the effectiveness of the closing order. Without It, Kansas would be reporting now between six and seven thousand cases a day, and the death rate would be higher than it is estimated."

Outdoor meetings may be permitted

In the state next week where necessary to hold them. The question of closing down entirely is going to be largely determined by the local health officials as the governor's proclamation left the matter of continuing the closing to the local officials.

Doctors Are Busy.

The state board of health has been authorized to order volunteer medical reserve doctors to any localities where they are needed, but indications today were that no aid from other states could be expected. Also, reports from practically every locality in the state show that all doctors and nurses are working night and day and that they cannot be spared for emergency calls.

Must Have Aid.

However, it is imperative that aid is sent to Crawford and Thomas counties, and it is probable that the state officials will simply go over their lists and select doctors for these counties from localities where their leaving will be likely to cause the least amount of uneasiness and hardships.

Nurses are Just as scarce as doctors, it Is said, and their services are Just as much in demand In places where the disease has not been gotten under control.

KEEP WINDOWS OPEN

Fresh Air Is Best Influenza Preventive, Dr. Clark Says.

TOPEKA NEWS JOURNAL Oct. 17, 1918

"Keep- every window In Topeka open."

This is the appeal made today by Dr. H. L. Clark, city health officer, in an effort to check the spread of influenza, "Fresh air is one of the best things to keep a person from catching influenza or to cure it after it develops.

Pneumonia patients have a better chance to recover if all windows and doors of the sick room are kept wide open, except when the patient is being bathed.

"The health authorities in Massachusetts, where influenza has been causing nearly a thousand deaths a week for the last month or two," says Doctor Clark, "have found that moving their' influenza -pneumonia case out of doors, into the open air and exposing them to the direct rays of the sun, reduces the mortality in these pneumonia cases from forty percent under the indoor treatment, to thirteen percent. This shows that a pneumonia patient has three times as good a chance to get well if placed outdoors in the sun as he has if kept in a room, "The street railway company is cooperating in the fresh air measures by instructing its conductors to- keep every window and ventilator open on their cars, rain or shine, during the influenza outbreak."

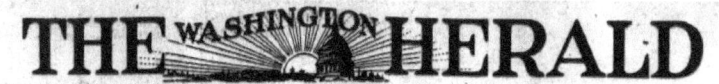

Flu Delays Death Till Representative Marries.

A death bed marriage between Congressman Jacob Edward Meeker and Mrs. Alice U. Redmond, his former secretary, was celebrated in St. Louis Tuesday nightt.

Congressman Meeker, Republican representative of the Tenth District of Missouri, is also the first member of Congress to succumb to pneumonia. His death was a shock to his colleagues.

Mr. Meeker was a graduate of the Oberlin Theological Seminary at Oberlin, Ohio. Before his entrance into politics he had served as pastor of the Compton Hill Congregational Church in St. Louis. During his Congressional term Mrs. Meeker was prominent because ofthe stand he took against probibition.

First member of Congress to die of Spanish Influenza.

Congressman Dies

ST. LOUIS, MO., Oct. 17, 1918 – Jacob Meeker, a congressman from the Tenth District, Missouri, died of Spanish influenza in the Jewish Hospital here. He had been ill since Monday.

Congressman Killed

BLOOMINGTON, ILL. Oct. 17, 1918 – Congressman John A. Sterling of this city was killed in an automobile accident two miles south of Pontiac today.

The Topeka State Journal.

TOPEKA, KANSAS, MONDAY EVENING, JANUARY 28, 1918 — EIGHT PAGES

THE TOPEKA DAILY STATE JOURNAL THURSDAY EVENING, OCTOBER 17, 1918

USE THE VACCINE

Chicago Will Try New Discovery on Flu Victims.

Chicago, Oct. 17. 1918, Vaccine originated by Dr. E. C. Rosenow of the Mayo Clinic, Rochester, Minn., will be used in Chicago's campaign against Spanish influenza.

Doctor Rosenow told the Chicago Influenza Emergency Commission of his experiments with the vaccine with which he has treated 20,000 persons. The commission at once named a commission of physicians to take charge of the manufacture and use of all vaccines and sera in Chicago, including the Rosenow vaccine. Another commission was named to raise funds for its manufacture and distribution.

Five days will be required to begin the manufacture of the vaccine here; it was stated. Meantime, Doctor Rosenow will provide a supply sufficient for 100,000 doses from his laboratories at Rochester.

The vaccine is designed to provide immunity from the disease, though Doctor Rosenow is unwilling to make specific claims as to its value. He believes it aided greatly to suppress the spread of influenza at Rochester.

FLU INCREASING HERE; STORES TO CLOSE SAT. NIGHT

Seventy-Six New Cases Reported
Up to Noon Today.
High Record Set During Last
Thirty-Six Hours.

KEEP CLOSING ORDER IN FORCE

Little Chance for Schools To
Open Next Week.
Hospital Is Badly in Need of
More Nurses.

TOPEKA STATE JOURNAL – (Oct. 17, 1918)

It becomes evident that there is no abatement in the Influenza epidemic, which threatens Topeka with the gravest dangers. On the contrary, it would appear that the disease is spreading rapidly.

Up to 12 o'clock today, seventy-six new cases, all of which were diagnosed cases reported by attending physicians, were turned in at the office of the public health department. Wednesday, 100 cases were turned in. One hundred ad seventy-six new cases in one and one-half days are the alarming report given out today. The total number of cases that have been reported since the outbreak of the disease now stands at 709. This morning's report is the largest that has been made up since the outbreak of the disease.

Two more deaths occurring Wednesday night bring the total number of deaths from influenza up to nineteen.
Mrs. Elsie Day, of 456 Freeman, and Miss Doris Hanson, of 410 Clay street, are the latest unfortunate victims of the disease. Neither of

these women was sick very long. But in the opinion of authorities, their lives might have been saved had care been given them in time.

Influenza works with great rapidity, says Dr. H. L. Clark, and it is often the attention given in the first days of the sickness, which determines whether or not the patient will live. If the case is neglected until a good start has been obtained, recovery is always doubtful.

Keep Closing Order In Force.

It is practically a foregone conclusion that the closing order will be in force all of next week. The city authorities could not lift the order under any circumstances until the statewide closing order is lifted. However, should conditions demand the continuation of the closing order in Topeka even after the state order had been lifted, it will be continued.

Close Stores Saturday Night.

This morning, Doctor Clark, city health officer issued a new closing order which is as follows:

Because of the continuance of Influenza in Topeka, and of the usual Saturday night crowds in the downtown district, all clothing, shoe, dry goods, department, and general stores, and all ice cream and soda fountains on Kansas avenue from Twelfth Street on the south to Fairchild on the north, and all such places of business on Sixth Avenue between Van Buren Street on the west and Monroe Street on the east are at this moment ordered to close not later than 7 o'clock on the evening of Saturday, October 19, 1918. Cigar stores will be allowed to remain open later than 7 o'clock if not more tuna, ten persons are allowed inside the doors at one time. Grocery stores, meat markets, restaurants, auto supply dealers and garages, and drug stores are not included in this closing order, but soda fountains in drug stores and cigar stores must be closed not later than 7 o'clock.

No individual notices will be issued; publication in the newspaper will be considered sufficient notice.

H. L. CLARK
City Health Officer, Topeka

SPANISH INFLUENZA

Many Cases at Hospital.

The emergency hospital was caring for seventy-one patients this morning. Thirteen have been released. Today several more patients will be released.

Another room in the hotel building now being used as the emergency hospital was to be opened up on the second floor of the building this afternoon. This is the first room on the second floor to be put into use for influenzas patients. Most of the rooms on the second floor have been used as sleeping rooms for the nurses who have handled the night shifts. According to Commissioner Porter, the hospital is now working at practically its greatest capacity, not that there is no more room there but for the reason that more patients cannot be handled with the staff of nurses now on hand. If the hospital is to be enlarged to care for the rapidly increasing numbers of cases, it will be necessary to first enlarge the staff of nurses

The city authorities have been sending out constant appeals for more nurses. They are still calling. Three nurses reported this morning, but nothing is known of the experience of these women until they report for an interview. It is not believed, however, that they are graduate nurses. This morning the hospital lost one of Its best nurses, a graduate nurse, who was called away by the government. She left at once. The authorities are striving both through the publicity given by the press and by carrying paid advertising to obtain nurses at once. Their success is anything but gratifying. If there are any women who can be of service in this emergency, no better time will ever come for them to report than right at present. The epidemic is at the highest point yet attained in Topeka.

Death Rate 3 Percent.

According to the figures compiled by Commissioner Porter, the death rate in Topeka is 3 percent. Three persons out of every 100 contracting the disease are dying.

There is a rumor current, which has been reported in the offices of the public health department, which it is thought may have tended to Influence people in not reporting cases. As telephoned this morning, it was to the effect that people believed that the city was making a charge of $5 for putting up the notices warning visitors of the presence of influenza. This is an erroneous impression. The city authorities gladly tack these cards up entirely free of charge. The case only has to be reported. There is a law, carrying a heavy penalty, which demands an immediate report on all cases.

One of Porter's inspectors in reporting hostilities among the Mexican population said the Mexican woman could "No know anything." But when the Inspector called another Mexican woman who understood better, mention of the "jailhouse" provided an instantaneous understanding. Her children had influenza, and cards were placed on the house.

Notes and Personals.

Henry Dietrich, who has been sick with influenza at his home on Central Avenue, has recovered and can be at his work at the Sheetz grocery again.

Doctor and Mrs. Thompson and their two children are sick with influenza at their home, 1015 Jackson Street. Mrs. Thompson and the children, who have been ill several days, are improving. Doctor Thompson was taken sick last night.

- It cannot be said that America Is not sending her best to France. In one colored regiment, the following answer to roll call: Alexander Hamilton, Horatio Seymour, George Washington, Cotton Mather, Benjamin Franklin, Thomas Jefferson, Paul Revere, John Quincy Adams. Phil Sheridan and Patrick Henry.
- And again, we recall the words of a certain august personage during a summer conference at great headquarters: "Us emperors must together hang." Prophetic words.
- Spanish influenza shows signs of following the lead of Bulgaria in effecting a separate peace.

TOPEKA SOLDIER DIES
Frederick N. Joseph a Victim of Pneumonia

at Fort Riley Camp.

Frederick N. Joseph, 823 North Kansas Avenue, a soldier in the medical officers training camp at Fort Riley, died Tuesday night of pneumonia, following an attack of influenza. The funeral will be held from the Penwell undertaking parlors at 10:30 o'clock tomorrow morning. Burial in Topeka cemetery.

Frederick Joseph, before his entrance into the training camp one month ago, was with the Badger Bag & Paper Co. here. He was 32 years of age. He leaves a brother in New York City

Indian Reservation Flu Shack

PYRAMID LAKE RESERVATION - Another type of dwelling in Virginia City. In this shack, I found four people on the dirt floor wrapped in rags: apparently, all suffering from influenza. I was told they had refused medicine from the white doctor, and Dick Mauwee, a Paiute enrolled at Pyramid Lake Reservation, was the doctor. The small four-light window admitted the only light. It was nailed tight; the only door was kept shut tight, and no ventilation was attempted or was possible. The stench which greeted us when we entered was most horrible and could be endured but a short time. An Indian had just been taken from this structure for burial. The father of the family was the Indian alluded to on another page as a "walking case."

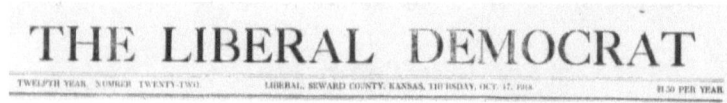

The Liberal Undertaking Company reports the following deaths:

The Russel brothers of near Tyrone, who died last week, one of blood poisoning and the other of pneumonia.

Mrs. Dubbs of near the same place also passed away last week, having had an attack of influenza.

ELMER WILBUR SHELTON

Son of Mr. and Mrs. Isaac Shelton of near Lorena, Oklahoma, a member of Motor Truck Company No. 21, died in the Base Hospital at Fort Bliss, Texas, on October 12, 1918, of pneumonia following an attack of influenza.

Wilbur, as he was known to his friends, was an employee of the Standard Oil Company of this city.

He was 24 years of age, a young man of excellent character, and of a disposition that made him friends wherever he went. Although he had been in the service for over a year, he had not been sent to France and was anxiously awaiting the day when the order would come for him to embark.

He returned during the month of July to assist his father in the work of the farm and seemed to enjoy his life in the army. A message came Sunday evening that he was seriously ill, and his father left Tuesday evening for his bedside, arriving there Wednesday evening. He died the following Saturday evening at 4 o'clock.

The remains arrived here on Train No. 4 Tuesday morning, and the funeral services were held at home Tuesday afternoon, conducted by M. M. Maricle, Co. E. National Guards, who had charge of the body. He was buried with Military Honors in the Lorena cemetery.

A beautiful floral piece representing an American flag was a contribution of his comrades in the Camp, as well as many beautiful pieces from friends here. He leaves to mourn his loss his father, mother, two brothers, and two sisters.

PAUL M. BENNETT

Youngest son of Mrs. Marv Bennett j formerly of Liberal, but now a resident of Whittier, California, is among those who have fallen a victim of pneumonia following influenza. Paul was transferred from a Camp in California to Camp Taylor, Kentucky, about five weeks ago, where he died October 12, at the age of 23 years. Paul was a Christian young man and stood for the highest principles of manhood and was of exceptional scholarly ability.

Paul spent his boyhood days in Liberal, being a graduate of Liberal high school, class of 1912. After graduating here, he went to Kansas Wesleyan College at Winfield, finishing a four-year course. He was a member of the College Glee Club and having an excellent tenor voice, and he was in demand in musical circles of the college. After graduating, he accepted a position as principal of schools at Cassady, Kansas. At the close of the term, he went with his mother to California. He enlisted in the officers' training reserve in the artillery section, where he remained until the time of his death.

The remains were shipped to Whittier, California, where the funeral services were held. His brother Gordon, of Haviland, Kansas, passed through Liberal Monday on his way to attend the funeral.

His mother, Mrs. Mary Bennett, brother, Gordon, and his grandparents, Mr. and Mrs. W. P. McClure of Whittier California, remain to mourn his death.

It is a sad duty on the part of the Democrat to chronicle the passing of these three most excellent young men. They were the very cream of the young manhood of the town and country. No cleaner, more honorable boys could have been found than these. We are proud that we have known them to be numbered among their friends. They have sacrificed their lives at the call of their country, that it might stand for all time to come as the protector of the weak and oppressed, a country embodying the highest ideal of Christian brotherhood. Such as may die in so noble a cause do not die in vain, and while the pages of history cannot contain the names of all who help make it nevertheless they shall not be forgotten, for their memory shall live in the hearts of the men and women who knew them and loved them for their true worth as men, and for their noble sacrifice in helping to build a nation whose ideals shall be the guiding light for the nations of the world.

To the parents and relatives of each, we join with the entire community in expressing the deepest sympathy. May they receive some measure of comfort from the fact that their loss and their sorrow is nationwide, and that they have contributed their utmost to the glorious cause of Liberty and righteousness.

The remains of Freddie Massie, age 27 years, who was a horse-shoer in the Medical department, arrived in Tyrone yesterday, from Fort Bliss, Texas, where he died October 13th, as a result of pneumonia. Private Warner, a member of the same company, accompanied the remains. Funeral services will be held in Tyrone today. A wife and baby are left to mourn his departure.

MATTIE COURSEY

Mrs. Mattie Coursey, the wife of E. E. Coursey, passed away at home in south Liberal Tuesday morning at 5 o'clock, following an illness of influenza and pneumonia, which were of about a week's duration.

Mrs. Coursey was only 24 years of age at the time of death. Her friends are many, as she was an industrious woman and of pleasant and likable disposition.

Funeral services were held at the Liberal Cemetery yesterday afternoon at 2:30, Elder Jas. M. Taylor in charge. A husband, three children, and a brother who is with Uncle Sam's men in France, and a sister, Mrs. Miller, of Oklahoma, who was present at the funeral.

The Democrat joins with the many friends in extending their heartfelt and motherless children who will so greatly miss her loving presence and tender care.

LILLY ALLEN THOMAS

Mrs. Lilly Allen Thomas of Ochiltree died at a local hospital on October 15, at 5:30 p. m., with pneumonia, which came as a result oi influenza with which she had been ill about a week. She was born in Colorado City, Texas, on July 22, 1892.

Mrs. Thomas is the only daughter of Mr. and Mrs. Allen of near Ochiltree, who, with her husband, was with her at the time of her death.

The remains, accompanied by the relatives, were taken to Colorado City, Texas, yesterday where funeral services will be held and interment will be made October 19th.

Robert Storms, another Tyrone boy, was a victim of influenza and pneumonia, and his remains were expected to arrive in Tyrone last night from Camp Meade, Maryland, where he died a week ago.

GETTING READY FOR ANY EMERGENCY
State Board of Health, Council of Defense, and Red Cross Guard Against "Flu."

That there might be a working organization in readiness in the event of a more serious outbreak of Influenza, acting under the orders of the State Board of Health, Dr. Geo. S. Smith, County Health Officer, called a conference with the heads of the Council of Defense and the Red Cross, and plans were made, which will no doubt prove of great benefit should the disease become as prevalent here as it is in some sections. A committee was appointed consisting of Dr. Smith, representing the Board of Health; Ray Millman, the Council of Defense; T. B. Moore, Miss Kate Wright, and Frank Summers representing the Red Cross. This committee may list nurses and physicians available, secure Hospital conveniences, and take charge of the situation should conditions become critical.

This is not expected but is a precautionary measure.

QUARANTINE WILL LAST ANOTHER WEEK ANYWAY
Schools, Churches, and Public Gatherings Prohibited Until Influenza Is Abated.
THE LIBERAL DEMOCRAT

Liberal, Kansas – (Oct. 17, 1918)
At a meeting of those in authority held Wednesday, it was decided best to continue the closing order at least another week, so the order will be continued in force.

There are several cases of Influenza in the city, but most of them are getting along very well. There has been but one death in the city, as a result of the disease. However, the health authorities thought it wise to not open up until the number of new cases reported had begun to diminish.

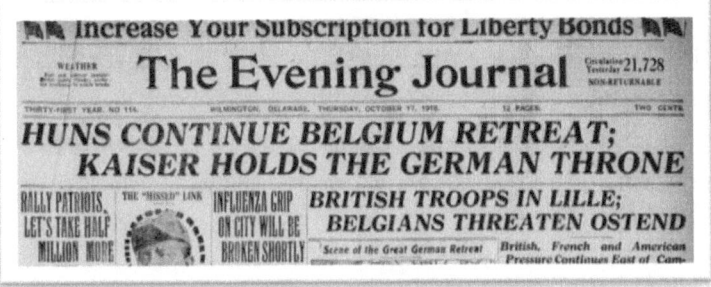

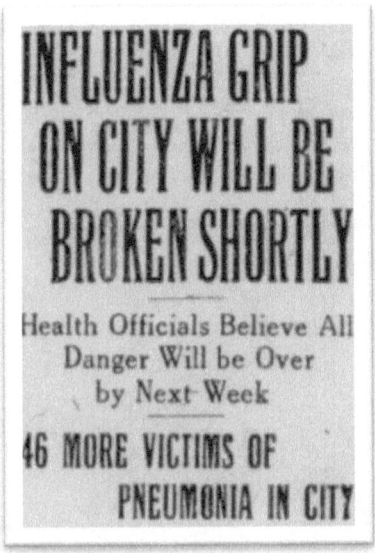

THE EVENING JOURNAL

Wilmington, Delaware (Oct. 17, 1918)

One week more and the epidemic Influenza will be nearing the end of its course In Wilmington.

This Is the expressed opinion of the city and State Board of Health officials.

There is an all-important "if" attached to this encouraging statement. If the citizens continue as careful of their health and of exposure to contagion as they have been during the past fortnight, the epidemic will soon become history, if people get the false idea that the danger is now all over, the disease Is likely to break out with renewed violence.

The City Board of Health has not set down any probable date for lifting the closing order, even in its own mind. |

"Positively, the order will not be rescinded until the death rate of the city has gone back to normal. That Is all we can say at present," is the statement made by Dr. R. E. Ellegood.

Dr. E. W. Scott, who has been in charge of the situation locally for the United States Public Health Service, received orders today to report at once in Columbus, Ohio. Dr. Scott made a trip to Washington yesterday to report on the Wilmington situation.

There were forty-six epidemic deaths in the city recorded at the Board of Health from yesterday noon up to 10 o'clock this morning, a much larger number than the twenty-three deaths for the previous twenty-four hours, but most of these deaths occurred two j

Dr. Scott will leave today for Columbus, Ohio, taking with him three of the government physicians who have been stationed in this city. Dr. B. O. Woodward, Dr. Stephen W. Weyer, and Dr. Helene Ratterman. Dr. Richards, of the Public Health Service, will be put in charge in Wilmington, assisted by Dr. A. S. Warder. Dr. W. F. Dolan, Dr. Van Stone, Dr. Ida McCormick, Dr. Ella Hunt, Dr. H. M. Stang, a government doctor to be transferred from Carney's Point, and two interns sent from outside.

This will mean that ten government physicians will continue to work in Wilmington. Dr. Scott has arranged with Dean Pierson, of the

Hahnemann Hospital, Philadelphia, for the twelve doctors who were to be recalled to the hospital from Carney's Point to remain at Carney s Point until Monday,

There are also three government physicians at that place, making fifteen doctors in all.

Dr. Scott has made further arrangements with the Ley Construction Company, erecting munition works at Port Penn, to send a number of their company nurses to help out In Wilmington for a while, until the number of pneumonia cases lessens. They will help at the emergency hospitals.

Dr. Scott said this morning that the one thing now necessary is for Wilmington people to keep up all their precautionary methods, and not to relax in the least. He said that the local situation Is very' encouraging, and it remains with the public to keep it so by co-operating in every way with the Board of Health. Dr. Scott has several times spoken in high praise of the way The Board of Health has handled the situation and gives the board a great deal of credit for measures which have checked the epidemic in this city more quickly than in most other places where It has flourished

The chief responsibility has fallen upon the Board of Health, and its officials have been on the Job ceaselessly and self-sacrificing during the epidemic. Wilmington may well be grateful to the Board of Health for its promptness and efficiency in taking care of the situation.

The United States Public Services Director, Dr. Scott, and his assisting government doctors have cooperated thoroughly with the Board of Health of this city and State. They have gone to work with a thoroughness that has helped greatly in putting the epidemic on the downgrade.

Today, the Wilmington Country Club Hospital reported forty empty beds, and the New Century Club Hospital reported thirty-five empty beds. Dr. Scott stated that a few new cases reported are of a mild form of influenza, practically all the severe cases being old ones. Among these early cases, there are pneumonia cases in very large numbers, the most serious element of the local situation today. Pneumonia arising from influenza is an insidious disease of a serious nature and requires the utmost care in nursing.

Convalescent patients are warned against getting about too soon, as many of the pneumonia cases have been a relapse of partially recovered influenza patients.

The Board of Health will ask physicians to prescribe only as much liquor as is necessary for treating a patient. By state law, the wholesale dealers may not sell liquor in less than a quart, to be consumed off-premises. One quart of whiskey can make a man drunk unless he spreads it over a reasonable length of time. Three individuals who had evidently had their quart within a brief period were seen careening down Market Street last night. The state law also requires that retail dealers may sell liquor only to be drunk on their premises.   The Board of Health's closing order forbids the retail dealers to have drinking on their premises during the continuance of the order. The request of the board that doctors shall not prescribe more than is necessary for a patient will mean that neither wholesale men nor retail men can flit the doctors' prescriptions, but that patients will have to get them filled at a drugstore. There are several druggists in the city who are licensed to sell liquor.

Dr. Franklin B. Royer, acting state health commissioner of Pennsylvania, who several days ago sent a telegraphic complaint that Coatesville negroes were bringing back large quantities of liquor Wilmington, has sent a congratulatory telegram to Mayor Lawson which reads:

Thank you for your telegram. Delighted to know you have discontinued the sale of liquor, and it is showing such splendid results."

***

Joseph Cohen, who lives at Eleventh and Tatnall Streets, is very sick with influenza.

Mrs. Jacob Rosenblatt, and little daughter Judith, are recovering from influenza and can be outdoors. They live at No. 312 West Fourteenth Street.

Henry R. Isaacs, No. 223 West Fourteenth Street, is ill with Influenza.

Mrs. Maud A. Bratton, a teacher of English for the past four years In the Wilmington High School, died this morning from Influenza-pneumonia, at the home of Harry Betts. No. 1210 Tatnall street. Her home is in Skowhegan, Maine. She is survived by her mother, Mrs. Marian Merrill, and a little son. She also has two sisters and a brother in France. The High School faculty and pupils regret the death of Mrs. Bratton greatly.

 Mrs. Mattie Cox Zebley, the wife of Patrolman Thomas Zebley, died at her home, No. 404 Walnut Street, this morning from pneumonia. Mrs. Zebley had been ill for several days.

Ferris Giles, who has been working for the Attorney General's office since the influenza epidemic started, burying those who were unable to secure undertakers, on Tuesday evening, found a seventeen months old child in at east side home. At the same time, in an upper room, the mother was seriously ill. The father was Intoxicated, and the renditions prevailing in the home were filthy.

Yesterday Mr. Giles had the woman removed to an emergency hospital, the attending physician claiming that sanitary surroundings were needed as much as attention.

The. Attorney's General's office had only one appeal sent in for an undertaker yesterday. The undertakers are now handling the burials more adequately.

Stella Dorsey, a Negress, aged 23 years, of Fifteenth and Scott streets, died at her home yesterday from influenza. The woman was not attended by a physician, and her death was reported to the coroner's office.

Richard Grieneisen, Jr., aged 26 years, and his wife Nellie M. Grieneisen, aged 24 years, died of influenza-pneumonia – one on Monday and the other two days later. The funeral, which will be private, will be held this afternoon at 4:30 o'clock, at their late home, No. 110 Ashton Street.

This morning there were only twelve patients In the Emergency Hospital of the Lynch Construction Company. Three patients were discharged yesterday as cured, and one new case was admitted. The total number of influenza cases at this hospital is 112, but there were never more than 40 patients at one time. There have been three deaths, the most recent being on Saturday.

There are now 2,500 men working at Union Park Gardens. Several of the houses would now be finished but for the failure of materials to arrive.

Two influenza patients were discharged from the New Castle County Hospital this morning. The remaining twelve patients are progressing rapidly toward recovery. None of the nurses is sick, and no new cases have been reported.

The State Hospital for the Insane reported 92 influenza patients this morning. None of them are dangerously ill. Six of the nurses are on the sick list, but their condition is favorable. There was one death from pneumonia yesterday, but the woman also suffered from a complication of diseases.

Outgoing Telegram Reporting Staffing Crisis at the Philadelphia Quartermaster Depot due to the Spanish Influenza Epidemic:

EPIDEMIC SPANISH INFLUENZA HAMPERING OPERATIONS OF DEPOT

ELEVEN COMMISSIONED OFFICERS, AND FOURTEEN HUNDRED AND EIGHTY-FIVE EMPLOYEES ABSENT TODAY. OF THE LATTER ELEVEN HUNDRED SEVENTY-SEVEN WORK IN FACTORIES. SITUATION NOT IMPROVING.

New Castle Situation Improves

The New Castle County Workhouse reports no new cases today, and their few patients are well along the road to recovery. New Castle, which together can accommodate seventy patients, had a combined total of thirty-four patients this morning. The situation seems to be much better in New Castle than it was two days ago.

It is reported that from fifteen to twenty new cases of influenza developed in Smyrna yesterday.

Lieutenant Ephraim Jolls, of Middletown, who has been ill from influenza at an embarkation hospital in Newport News, reached the home of his parents in Middletown yesterday. He has not fully recovered and has lost twelve pounds in weight as a result of his sickness.

DEATH ENDS HIS LIFE SENTENCE

THE EVENING JOURNAL

WILMINGTON, DEL. (Oct. 17, 1918) – Ernest Holley, Negro, aged 17 years, serving a life sentence at the workhouse on a charge of murder, died at that institution last night. The workhouse officials gave the cause of death as tuberculosis. The coroner's office, however, said Holley died of influenza.

Holley was sentenced by the New Castle County Court on May 17, last year. The body was removed to the morgue.

CAR HITS HEARSE: CORPSES IN STREET
W. F. Lynn, Undertaker, and Richard Campbell, Driver, Hurt
BLAME ACCIDENT TO LEAVES ON TRACK

THE EVENING JOURNAL

Wilmington, Delaware (Oct. 18, 1918)

Crashing into a hearse owned by William F. Lynn, undertaker, of No. 206 West Sixth street at Woodlawn and Lancaster avenues at 8.50 o'clock this morning, trolley car No. 329 of the West Fourth Street line demolished the hearse and threw to the street a casket containing the remains of a woman who had died of pneumonia, and the body of a small child. The remains were being removed to the Cathedral Cemetery for interment.

Richard Campbell, the driver of the hearse, was thrown from his seat and had both legs broken. Mr. Lynn also was thrown to the ground and had his ankle and knee badly injured. Mr. Campbell was taken to the Delaware Hospital In a passing automobile, and Mr. Lynn was removed to his home.

The trolley car, which escaped damage, was in the charge of Conductor J. R. Hutchinson of No 915 Clayton Street and Motorman E. Hinson, of No. 203 Monroe Street. They were not injured.

The trolley car was proceeding westward at the time of the collision, and when the hearse pulled onto the tracks ahead of it, Hinson applied the brakes.

The car slid. However, the rails being covered with wet leaves, the impact of the collision tore the lid from the casket, exposing the remains of the dead woman.

Another hearse was sent to the scene, and the remains of the dead woman and child were placed In it and taken to the cemetery.

Officials of the local traction company, after making an investigation, stated that the driver of the hearse pulled onto the tracks when the trolley car was but 10 feet away. The car was traveling slowly at the time, and the speed was reduced by the applying of the brakes, but the wet leaves on the tracks allowed the car to slide some distance.

H. M. BARKSDALE
DIES OF PNEUMONIA
DuPont Co. Vice President
and Greatest Dynamite
Expert Succumbs
WAS FAMOUS IN
U. S. AS ENGINEER

Hamilton M. Barksdale, vice-president, and director of the E. I. DuPont de Nemours and Company, and recognized as the greatest dynamite expert in the world, died shortly before 12 o'clock today, a victim of influenza at his home "Wynderest," Pennsylvania Avenue and Mt. Salem Lane. Mr. Barksdale became ill on Sunday, and several days ago, pneumonia developed.

His condition gradually became worse, and death came this morning.

Mr. Barksdale was a noted engineer before he became connected with the duPonts some years ago. He was born June 30, 1861, at Richmond, Va., the son of Dr. Randolph Barksdale, who was a distinguished physician at Petersburg. Va. He was a grandson of William H. McFarland, who, at the of the Civil War, was one of the leading attorneys of Virginia.

The deceased graduated from the University of Virginia in civil engineering and soon made a national reputation as an engineer. After leaving college, he went to the State of Mississippi on construction work and then to Colombia, South America, where he remained for several years on important construction work.

On his return to this country, Mr. Barksdale went with the Baltimore & Ohio Railroad, which was just starting the construction of its line from Philadelphia to Baltimore. He was an engineer in charge of the division that included the section through Delaware and made his headquarters at Newark, this State, for some months. There were connected with him in the engineering branch of this work, several men who have since become noted in the railroad world, including Gamble Latrobe, now with the Pennsylvania system.

Mr. Barksdale went with the duPonts some years ago, long before the present large company was organized. He specialized in dynamite and became known as the best known and greatest dynamite expert in the world. He Is given credit for the building up of the immense dynamite trade that the company has and for years was director of now the high explosives department. He is survived by his wife, who was Miss Ethel Dupont, daughter of Victor DuPont Two children, Mrs. Greta DuPont Brown, wife of F. D Brown, treasurer of the DuPont Company, and Miss Ethel DuPont Barksdale.

Mr. Barksdale was appointed a trustee of Delaware College by former Governor Charles R. Miller about four years ago.

He was chairman of the finance committee of the board and took and took an active part in the development of that college during the past few years.

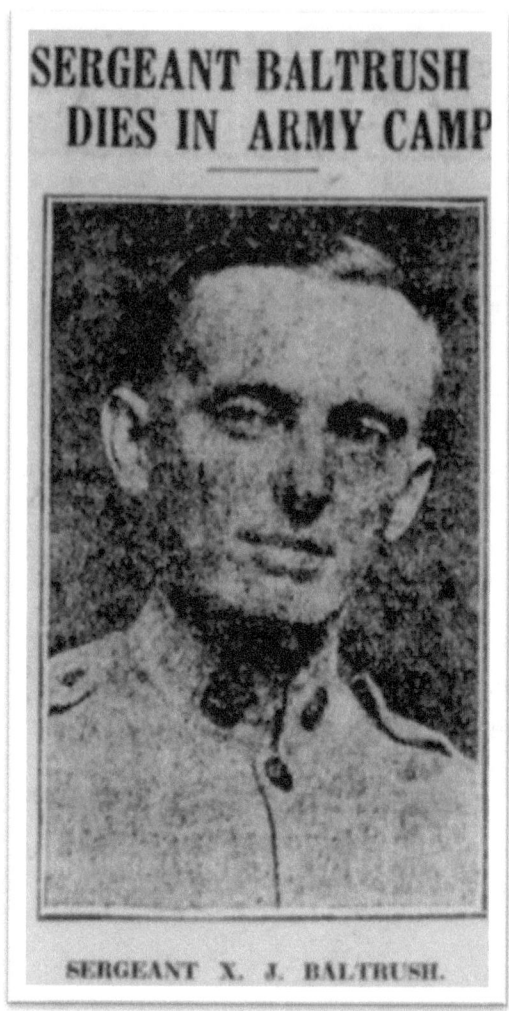

SERGEANT X. J. BALTRUSH.

SERGEANT BALTRHSH DIES IN ARMY CAMP

Sergeant Xavier J. Baltrush died at Camp Joseph E. Johnstone. Florida, yesterday of pneumonia following an attack of Influenza. His mother, Mrs. Veronica Baltrush of No. 412 Lombard Street, received a telegram yesterday from the camp announcing the death of her son. Sergeant Baltrush was a member of the Motor Transport Corps.

Before being sent to camp last May, he was a traveling truck inspector for the Atlas Powder Company.

Nurses Are Recovering

One of the best and happiest places of news regarding the epidemic situation is that the heroic nurses who have been stricken down while ministering to others suffering from Influenza, are now getting well, and the number of sick nurses is rapidly lessening. No more have been added to the pathetic list of nurses who have died as gloriously as any soldier on the battlefield.

In place of thirty-six, the Delaware Hospital last night reported only fifteen of the nurses on the influenza list, and none of them is in a critical condition.

The Physicians and Surgeons Hospital last night had only two nurses who were Influenza patients. One of them has gone home, convalescent, and the other can be up and about,

At the Homeopathic Hospital, the word was given out that none of the nurses were sick. There have been no deaths from Influenza among the Homeopathic Hospital nurses.

The Holiday House of the Young Women's Christian Association, which given as a convalescent home for nurses, now has only three patients left.

INFLUENZA TAKES HUSBAND AND WIFE; SOLDIER DIES AT CAMP EUSTIS

Just one day after his wife was buried, William Campbell, aged about 35 years of No. 2204 Jessup street, an employee of the DuPont Powder Company, died of influenza. His wife, Mrs. Margaret Campbell, who died at their home early this week, was buried on Thursday. The husband was ill at that time and was removed to the home of his mother, No. 403 East Eighth Street, where he died yesterday. Influenza was the cause of both deaths. Mr. Campbell was popular and had a host of friends. He held a responsible position with the DuPont Company at

Deep Water Point. He was one of the most popular members of the Senate Club. Plans for the funeral have not yet been completed.

William M. Dole died this morning at his home in the Grantley Apartments. He died of pneumonia, following an attack of influenza, and had been sick only a short time. Mr. Dole's condition was very critical yesterday, but it had been hoped that he would pass the crisis safely.

Mr. Dole was connected with the Dupont Powder Company. He is survived by his wife, who was Miss Edith Raskob, a sister of John J. Raskob. There are no children. The funeral arrangements have not yet been made.

Andrew P. Hoodock, aged 26 years, son of Mr. and Mrs. Joseph Hoodock, of No. 1220 Apple Street, died at Camp Eustis, Va., yesterday of pneumonia.

The deceased was sent to FortDupont from Dover, where he was working, with other Kent county draftees last December. From that fort, he was transferred to Camp Eustis. Plans for

the funeral has not been completed as the body has not reached this city.

INFLUENZA GRIP IS NOW BREAKING
Health Board Reports 618 Deaths in City from Pneumonia in Five Weeks
REQUEST ALL TO FUMIGATE HOMES

The crisis has been passed in the Influenza epidemic In Wilmington, according to the United States Public Health Service officials, who have withdrawn all the government doctors from Wilmington.

The physicians have gone to places where there is more for them to do.

All but two of the government doctors left the city yesterday. These two, Dr. Ida McCormick and Dr. Ella Hunt, received word today to leave

Wilmington at once.

The local physicians are now able to handle all the cases without help from outside, and the Board of Health is receiving practically no appeals for their government doctors to attend.

The men and women physicians sent here by Surgeon General Rupert Blue wish to express their appreciation for the care taken of their comfort, and the courtesy shown them by the people of Wilmington. They thank especially Mayor Lawson, Dr. Robert E. Ellegood, and the other officials of the Board of Health, the Red Cross Motor Corps, and all who furnished automobiles and took them upon their errands of mercy in the city.

Health certificates filed at the Board of Health show a total of 618 deaths in this city from Influenza or pneumonia for

the past five weeks up to 10 o'clock this morning. Of the total of deaths due to the epidemic, there were 289 deaths recorded for the week ending today; 229 deaths filed last week; 57 deaths recorded the previous week; 10 deaths the week before that; and two deaths the fifth week ago. This week's list is not complete, as several additional certificates were brought in but not on file at 10 o'clock today. It will be noted that the past fortnight has been the death period of the epidemic, the city death rale Is still many times the normal rale.

Board of Health between yesterday noon and 10 o'clock this morning, of deaths in the city due to Influenza or pneumonia, with other death reports coming In.

That the death certificates filed within a given period are no indication of the number of persons dying within that period, may be seen from a study made last night of 28 city death certificates filed yesterday at the Board of Health office. Of 24 of these certificates showing influenza or pneumonia as the cause of death, only two of the victims died yesterday; six on Thursday; eight on Wednesday; five on Tuesday; two on Monday, and one last Sunday.

Fumigation is the point in which the city Board of Health urgently requests that all public gathering places which were ordered closed on Oct. 2nd be at once fumigated, cleaned, and thoroughly aired. There is an especially good chance to do this now without inconvenience to either patrons or proprietors, while the buildings are closed. It is a precautionary measure that will prevent any possibility of a return of epidemic conditions. Nobody desires this scourge to sweep over the city again, bringing sickness and death and making another shutdown of public gathering places necessary.

The Board of Health further requests that all sick rooms, where influenza patients have been cared for, be at once fumigated. No amount of scrubbing or cleaning will kill influenza germs.

The counsel given to private families by the Board of Health is to burn a formaldehyde candle, which can be purchased at a druggist, in every room in which influenza patients have been cared for. All bedding, clothing, furniture, everything which has been exposed to the contagion by contact with the sick, should be placed in the room to be fumigated, and the room should be closed tight with the formaldehyde candle is burning. This does not mean that closing all doors and windows is sufficient. All keyholes, spaces between doors and floors be stuffed tightly with cotton. The process of fumigation should go on in the room for five hours or so. No person should be in the room while it is fumigated.

There have been hundreds of mild cases that have not been given a doctor's attention, and in view of this, the Board of Health fears that families may not realize it is just as Important to fumigate after a mild case of Influenza as after a severe one. A severe case can be caught from germs left by a mild case. Hundreds of thousands of the germs wait in the sick room bedding and furniture and In the clothing of the recovered patient, ready to attack the healthy persons in the family.

Probably everybody in the city had noted the startling way in which the epidemic had spread through entire families when once it got lodging in a house.

Closing Order Continues

There is no telling when the closing order can be safely be rescinded, say the health authorities today. Certainly not when the death rate is as many times above normal as it is present, they add.

The Board of Health thinks an overlong closing better than a premature opening, which would bring back the epidemic and make a second closing necessary.

Newspaper office telephones, in this city, used to be bombarded with, "What's the score?" but the question now shot over the office phones at brief intervals is, "When will the closing order be lifted?"

Members of the Board of Public Education were observed at the Board of Health offices last night, inquiring, "When do you think ---?" but at that interesting point in the conversation, the door to the inner sanctum was shut.

The ministers of the city have displayed a commendable common sense, which should be an example to those of their Philadelphia authorities to open churches even though the epidemic is still at a high point in that city.

One man called up a local newspaper office so persistently to know when the churches and schools would reopen that he aroused the curiosity of the reporters as to his identity. They investigated and found that he was a saloonkeeper. Evidently, the man feared criticism if he inquired when the saloons could reopen and took this roundabout method of finding out.

The Board of Health announces that when the closing order Is lifted, all public gathering places will be opened at the same time. Churches and schools will not be opened any sooner than theatres or saloons. They would be equally dangerous as spreaders of infection.

Valuable aid in the fight against the epidemic has been given by the Wilmington Canteen Service of the Red Cross. The women composing the service have been kept busy supplying the three emergency hospitals with ice cream, fruits, jellies, fresh eggs, cigarettes, magazines, stationery, and stamps for the convalescents. This was undertaken in addition to the regular work of helping the soldiers at army headquarters and at Pigeon Point.

The number of Influenza cases in the city is still in the thousands, with pneumonia cases by the hundreds.

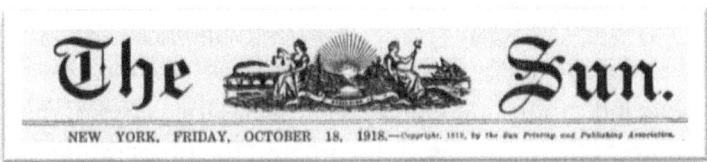

NEW YORK, FRIDAY, OCTOBER 18, 1918.—Copyright, 1918, by the Sun Printing and Publishing Association.

DRAFT HALTED
HERE TO ASSIST
FIGHT ON GRIP

Conboy Releases Doctors and
New Vaccine Promises Relief.

MANY HOUSES ARE LENT

Decrease Shown in New Cases as Business and Phones
Are Crippled.

THE SUN

New York, N.Y. (Oct. 18, 1918) – Three outstanding developments yesterday marked the light New York Is making against the epidemic of Influenza and pneumonia.

Martin Conboy, director of the draft here, stopped the operation of his machine, which has been busy In Its 189 local exemption boards classifying the men who registered for service last month. As a result, it Is expected that a large number of physicians who have been giving their time to the examination of registrants will be released to combat the local epidemic Also the mandatory order calling a registrant for examination Is done away with for a time, eliminating the possibility that responding registrants might spread the disease.

Vaccine Findings Presented.

The Department of Health presented the results of experiments conducted with the anti-Influenza vaccine prepared by Dr. William II. Park, director of the bureau of laboratories in the department. They Indicate that where the vaccine has been used, there has been a sharp decrease in the number of new Influenza cases. The report led Health Commissioner Copeland to say that inasmuch as immunity from Influenza has been produced by the use of the vaccine. It is the strongest possible indication that Pfeiffer's bacillus is the cause of the disease. On the strength of this report, ho ordered the preparation of sufficient vaccine to meet the demand of 30,000 doses a day.

The third development was the response of the general public to the appeals which have been sent out for aid,

Mrs. Louis O. Kaufman, the wife of the president of the Chatham and Phenix National Bank, donated to the Health Department for its use, a building formerly a private hospital, at Fifty-Seventh Street and Lexington Avenue.

Mrs. Kaufman has fitted up the building with the necessary surgical and nursing adjuncts at her own expense and simply asked the Health Department to assume the responsibility of providing physicians and the treatment of the eighty children and babies who can be cared for at one time. Many other prominent women offered their homes and other buildings to be used as temporary hospitals. One hundred percent of the post-graduate students in Teachers College who are studying nursing volunteered their services.

Homes Sought for Children.

An appeal was sent out to New Yorkers who have the room to take into their homes for a short period, the children of victims of the epidemic removed to hospitals to prevent the spread of the disease.

While these activities were in progress reports received, embracing the entire city indicated a decrease in the number of new Influenza cases.

Other developments showed that while the organization to fight the epidemic is rounding into shape, Influenza and pneumonia are making Inroads Into the forces of almost every Industry.

The New York Telephone Company issued an additional statement, which read in part:

"With the losses of central office operators In New York City through sickness increasing rather than decreasing the company today issued another appeal to telephone users, asking them voluntarily to restrict their telephoning to calls that are absolutely necessary.

"At the company's main office at 15 Day Street, it was said that the operators absent today due to Spanish Influenza totaled 1,600. Untrained employees cannot take their places."

The statement also said the company had sent cards to all telephone subscribers in the city, repeating the appeal and asking that the cards be placed beside the subscriber's telephone.

The Public Service Commission of the Second District reports from its headquarters In Albany that operating forces in the telephone offices under its jurisdiction have been seriously depleted.

Business houses and banks have begun to feel the effects. An official of the Federal Reserve Bank In this district said that 230 employees of that Institution were absent through illness.

This Is approximately 10 percent of the total force. The Federal Reserve Bank is particularly busy because of the full pressure of Liberty Loan week.

In making public, the report from the bureau of laboratories, Health Commissioner Copeland emphasized that Dr. Park, who perfected the vaccine, insisted on a conservative estimate of Its merits as a preventive. The report read:

"Camp A – Average hospital admissions before vaccination were 18 a day. After vaccinations, admissions to hospitals fell to 2 a day.

"Regiment B – Admissions rose quickly to 80 and above a day. Fell abruptly to 12 a day immediately after vaccination.

"Guard B – Total incidence before vaccination was 10 percent: 541 were vaccinated, and no cases appeared thereafter.

"Two Hospitals – Report practically no cases among doctors and nurses who have been vaccinated.

"Camp D – Reports a sharp fall in hospital admissions, after vaccination.

"Organization E – General 'very good.' sharp contrast between vaccinated and unvaccinated."

Arrangements were made yesterday through the cooperation of the American Red Cross and theatre managers to spread the appeal for more nurses. It has been reiterated by all of the agencies fighting the epidemic that the shortage of nurses must be met and the Red Cross in an effort to place the appeal before a larger number of persons will have its "Three Minute Men" address audiences in theatres asking tor this aid.

Red Cross Makes Appeal.

The Red Cross will also make possible the use of the residences donated for the care of convalescent victims of Influenza and pneumonia. One of the several homes and vacant houses turned over for use yesterday was the home of Mrs. James Madison Bass at 15 East Twenty-First Street.

The Health Commissioner's Emergency Advisory Committee has announced the opening of district headquarters in different neighborhoods in Manhattan.

Forty-two of these centers were put in operation, and all cases needed the care of physicians, nurses, domestic help, shelter, or food should be reported to them. They will forward such appeals to the proper authorities.

Lee K. Frankel of the emergency committee has appointed an executive committed on district work with central headquarters in Room 2208 Municipal Building. The members of the committee are John Collier, Chairman; Mrs. H. Foster Armstrong, Mrs. John Blair; Mrs. C. F. Simonson, Miss Estelle Deutsch, Miss Mildred Taylor, Mrs. G. Simkovitch, Walter Willis, C. Kemp Van Ee, Miss Frances Perkins, Miss Beulah Weldon, and Dr. Herbert B. Wilcox.

At each center, there are eight nurses under the direction of a supervising nurse, and orders were issued for these nurses to begin visiting in the homes where regular nurses are not in attendance.

Shortage of Gravediggers

It was reported that Calvary Cemetery has had to place bodies in temporary receiving vaults because of the shortage of gravediggers. Many cemeteries here applied to the United States employment bureau for laborers.

The figures reported yesterday to the Health Department, which are officially believed to represent about half the number of actual cases occurring in the greater city, show a decrease in the total number of new influenza cases amounting to 280, with an increase of sixty-six new pneumonia cases. Ten more deaths from both influenza and pneumonia were reported.

While the total new Influenza cases disclosed a big decrease over Wednesday, there was an increase In Queens of 196 cases. In Richmond, the increase was only one reported case. In Manhattan, Brooklyn, and The Bronx, substantial decreases were shown.

New pneumonia cases reported showed decreases in the Bronx and Richmond, while Increases were reported In Manhattan, Brooklyn, and Queens.

INFLUENZA NEW CASES

4,733 (Decrease 380)

PNEUMONIA – NEW CASES

646 (Increase 69)

DEATHS

336 (10)

At Camp Upton, the bulletin issued yesterday by the army, surgeons reported twenty-nine new influenza cases and thirteen deaths. The Y.M.C.A., and other welfare buildings, except for the large auditoriums, opened for general entertainment last night, which the Liberty and Buffalo theaters will reopen next Thursday. This would indicate that the epidemic has almost burned itself out in the camp.

100,000 SHOTS OF "ANTI-FLU" SERUM SET FOR EACH DAY

ROCK ISLAND ARGUS

Chicago. (Oct. 21, 1918) – The administration of vaccines as a preventive of influenza was begun today by the city health department. A shipment of 100,000 doses was received from Rochester, Minn., and other shipments are to follow. The health department also began the manufacture of the vaccine, and by Wednesday, it was said the city would be prepared to distribute 100,000 doses daily.

Treatment with the vaccine, which is supposed to be a preventive but not a cure for influenza, consists of three doses administered by subcutaneous inoculation.

To obtain the vaccine, the health departments of the various cities and towns of the state must apply to Dr. St. Clair Drake, head of the state health department at Springfield.

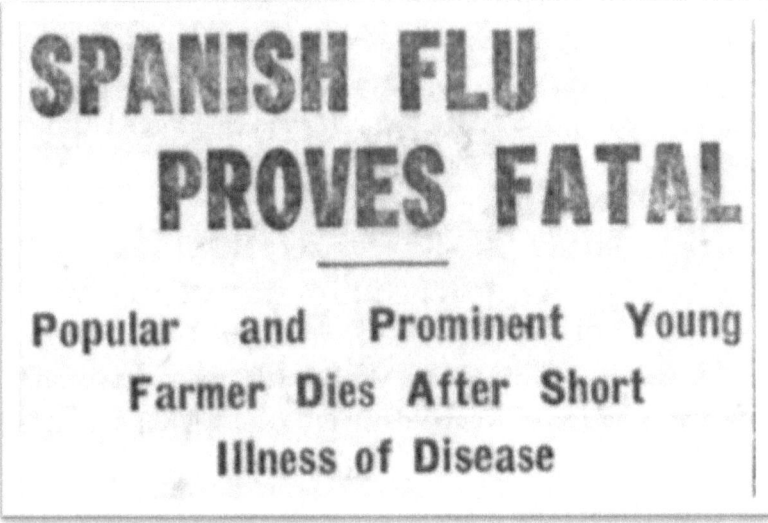

SPANISH FLU PROVES FATAL

Popular and Prominent Young Farmer Dies After Short Illness of Disease

MT. STERLING ADVOCATE

Mt. Sterling, Kentucky (Oct. 22, 1918) – Mr. Sam Duff, aged 34 years, died at his home near Spencer Station Sunday morning after a short illness of Spanish Influenza. Mr. Duff was one of the best-known young farmers of our county and was popular with a wide circle of friends, and the news of his death was quite a shock to all who knew him. He is survived by his wife, one daughter, Ruth, aged six, and one son, Roger, aged twelve, who is at present in a serious condition with pneumonia following an attack of influenza. He is also survived by one sister Mrs. Preston Belcher and three brothers, Tom, Boone, and Will Duff, besides many other relatives. Funeral services were conducted at the grave Monday morning at eleven o'clock with burial in Machpelah. The Advocate joins friends in tendering sympathy to the stricken family.

DIES AT MIDDLETOWN, OHIO

Mike Gibbons, son of Mr. and Mrs. Frank Gibbons, formerly of this city, but who have been living in Middletown, Ohio for some time, past died at the home of his parents last Thursday of pneumonia following an attack of the Flu. Ho was called "Little Mike" by a host of friends, and the news of his death was received with sorrow by all who know the genial, good-natured young fellow. His remains were brought to this city Saturday and interred in St. Thomas Cemetery. Besides his parents, Mr. and Mrs. Frank Gibbons, he is survived by two sisters, Mrs. S. P. Greenwade, of this city, and Mrs. Elizabeth Lamm, and three brothers, Millard, Bernard, and Cardinal Gibbons.

ARMY STUDENT DIES FROM FLU
Popular Local Boy and Son of Prominent Farmer, Dies at Danville Wednesday

Mr. Cecil R. Skidmore, son of Mr. and Mrs. Daniel B. Skidmore, of this county, died at Danville last Wednesday after a short illness of pneumonia following an attack of Spanish Influenza.

Mr. Skidmore, familiarly called "Skid" by his host of friends, was a jovial, happy, carefree young fellow who always had a smile and pleasant greeting for everyone. When it became known that he had died, expressions of sorrow and of sympathy for his parents could be heard on all sides. Deceased was a graduate of K. M. I. and during his college clays was quite an athlete. He entered the Students Army Training Corps at Danville a few weeks ago and was studying hard so he could be of some real service to his country when overtaken by the illness that caused his death.

The funeral services were conducted by Rev. Clyde Darsie of the Christian Church Friday morning with burial in Machpelah Cemetery. We join friends in tendering sympathy to the bereaved family.

PHYSICIANS GIVEN ANTI-FLU VACCINE
Local Practitioners Say They Are Certain It Works
THE WEST VIRGINIAN

Fairmont, West Virginia (Oct. 23, 1918) – Quite a number of local people have been "shot" with the anti-flu serum since the epidemic began in this city with what is believed to be good results. Many of the leading physicians of the city are advocating its use not only as a means of protecting the individual but as a means of preventing a further spread of the malady.

Local druggists and physicians in discussing the matter state that so far as can be ascertained, beneficial results have been obtained from the use of the vaccine.

While the vaccine has been used to a considerable extent by leading physicians of the city yet, quite a number of the fraternity have been rather slow in experimenting with the serum.

Local drug stores have on hand quite a quantity of the serum and believe that in case there should be demand for its use, that they will be able to secure an adequate supply.

Some physicians who are using the serum obtain it in three-shot cases while others secure it in cases that require four shots.

One physician of the city who has by reason of experiment been convinced that the serum has merit has not only taken the shots himself but has had other members of his family inoculated.

No sickness follows the shots, and the patient goes about his duties as usual.

The serum has the endorsement of the U.S. Government and is prepared and sold by all the leading drug houses in the country.

A number of the larger cities in the United States are strongly recommending its use.

So imbued have the physicians of Clarksburg become with the good results of the vaccine that 3,000 industrial workers of that place, employees of the Weirton Steel Company. The Hazel Atlas Glass company and the Owens Bottle Machine company have consented to be inoculated with the serum, and the amount of serum necessary has been ordered shipped from Philadelphia.

 The state of Massachusetts through its health commissioner recently appointed a committee composed of the leading research physicians and authorities of the world to Investigate the serum prescribed to allay the malady with the result that the following recommendations were made:

"That the state encourages the distribution of influenza vaccine intended for prophylactic use, but in such manner as will secure scientific evidence of the possible value of the agent. The use of such a vaccine is regarded as experimental.

"That the state shall neither furnish nor endorse any vaccine at present in use for the treatment of influenza."

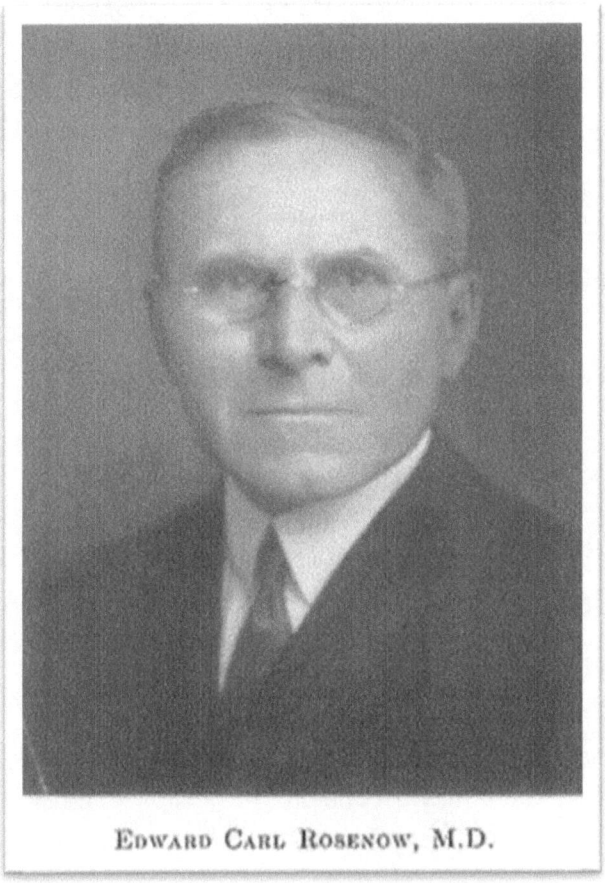

EDWARD CARL ROSENOW, M.D.

The committee appointed was composed of such men as Drs. E. C. Rosenow recognized as the greatest research expert in the United States, Frederick P. Gay. George W. McCoy, George C. Whipple, William Davis, and F. C. Frum.

These recommendations, as well as other comments concerning the use of the serum, is contained in the current issue of the Journal of American Medical Association.

10,000 FLU CASES IN PITTSBURGH TO DATE

PITTSBURGH, (Oct. 23, 1918) – A total of 1,043 new cases of Spanish Influenza were reported by the Health Department in the last 24 hours ending at noon. This is the largest number of cases reported in a single day since the epidemic began. The cases recorded here have passed the 10,000 mark.

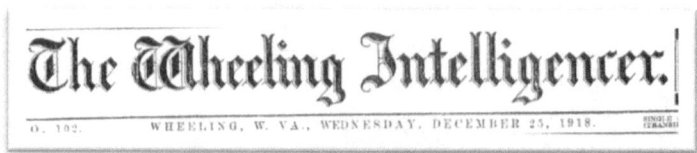

Slight Improvement in the Influenza Epidemic Situation Is Reported

THE WHEELING INTELLIGENCER

WASHINGTON, Oct. 23, 1918) – A slight improvement in the Influenza situation over the country was Indicated by reports received today by the public health service. Still, in many places, the epidemic apparently has yet to reach its crest. In the far west and on the Pacific coast, the situation as not yet proved nearly as serious as It did in the east and south.

Continued abatement of the epidemic in army camps was reported today in the office of the surgeon-general of the army. New cases during the 24 hours ending at noon today totaled 2.773 against 3.007 the day before, while the deaths decreased from 404 to 392. There was a slight increase in the number of pneumonia cases.

Army medical officers said influenza may now be said to be epidemic in only five camps.

In the east and south, generally, conditions among the civilian population are rapidly Improving.

CLEVELAND, OHIO, (Oct. 22, 1918) – Emergency bureaus to assist civilian communities and slate boards of health in combating the Spanish Influenza epidemic are to be Immediately established at Columbus, Indianapolis and Louisville by the lake division Red Cross committee on influenza.

EVERY RESIDENT OF PITTSBURGH MAY BE VACCINATED

PITTSBURGH, PENN. (Oct. 22, 1918) – The advisability of inoculating every resident of Pittsburgh with a newly discovered serum as a preventative of further spread of Spanish influenza was discussed at a conference today of health department officials, members of the Allegheny County Medical Society, and the Pittsburgh chapter of the Red Cross.

Following the conference, this afternoon, Health director Davis said no decision had been reached on the plan for general anti-influenza Inoculation. After the meeting, it was reported that a new kind of serum had been discovered and is being manufactured in Pittsburgh. There was no official confirmation of this report.

TOLDEDO, OHIO (Oct. 22, 1918) – With eighty-six, deaths and three thousand cases reported to date, and health authorities announced that the crest of the Spanish Influenza epidemic here had passed.

NEW YORK. Oct. 22, 1918) – The New York Telephone company today suspended service 1b half of the public booths hire because of a shortage of operators caused by the Spanish influenza epidemic. It was said that 200, or about 25 percent of the operators, are ill.

BALTIMORE. Oct. 22, 1918) – With less than 200 new cases of influenza and 170 deaths reported during the last 24 hours, the health authorities of the city are more encouraged.

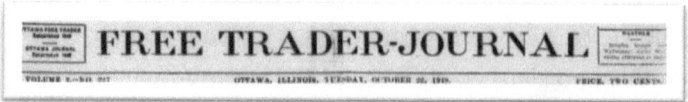

TO IMMUNIZE MCARTHUR DRAFTEES
AS SOON AS VACCINE ARRIVES
STATE IS SENDING NEW
INFLUENZA PREVENTATIVE TO OTTAWA
LOCAL BOARD CALLS FOR 550
MEN 19 TO 37 TO REPORT
THURSDAY AND SATURDAY.

FREE TRADER-JOURNAL

Ottawa, Ill. (Oct. 22, 1918) – The Ottawa contingent of 125 men whose trip to Camp McArthur was deferred on account of the prevalence of influenza will be Immunized just as soon as the vaccine can be received from Springfield.

The local board sent a telegram to Springfield asking for a quantity of vaccine with the result that a sufficient quantity will be received here for the use of the 125 members of the camp McArthur contingent.

State Department of Health is prepared to distribute limited quantities Influenza Pneumonia Vaccine to Draft Boards for immunizing men of Class 1, who have not yet developed Influenza, and who will be inducted the first call. This particular vaccine for prevention and Is not recommended for the treatment of those who have developed the disease. Order no more than absolutely required and direct order to C. St. Clair Drake, Sherman Hotel, Chicago, Ill., stating the number of men to be immunized. No charge for vaccine and suggest no charge for immunization of draft men.

No positive assurance can be given as to the effectiveness of vaccines but deemed worthy of trial by Influenza Commission. Board now conducting physical examinations can conveniently administer this vaccine at the examination. The administration is not compulsory but should be offered to all men called and administered to those of them who may voluntarily desire it.

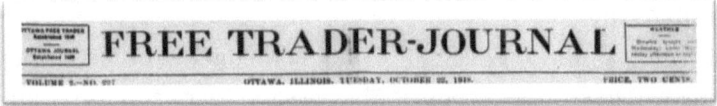

INFLUENZA EPIDEMIC IS NOW SUBSIDING SAY PHYSICIANS
FIVE DEATHS REPORTED IN OTTAWA TODAY— RELAPSE CASES THE ONES TO BE FEARED THE MOST.

FREE TRADER-JOURNAL

Ottawa, Ill. (Oct. 22, 1918) – Only four deaths from influenza and one from a complication of diseases were reported In Ottawa today, and physicians and the local health department report the backbone of the epidemic is broken. Practically no new cases were reported today to Health Officer Pike.

Physicians declare that even though the crest of the epidemic has passed, there will be more deaths, the most serious they have to battle now is the large number of relapse cases, people who went out too soon and are now suffering from setbacks.

This morning there were twenty-five patients at Ryburn Memorial Hospital, and several more were expected during the day.

Today's death toll included the names of Frank Holmes, Charles Monroe, Leo Duffy and Bothwell

Leo Duffy.

Leo Duffy of 1507 Sycamore Street died at the Boat Club emergency hospital Monday evening at 6 o'clock after a couple of weeks' illnesses of influenza and pneumonia, at the age of 24 years.

The deceased was a native of this county and was a graduate of St. Cojuma School. He leaves surviving his widow, Julia M., and one son, Leon, his mother, Mrs. James Duffy; five brothers and three sisters, John M. of Wallaceburg, Ontario; William P. Frank and Edgar at home, James T. with Company C in France, Agnes of Chicago and Mary and Gertrude at home.

The funeral will take place from St. Columba's church Wednesday forenoon at 0 o'clock.

Frank Bothwell.

Frank Hackman Bothwell, aged about 23 years, died this morning at 2:30 o'clock at the home of his sister, Mrs. Maurice Wolfe, 828 Joliet street; after an illness lasting ten days, of Spanish influenza and pneumonia.

Mr. Bothwell resided in South Ottawa township, mil when taken ill he was removed to the home of his sister. His wife and children are sick at their home, suffering from influenza.

The decedent was born in Ottawa and had resided here during his entire life. He had been employed at farming at the Stevens dairy farm in South Ottawa for several years.

Surviving, he leaves his widow, three children, Francis, John, and Elizabeth: his parents, Mr. and Mrs. James Bothwell, and three sisters, Mrs. Elmer Allbee of Livermore, Iowa, and Mrs. George Sampson and Mrs. Maurice Wolfe of this city.

The funeral arrangements will be announced later.

Charles W. Monroe

Charles W. Monroe. 412 Third St., died last evening at 7:40 o'clock at the family home, following a ten-days illness of Influenza followed by pneumonia.

The deceased was thirty-three years old in July and had resided in Ottawa practically all his life. He was born in Wallace township and moved into town when a small boy.

His marriage to Miss Hattie Goetz took place in this city.

Surviving, he leaves his wife and five children, Francis, George, John, Marie, and Lucile. He is also survived by his parents, Mr. and Mrs. Henry Monroe of this city, three brothers John, Henry, and James all residing In Ottawa, and five sisters, Mrs. Ed. Keleher of this city, Mrs. L. D. Lowe of St realtor and Mrs. John O'Kane, Mrs. Harry Kelly, and Mrs. J. P. Lavello of Chicago. The funeral will be held tomorrow morning at 11:30.

Frank E. Holmes

Frank Edward Holmes, the only son of Mr. and Mrs. Jesse Holmes, Superior street, a well-known young man, died at his home last evening at 8 o'clock, following an illness of one week, from pneumonia. He had resided in Ottawa during his entire life and ha many friends in this city.

Mr. Holmes was horn In Ottawa in July 1897. He attended the Ottawa public schools and the High school and later went to work at. Brickton, where he was employed as an engineer.

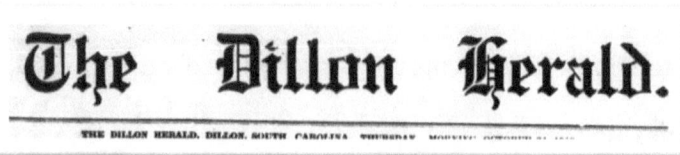

INFLUENZA EPIDEMIC ON THE DECREASE
DISEASE TOOK HEAVY TOLL OF HUMAN LIFE LAST WEEK
Citizens Met and Appointed Committee to Co-Operate With Health Authorities

THE DILLION HERALD

Dillion, S.C., (Oct. 24, 1918) The influenza epidemic which has had Dillon in its grip for the two weeks showed signs of abatement Monday. There are still a number of serious cases, but the physicians say the epidemic reached its crest Sunday, and Monday then were signs of an improvement in the situation.

The disease has laid a heavy hand on Dillon County. It Is impossible to secure a correct list of the dead, but up to Sunday, there were twenty-one deaths reported, and a conservative estimate places the total dead at twice this number. Up to Saturday, 600 cases had been reported within a radius of five miles.

The citizens held a meeting at Red Cross rooms Thursday afternoon and appointed a committee to cooperate with the health authorities in fighting the epidemic. The committee is working in conjunction with the Red Cross, and everything that can be done is being done to relieve the sick and suffering. Nourishment is being sent out to homes where all the members of the family are sick, and special nurses are assigned to places where there is no one to wait on the afflicted members of the family.

The Red Cross has worked heroically in relieving distress and suffering. If it had not been for the assistance rendered by the concentrated and systematic efforts of this organization, the suffering would have been terrible, and the number of deaths would have been larger. Red Cross rooms have been kept open day and night, and all calls for help have met with a ready response.

The home of the late W. L. Bethea on East Main street has been equipped with beds and other necessary articles and is being used as a temporary hospital. By concentrating the cases, the nurses and physicians can give the patients better attention with less exertion.

The Deaths.

Frank M. Page, a prominent citizen of the Pleasant Hill section, died Friday after a week's illness from pneumonia following an attack of influenza. Mr. Page was a strong, robust man and had always enjoyed the best of health. He was a leader in his community and will be greatly missed in the many fields of endeavor in which he was very active. His wife was taken down with pneumonia the day before he died, and grave fears are entertained for her recovery.

Another prominent citizen who succumbed to the disease was W. B. Gaddy, who died at the home of his son in Dillon Tuesday night. Mr. Gaddy came up from his home near Gaddy's Mill the week before to nurse his son, Ralph Gaddy, who was seriously ill with pneumonia. He stayed at the bedside of his son night and day, and his vitality was at a low ebb when he was stricken. While Mr. Gaddy was seriously ill, his mother, who had been ill only a few days, passed away in an adjoining room. The son, Mr. Ralph Gaddy, is improving, but his condition has been serious. Mr. Gaddy was one of the most prominent and progressive farmers of the Gaddy's Mill section. He was serving his second term as county commissioner from his district, and as a county official, he was diligent and painstaking in everything he undertook. He was prominent in church, and fraternal wor, and his death leaves a vacancy in the social and religious life of his community, which will be hard to fill.

Dick Dewey Stanton, one of the town's most promising young men, fell victim to the disease at one o'clock Friday. He had been sick about ten days, and the cause of his death was pneumonia following an attack of influenza. Mr. Stanton's death cast a gloom over the entire community. He held the position of assistant cashier at the First National Bank, where he was held in the highest esteem by the Bank's officials and his fellow-employees. Kind and courteous, affable, and generous and a gentleman at all times, he was greatly beloved by a large circle of friends by whom he is deeply mourned.

There was no more promising life In Dillon than Dick Stanton's.

Government Officials Arrive

The influenza situation had become so serious Sunday that the State Board of Health was asked to send government help and Monday night Dr. A. E. Schweitzer and nurse E. I. McCune arrived on Train No. 82. Immediately after their arrival, they held a brief conference with the health authorities, and tentative plans were mapped out for directing the work of stamping out the epidemic. Another conference was held at Red Cross rooms Tuesday morning, and plans were adopted for systematizing the relief work. Dr. Schweitzer and Miss McCune have been at Newberry, where conditions were so bad that federal aid had to be secured to check the disease. Conditions at Newberry are much better. Dr. Schweitzer has the authority to enforce any orders she sees fit to issue, and at Tuesday's conference, she was requested to take full charge of the situation and handle it in her own way.

No Services Sunday.

Tryon, N. C., Oct. 21, 1918.

Editor Herald: - Please announce there will be no services at Bermuda and Piney Grove churches next Sunday on account of the epidemic.

The pastor requests we use the hours, respectively, in earnest prayer to God that he may stay the deadly malady.

Respectfully,

J. A. LANGLEY

Woman Found Dead.

A colored woman was found dead in a house near the oil mill Monday morning. The woman had been ill for some time with tuberculosis.

She had no relatives in town, and the neighbors had been waiting on her. No one thought the end was so near, and as she was alone at the time of her death, the body was not found until Monday morning.

Enforce the Ordinance.

One thing we would like to call the attention of the town authorities to is the way some of the merchants leave their boxes, barrels, and carts on the sidewalks at night to be run over by pedestrians at night when the lights are out. It dangerous, and sooner or later, someone will have a broken leg or arm as a result. This should be looked into by the authorities and request the merchants to leave their boxes, etc., off the sidewalks.

Mills Running Half Time.

There has been a decided improvement in the "flu' situation in the mill villages. Dillon and Maple Mills are running again, but only half the machinery is in operation. Hamer Mill will start up again today or tomorrow. The epidemic got a stronghold on the mill villages, and for several days the situation was serious.
There are no new cases, however, and the old cases are doing well. The mills will be in full operation again in a week.

Mr. and Mrs. Ralph Little Bereaved.

G. Ralph Little, Jr., the five-year-old son of Mr. and Mrs. G. Ralph Little of Columbia, died Sunday night after an attack of influenza. The remains were brought to Dillon Monday night and taken to the home of the grandparents, Mr. and Mrs. E. R. Hamer, and the interment was made at the Little Rock cemetery Tuesday morning.

M. J. Jackson.

M. J. Jackson died at his home near the cotton mills last week. Mr. Jackson was a farmer and a hard-working man. He was aged 50 years. Mr. Jackson leaves a wife and three sons besides hosts of friends to mourn his death. – *A FRIEND*

Mrs. F. M. Page Dies.

Mrs. Frank M. Page, who has been critically ill with pneumonia since the death of her husband last Thursday, died Tuesday night. Mrs. Page leaves six small children, the youngest being only two days old.

W. W. Hamilton.

Pneumonia following influenza claimed another victim Tuesday morning when Mr. W. W. Hamilton, better known as "Bud" Hamilton, passed away at his residence two miles west of Dillion. "Bud" Hamilton had been ill only three days. His entire family has been down for a week, and Mr. Hamilton contracted the disease while staying at their bedside day and night. He was a strong, robust man, but he developed pneumonia a few hours after being attacked with influenza and declined rapidly. The interment was made at the Hamilton burying ground near Dillon yesterday afternoon.

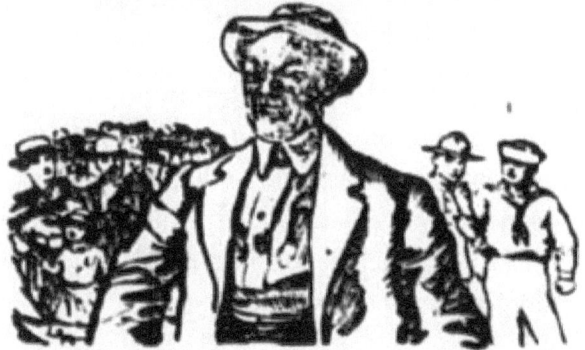

Coughs and Sneezes Spread Diseases

As Dangerous as Poison Gas Shells

EVERYBODY URGED TO COOPERATE WITH HEALTH AUTHORITIES IN FIGHTING INFLUENZA

Dillon and Dillon County are facing a grave situation. Influenza is taking a heavy toll on human life. There does not appear to be any abatement of the epidemic. The town and health authorities are using every means in their power to check the disease, but it is still spreading.

The public must come to their assistance, or the mortality rate will be something fearful to contemplate. It is a time when every person must, in a sense, be their own physician. Every precaution must be taken to keep from contracting the disease. Every person not afflicted must help those who are afflicted. Not only is it a Christian duty, but it is a duty you owe your community as a citizen. The disease is likely to strike your home at any moment.

The Board of Health has laid down certain rules to be followed. Read them. Obey them. Do your part in helping to stamp out this terrible scourge, which has laid such a heavy hand on your community.

The rules are as follows:

- All stores must open at 9 o'clock and close at five.
- No loafing or loitering will be allowed on the streets. Parents are warned to keep their children in their back yards.
- Persons coming to town on necessary business are asked to transact their business as quickly as possible and return home.
- Persons entering sick rooms are required to wear masks. Masks can be obtained at Red Cross headquarters.
- Precautionary Measures Advised by Physicians:
- Fresh air in rooms for sick and well persons.
- Do not allow a well person to sleep in a sick room.
- All persons who are nursing the sick must keep a cheesecloth or handkerchief tied over mouth while in the sick room.
- Never stand near any person who is coughing or sneezing.
- Do not go near any person while talking.
- Do not put more than one sick person in the same bed.

- Take turns staying up night and day so one person will not lose too much sleep.
- Eat plenty and sleep plenty when you are well, and it will protect you.
- Do not visit people sick with the disease unless you are going to help and always wear a mask.

BE ON YOUR GUARD

The influenza epidemic, which has taken such a heavy toll of life in the last few weeks, seems to be subsiding, but the danger period is not over. According to experts who have studied the disease, there will be frequent outbreaks during the winter months, and the public is advised to exercise extreme caution in the protection of health.

The epidemic had its origin in the poverty-stricken districts of Spain and was carried to Germany in submarines.

From there it was transmitted to the United States by prisoners of war. "Contrary to popular belief," remarked a government health expert who spent several hours in Dillon Tuesday, "the germs are carried quite a distance by strong winds."

The measle germ is the only known germ that has a longer life. The disease is transmitted by contact.

Coughing and sneezing are one of the most prolific sources of infection. An infected person should be kept isolated for ten days after the fever leaves them. If proper precautionary measures are taken, the disease can be confined to one person in a home.

Four-ply gauze masks or some mouth covering should become be worn when one enters the sick room, and the masks should be sterilized after two hours of use. All vessels used in the sick room should be sterilized. If these simple precautionary measures are used, the spread of the disease can be reduced to a minimum. To prevent contagion, plenty of good wholesome food should be eaten; the body should be kept clean, and intoxicants should be kept out of the system. Sleep-in well-ventilated rooms and stay out of doors as much as possible. A person who had been infected is not immune. There will be a recurrence of the epidemic in certain communities during the winter months, and every town should adopt and enforce strict sanitary laws.

The protection of one's health is largely an individual matter, and those who fail to recognize the simple law of hygiene and sanitation are more susceptible to the disease. In other words, every man must be his own doctor. *Your health is in your own hands.*

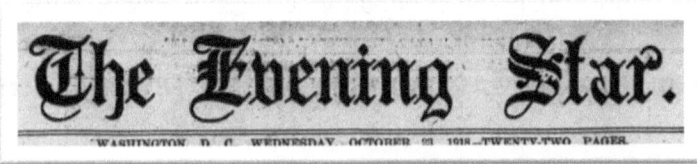

THINK INFLUENZA IS RECEDING HERE
Health Authorities Report Fewer Deaths
And Decrease in New Cases.
CAUTION IS STILL NEEDED

THE EVENING STAR

Washington, D.C. (Oct. 23, 1918) – Only forty-five deaths from influenza were reported to the District health department in the twenty-four-hour period ending at noon today, which led officials to believe that the epidemic has passed its crest here. This was a decline of twenty-six from the seventy-one deaths reported in the preceding twenty-four hours.

A decrease of 3S6 in the number of new cases reported in the last twenty-four hours was even more encouraging to Health department officials. Today's report shows 392 new cases, as compared with 778 yesterday.

Health Officer William C. Fowler expressed gratification at the decline but warned that precautions should not be cast aside because of an indication that the disease is being checked. Health officials believe that new cases now being reported are of a milder type than the cases which occurred in the early days of the epidemic.

Appeals to Motorists.

Lieut. Howard S. Fisk, in charge of transporting nurses to the homes of the sick, appealed to the motorists today not to let up in their volunteer work. While the disease is under control, he said, every agency should keep up its relief work to stamp it out completely.

Lieut. Fisk now has 150 automobiles at his command but should have at least a hundred more. The greatest need for cars is at 9 o'clock in the morning when nurses must be dispatched to all parts of the city to relieve those who have been on duty throughout the night with critical patients.

Surgeon General Blue of the United States public health service has visited the Webster School headquarters on a tour of inspection and was pleased with the progress made and the perfect harmony in which the organization was operated under the direction of Lieut. Fisk and Dr. C. B. Herdliska.

 G. M. Minot, R H. Skeels, and R. W. Bone, who has been running the ambulance, have put in from fourteen to sixteen hours every day, which further emphasizes the need for autos and drivers.

Emphasizes the Need for Caution.

While assurance is felt by Health Officer Fowler that the critical point has been passed in the influenza epidemic, he is fearful that the general public may become careless in taking precautions against the contagion, with the result of an increase in both mortalities and the development of new cases.

Dr. Fowler today emphasized the necessity of continuing every precaution now in force to prevent the spread of the contagion.

In this instance, he said that strong influences are being brought to bear upon him to recommend to the Commissioners the raising of the ban on public gatherings. Despite these influences, he says, he will not make recommendations for the opening of schools, theaters, moving picture houses, churches, public dancing places and other places where there would be large gatherings of persons.

He is of the opinion that the closing of these places was a necessity for public safety and that the ban has been a major aid in keeping down the spread of the contagion.

Acknowledges Valued Aid.

Dr. H. S. Mustard of the United States public health service, working in conjunction with the District of Columbia health department in the fight against influenza, said this morning that Red Cross activities and those of the Associated Charities, Central Union Mission. Salvation Army, Gospel Mission, and other charitable and religious organizations are proving of great assistance to the health authorities.

Cases have been found by these organizations where whole families, father, mother, and children, were down with influenza and not only needing medical attention but the necessities of life, which have been promptly furnished.

One hundred and fifty-eight quarts of hot broth and 101 pints of milk were donated by different churches and private families yesterday and were delivered to influenza patients through the public health service.

Still In Need of Nurses.

The need for more graduate nurses and aids is great. There are enough doctors to handle the situation. Dr. J. G. Wilson of the public health service, in charge of the influenza emergency hospital, stated that there were 186 patients in the hospital at the present time, sixteen having been admitted during the night.

Thirteen doctors are in constant attendance, but out of forty graduate nurses register there, only about twenty-five are on duty, the rest have failed to report.

There were two deaths at the hospital yesterday, and six patients were discharged. Many of the patients were improving and will be able to leave the latter part of this week.

Three more good chefs are needed and one high-class waiter to direct the dining room force. These men will be paid good salaries and will, at the same time, be performing a patriotic duty.

INFLUENZA DEALS BLOW TO STATE DEPARTMENT

THE EVENING STAR

Washington, D. C. (Oct. 23, 1918) – About thirty-five employees of the Department of State have been incapacitated for several weeks past by influenza. Two women clerks died in the early days of the epidemic.

Assistant Secretary Phillips had a mild attack of the disease but has recovered sufficiently to be able to resume his official duties. Breckinridge Long, third assistant secretary, and Glenn Stewart of the Latin American division suffered from the disease in a more severe form and still are confined to their homes. The wife of Mr. Stewart died from the disease during his illness.

STEAMER ST. JOHNS SUNK FOLLOWING A COLLISION

Former Excursion Boat, Now Operated by Navy Department, in Accident Near Norfolk.-

THE EVENING STAR

Washington, D.C. (Oct. 23, 1918) – The steamer *St Johns,* plying for years between Washington and Colonial Beach, Virginia, and recently chartered by the Navy Department, was sunk yesterday morning in a collision with the steamer *Princess Anne*, owned by the Old Dominion Steamship Company, off Lambert's Point, near Norfolk. Va.

No lives have been reported lost. The damage done the *Princess Anne* has not been learned.

The *St. Johns* was in command of Capt. Bailey Reed and operated for the Navy Department between Norfolk and a naval operating base near there. Her tonnage was 1,800, and she was 250 feet long.

The *St. Johns* was built in 1878 and was known for years along the river. Capt. Reed is almost as well known here as the boat he commanded.

EPIDEMIC ABATES ONLY IN SECTIONS
Authorities Report the Crest Among Civilians Is Not Yet Reached

THE EVENING STAR

Washington, D. C. (Oct. 23, 1918) – Improvement In the influenza situation among civilians in several districts and Army camps of the country is Indicated by reports from both the public health service and the office of the surgeon general of the Army.

However, the epidemic has not yet reached its crest among civilians. In the far west and on the Pacific coast, the numbers of cases in various states have been fairly numerous. Still, the situation was not so serious as in the east and south, where conditions generally are rapidly improving.

In Middle West States.

In the middle west and in the states bordering the Mississippi and Missouri rivers abatement of the disease has been noted, although many new cases still are being reported daily.

Continued abatement of the epidemic in Army camps was reported today to the office of the surgeon general of the Army. New cases during the twenty-four hours ending at noon today totaled 2,773, against 3,007 the day before, while deaths decreased from 404 to 392. There was a slight increase in the number of pneumonia cases.

Still Epidemic in Five Camps.

Army medical officers said influenza may now be said to be epidemic in only five camps, the others reporting less than 50 new cases each daily.

The total cases since the disease became epidemic number 292,770, with 15,497 deaths.

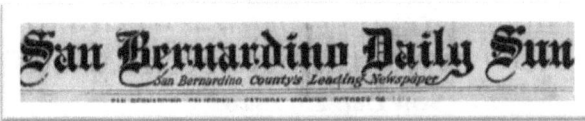

FLU SITUATION BETTER IN THE EAST, BUT WORST ON THE COAST

SAN BERNADINO SUN Oct. 25, 1918

WASHINGTON, Oct. 24, 1918 – Further subsidence of the influenza epidemic over the country was indicated in reports today by the public health service from 44 states. The situation still is serious in many localities, however, and more particularly in the larger cities.

There was practically no change in army camps, 2772 new cases being reported, a decrease of one from yesterday's total. Pneumonia cases decreased from742 yesterday to 699 today, and deaths were 307 against 327 the day before. The total of influenza cases reported now is 298,275, pneumonia cases 48,328, and deaths 16,174.

Camps Dix, New Jersey, and Grant, Illinois, where influenza epidemics have been particularly serious, did not report a single new case, while only seven were reported from Camp Devens, Massachusetts. The largest number of new cases reported today was from Camp McClellan, Alabama, with 123.

Arkansas reported today that the peak had been passed in the larger towns, but that conditions were more serious in the rural districts.

In Florida, deaths in the cities and towns increased rapidly early this month, but they now show a sharp decrease. In Arizona, the disease is spreading to some extent in the mining districts, but elsewhere is on the decline. The total cases reported in Colorado are 11, 432, while in other far-western states, the disease is epidemic in most cities.

Improvement is shown in Washington and Oregon as well as California. In the northwest, conditions continue to be serious, particularly in Minnesota, but in the states bordering on the Mississippi River, there is a decline in the number of new cases.

Over the south and east, generally, improvement is shown, but the disease still is active in most of the large cities.

INCREASE IN LOS ANGELES
SAN BERNADINO SUN Oct. 25, 1918

Los Angeles, Oct. 24, 1918 – More new cases were reported to the health department here for the 24 hours ending at 5 o'clock tonight than for any similar period since the malady became epidemic in California. There were 1,39 cases of influenza and 31 other cases in which disease was complicated with pneumonia. Deaths from influenza numbered 16, from influenza-pneumonia 24, and from pneumonia alone 3.

IN SAN FRANCISCO
SAN BERNADINO SUN Oct. 25, 1918

SAN FRANCISCO, Oct. 24, 1918 – The Board of Health announced tonight that 1,407 cases of Spanish Influenza had been reported up to late today, bringing this city's total to 10,283 cases. Eighty-two additional deaths were reported, making a total of 385.

MASKS IN SAN DIEGO
SAN BERNADINO SUN Oct. 25, 1918

SAN DIEGO, Oct. 24. – The city board of health today drew up an order making it compulsory for every individual appearing on the streets or in places where the public is met to wear a gauze mask.

IN SAN FRANCISCO, TOO
SAN FRANCISCO, Oct. 24, 1918 – At the request of the board of health, the board of supervisors at a special meeting here today passed an ordinance compelling every person in the city to wear a gauze mask as influenza preventative.

People of Bear valley are looking for the man who dared to go into the valley and spread influenza. Fifteen cases have developed in the valley within the last week, and although none of them have resulted, fatally, several people have been very ill with the malady.

When the courthouse closes at noon Saturday, it will be sealed, and wholesale fumigation of all offices will begin to last until Monday morning. The fumigation is ordered as a hearth measure, for there have been many cases of Influenza, among the employee.

Mrs. Joseph Dempsey was critically ill last night from pneumonia. Relatives were summoned.

'FLU' SITUATION IS GROWING BETTER

Less Number of Cases in Los Angeles and More in San Francisco

WASHINGTON, Oct. 25, 1918 – Three army camps did not report a single new case of Influenza today, and only two, Kearny, California, and Lewis, Washington, reported more than 100 cases. The total of new cases for all camps, a statement from the office of the surgeon general said, was 2,375 against 2,772 the day before. Pneumonia cases decreased from 699 to 500 and deaths from 307 to 241.

FEWER CASES

LOS ANGELES, Oct. 25, 1918 – New cases of influenza reported today to the Los Angeles Board of Health numbered 806 with 46 additional cases of influenza-pneumonia. This was 224 under the number reported during the preceding 24 hours. There were 13 deaths from influenza, 24 from pneumonia-Influenza, and seven from pneumonia.

There have been 10,602 cases reported since October 1, with 378 deaths, of which 127 resulted from influenza, 79 from pneumonia-influenza, and 172 from pneumonia.

REACH HIGHEST POINT

SAN FRANCISCO. Oct. 25, 1918 – The Spanish influenza epidemic reaped its greatest toll of victims today, with 2,007 new cases reported up to 5 p. m., according to the board of health. Ninety-six deaths had been reported up to that hour.

"SHOOT HIM AT SUNRISE"

SAN FRANCISCO, Oct. 25. The dates of the present Spanish Influenza epidemic, which he said was now in decline, and the temblor, which shook the Grecian archipelago on October 21, was accurately forecast by Professor Albert F. Porta, an Oakland scientist, it developed here today. The influenza epidemic was related to certain conjunction of Jupiter with other planets, according to the forecasts and explanations of Professor Porta. This planet arrangement is now passing, indicating that the epidemic is on the wane, he said.

HELP TO BURY DEAD

NEW YORK, Oct. 25. Mayor Hylan tonight called on presidents of the five boroughs of New York to provide laborers, equipped with picks and shovels, to help bury persons who have died of influenza.

Little Change Comes in the Influenza Situation With Less of New Cases

There was little change in the influenza situation yesterday. Five deaths in the city, four of them Mexicans, brought the total to 27 for the epidemic.

A decrease in the number of new cases continued yesterday, but there are scores of serious cases in the city. The disease seems to have become more severe as the epidemic continues.

MRS. ANDREWS A VICTIM OF THE EPIDEMIC

Last Rites for the Late G. W. Leonard Will Be Held This Morning

THE SUN'S Staff Correspondence.

COLTON. Oct. 25, 1918 – Sinking wearily into the Everlasting Arms after less than a week's battle against the dreaded malady that is casting Its pall of sorrow over the city, Annie Elizabeth Andrews, wife of Dwight Andrews, passed away at 11 o'clock this morning at the family residence On West H Street. With her passing, all the sunshine has gone from the home, and two little sons, one-two years of age and the other a baby of only seven months, are left motherless. In addition to the husband and babies, a mother and sister survive, Mrs. Wilcox and Miss Ivy Wilcox. Just about three months ago they came out from Ohio and had since been residing at the Andrews home. The deceased was a native of England and 29 years of age. Gentle of nature and possessing true womanly qualities, she won many friends during her residence in Colton. In 1914 she became the wife of Dwight Andrews, and two years and a half ago, they came west and settled here. Mr. Andrews Is a baker by trade, and part of the time has been connected with the bakery of his brother, J.H. Andrews, having been employed for a while In Riverside.

RUTGERS TO PLAY LEHIGH
Game Will Be Staged at New Brunswick Tomorrow
THE SUN (Oct. 25, 1918) SPECIAL DISPATCH TO THE SUN

New Brunswick, N. J. Definite announcement was made today that Lehigh and Rutgers will meet in football here on Saturday afternoon. The game originally was scheduled for last week at South Bethlehem but was postponed because of the Influenza epidemic.

After the hard workout against the Pelham Bay team, the Rutgers squad has begun to find Itself. Foster Sanford has spent several afternoons correcting the faults manifested in that contest and in smoothing out the Rutgers defense.

The Rutgers players were vaccinated this afternoon and were a mighty sore lot. There was no practice, but a short drill will be held tomorrow. Sanford was further handicapped when It was learned that Francke, who sprained an ankle yesterday, would be out of the game for ten days.

'FLU' EPIDEMIC FAST IMPROVING
Seven More Local Boys Are Now on Their Way to War Front in France
THE SUN'S Staff Correspondence

HIGHLAND, Oct. 25, 1918 – While the number of cases of influenza in the Highland district has slightly increased, the general situation may be said to have Improved. New cases are not so severe, and old ones are all Improving.

In the C. D. Hathaway family, five members were ill at one time early in the wee, and outside assistance was necessary. For this, Mr. and Mrs. Hathaway desire to express their gratitude. All members of the household are now convalescent.

At the Churches
Silence and emptiness will reign by the adamantine order of Health Officer Dr. J. H. Evans.

The only sermon to be preached in Highland next Sunday will be by Rev. F. E. Dell in THE SUN, by request of the editor. It will be one of several short sermons, with San Bernardino County for an audience. Everybody can go to church Sunday.

276 Cases in Kern
BAKERSFIELD, Oct. 17, 1918. —Two hundred seventy-six cases of Spanish influenza have been reported to date in Kern county, the health officer * announced today. All of the cases, it was said, have been light.

There have been three deaths, Chicago Tries Vaccine

CHICAGO, Oct. 17. —Vaccine originated by Dr. E. C. Rosenow of the Mayo Clinic, Rochester, Minn., will be used in Chicago's campaign against Spanish influenza.

Dr. Rosenow told the Chicago influenza emergency commission of his experiments with the vaccine, with which he has treated 20,000 persons. The commission at once named a committee of physicians to take charge of the manufacture and use of all vaccines and serum in Chicago, including the Rosenow vaccine. Another committee was named to raise funds for its manufacture and distribution. Five days will be required to begin the manufacture of the vaccine here; it was stated. Meantime, Dr. Rosenow will provide a supply sufficient for 100,000 doses from his laboratory in Rochester. The vaccine is designed to provide immunity from the disease, though Dr. Rosenow is unwilling to make specific claims as to its value. He believes it aided greatly to suppress the spread of influenza at Rochester.

New Cases Fall Off

NEW YORK, Oct. 17.—A total of 1 1 33 new cases of influenza was reported today against 5113 yesterday. There were 336 deaths, against 317 yesterday. Pneumonia cases showed an increase, with 646 new cases, against 565 yesterday. Deaths totaled 287, against 316 yesterday.

RIVERSIDE DAILY PRESS Oct. 17, 1918

Except for Camp Dodge,
The disease was on the increase.
$10,000,000 to fight It

WASHINGTON, Oct. 17, 1918 —Ten million dollars to fight Spanish influenza is appropriated in an amendment to the pending six-billion-dollar army bill, introduced today by Senator Lewis, Illinois.

Chicago Tries Vaccine

CHICAGO, Oct. 17. —Vaccine originated by Dr. E. C. Rosenow of the Mayo Clinic, Rochester, Minn., will be used in Chicago's campaign against Spanish influenza. Dr. Rosenow told the Chicago influenza emergency commission of his experiments with the vaccine, with which he has treated 20,000 persons. The commission at once named a committee of physicians to take charge of the manufacture and use of all vaccines and serum in Chicago, including the Rosenow vaccine. Another committee was named to raise funds for its manufacture and distribution. Five days will be required to begin the manufacture of the vaccine here; it was stated. Meantime, Dr. Rosenow will provide a supply sufficient for 100,000 doses from his laboratory in Rochester. The vaccine is designed to provide immunity from the disease, though Dr. Rosenow is unwilling to make specific claims as to its value. He believes it aided greatly to suppress the spread of influenza at Rochester.

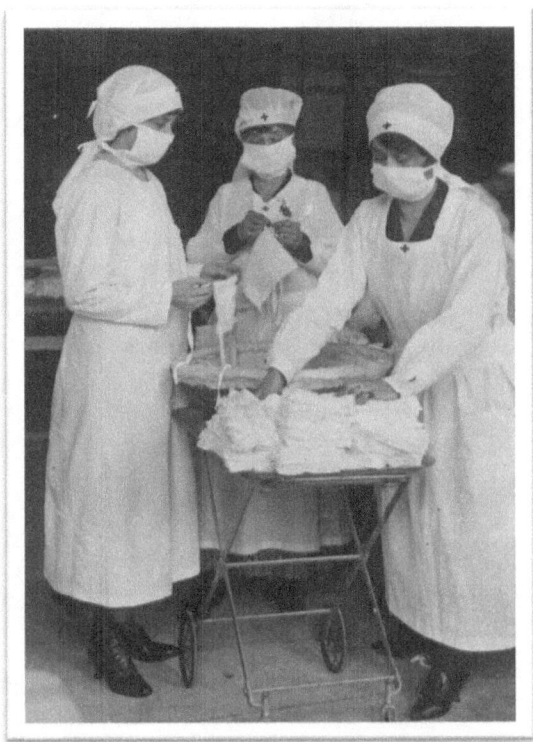

Red Cross workers in Boston process masks for soldiers made by women of the city. Photo National Archives.

PREVENTIVE OF PNEUMONIA IS PREPARED HERE

Vaccine Will Be Delivered to Doctors Free but is Not Intended as a Cure for Malady.

Omaha, Nebraska (Oct. 26, 1918) – A vaccine intended for the prevention of pneumonia is being prepared by a large number of doctors and scientists under the direction of City Health Commissioner Manning. These doctors are from the faculties of the University of Nebraska College of Medicine and Creighton Medical college, and they are engaged in studying the "flu," its causes, methods of propagation, and treatment.

"The vaccine will be ready probably the first of next week," said Dr. Manning. "It will be given free to all doctors in the city and state who apply for it. It is not intended as a cure but as a preventative. It is harmless, and no bad effects are felt from its use."

Cases Diminish.

The germs used in making the vaccine are taken from victims of the disease here. They are placed in a culture where they grow and multiply. Then they are placed in a salt solution where they die and form the vaccine.

The report of new cases of "flu" in Omaha showed that the daily number is still less than it was Thursday. Only 80 new cases were reported to the health commissioner in the 24 hours ending at 9 o'clock Friday morning. During the same period, 26 deaths were reported. A number of these, however, occurred several days ago and had not been reported.

More than 100 medical students are volunteers on call at the Visiting Nurses' Association and the Red Cross. They go out to attend cases of "flu," which are not very serious, but which require the attendance of a doctor. There are also several doctors who have medical students helping them in their regular work.

Dr. Manning again warned pool hall proprietors today that they must limit crowds in their places.

In several towns, the pool halls have been closed. Those in Omaha are said to be badly ventilated, unsanitary and crowded during many hours of the clay.

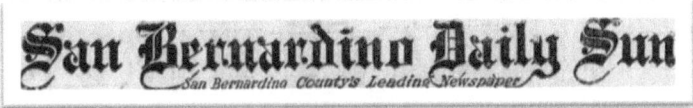

CAMPAIGN NOW ON IS STRANGE
"Flu" Situation Compels the Resort to Unusual Plans by the Candidates

San Bernardino Sun, Oct. 27, 1918

SAN FRANCISCO. Oct 26. Politicians and office-seekers, restricted by the Spanish influenza epidemic, are waging the strangest campaign in the history of California. For once the stump and soapbox are forsaken, of necessity, and those who are running for office, as well as those who are grooming them, are making their appeals by mail, by newspaper publicity and by means of advertisements.

The gubernatorial situation is typical of all the offices to be filled. Governor Stephens is in Sacramento and, according to his headquarters here, is not doing any campaigning for re-election, but is devoting his entire time to combating the epidemic. Miss Esther Rojuaro, the state organizer of the women on the governor's behalf, is sending letters throughout the state.

Theodore Bell, Democratic candidate for governor, who has been an Influenza sufferer for several days, was expected to be out tomorrow. It was stated that Bell will make his postponed trip through the southern part of the state but will not make any effort to speak in public.

PUBLIC WARNED AGAINST THE SURE-CURES
Influenza Situation in Both San Francisco and Los Angeles Improves

WASHINGTON, Oct. 26, 1918 – Use of vaccines in combatting or treating

Spanish Influenza has not gone beyond the experimental stage, so far as the United States public health service has learned. In a statement tonight, the service warned the public against any of the sure cures advocated for the malady, which, according to reports today, is subsiding rapidly In all army camps and showing a - lessening tendency in many states among the civilian population.

LARGE DECREASE

SAN FRANCISCO, Oct. 26. While there were seven more deaths' today from Spanish Influenza than were reported; yesterday, the number of new .cases reported fell away almost 700, and Dr. William Hastier, public health officer, declared tonight that the epidemic In this city -is on the decline.

For the 24 hours ending at 5 p. m. today there were 1,320 new cases reported and 100 deaths. At that hour yesterday, 2,006 new cases had been reported and 93 deaths.

"The disease Is disappearing," Dr. Hassler declared, "due to the fact that the people are taking care of themselves and wearing their masks. I am going to make the people wear masks until the situation returns to normal."

Practically all the San Francisco banks will close at 2 p. m. hereafter until the epidemic is pronounced abated. This determination was expressed today by the members of the California Bankers Association and the San Francisco Clearing House Association, which adopted resolutions of intention to close an hour earlier each day except Saturday, in order that their employees may have more time for exercise in the open air.

CONDITIONS IMPROVE

LOS ANGELES, CALIF. Oct. 26, 1918 – Continued decrease in the number of new cases of influenza in Los Angeles was shown by the report tonight of the city health department. There were 700 new cases today, compared to 846 yesterday and 1,070 Thursday. There were 16 deaths during the past 24 hours from influenza and 20 from influenza-pneumonia.

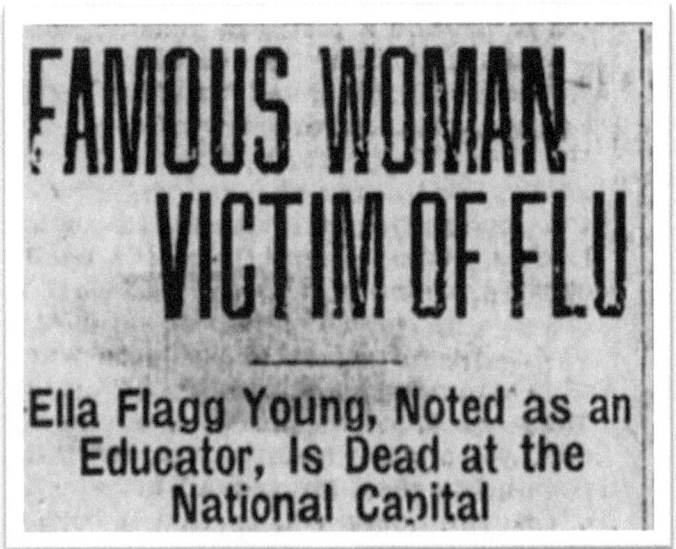

FAMOUS WOMAN VICTIM OF FLU

Ella Flagg Young, Noted as an Educator, Is Dead at the National Capital

SAN BERNARDINO SUN

WASHINGTON. Oct. 26, 1918 – Ella Flagg Young, chairman of the national woman's Liberty loan committee, died today of pneumonia following an attack of influenza.

Mrs. Ella Flagg Young was one of the best-known women educators in the United States. She was a leader of progressive educational ideas to which she devoted more than fifty years of her life.

She was chosen superintendent of Chicago's public schools in 1909 from a list of six candidates, five of whom were men educators of national reputation. She succeeded Edwin G. Cooley and was the first woman to be elected superintendent of schools in one of the largest American cities. As head of the public schools of Chicago, she was entrusted with the education of 300,000 children.

She inaugurated many Important reforms, among these being the teaching of sex hygiene, the enlargement of the kindergarten course, an increase in the scope of the vocational training department, and simplification of the curriculum of the primary grades. She was aggressive and possessed the great executive ability. She insisted upon the complete divorce of politics from the public schools and fought many successful battles in support of this principle.

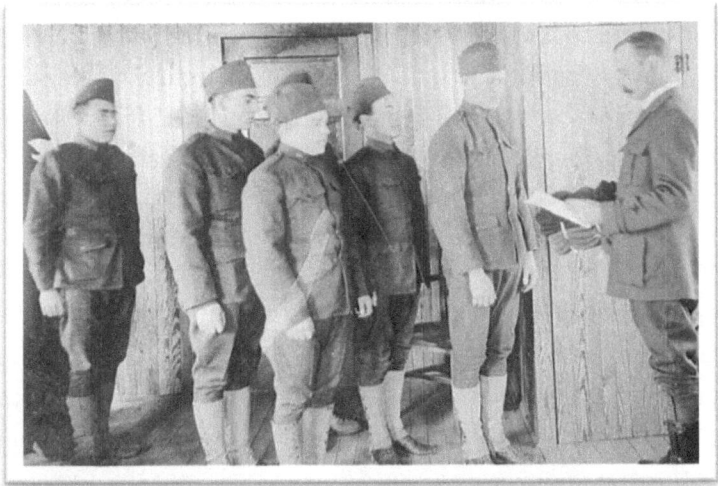

Soldiers at Camp Upton on Long Island, New York, volunteered to test the vaccine for the pneumonia-related Spanish Influenza.
Library of Congress.

THESE ARMY MEN DISCOVER PNEUMONIA VACCINE THAT HAS SAVED 10,000 TROOPS

Discovery Will Be Real Victory of War If Tests of New Vaccine Continue to Prove Successful, Army Physicians Say of New Cure Now Being Used on Washington War Workers with Excellent Results

THE WASHINGTON TIMES

Washington, D.C. (Oct. 27, 1918) – The story of how four army officers detailed to the task by Secretary of War Baker, discovered the vaccine that is being put into the veins of thousands of war workers in Washington to ward off dreaded pneumonia that has cost an untold number of lives during the epidemic of Spanish influenza came to light for the first time yesterday.

The application of the serum as pneumonia preventive is already considered a success in army circles. At Camp Upton, 10,000 soldiers volunteered to test the vaccine, with the result that not a single case of pneumonia was contracted. With the manufacture of the serum reaching a higher stage of production, its use has spread to the other camps, and members of the army medical corps are unanimous in its praise.

Great Achievement

Cloaked behind what they call professional ethics, the members of the board have succeeded until now in keeping secret their part in what army officials are calling one of the greatest medical achievements of the war. They have not only completed the work of many scientists of isolating the pneumonia germ, but within six months, they have discovered a serum which being successfully used.

The board is not making any claims for the serum. It must yet pass the final test – the test which comes with the long winter months when pneumonia ravages throughout the country. There are relatively few cases of the disease in the summer or the fall. It is the cold months that are feared, and the success of the serum will not be established until Secretary Baker receives the final report next spring.

Personnel of Board

The board is composed of Col. Dean C. Howard, Col. William Henry Welch, Col. Victor Clarence Vaugh, and Col. Frederick Fuller Russell. It was formed last winter when the medical division seemed to have lost all control of the situation, for pneumonia is a crowd disease, and with a million men gathered hurriedly into camps, it seemed impossible to halt its ravages.

Affords Protection

The board emphasized the fact that the vaccine is intended to afford a certain degree of protection to healthy individuals against pneumonia. It is not intended to cure those already sick. It is not advised for persons suffering from acute colds or fever.

The serum is a lipo vaccine preparation made by the Army Medical School. It is given in a single injection and contains three types of pneumococci. Reactions as a rule unpronounced.

The prophylactic vaccination against pneumonia is administered at the school, 462 Louisiana Avenue, between 4 and 4:30 o'clock. At present, about 200 persons a day take the treatment, but as soon as the facilities permit fully 500 a day will receive injections.

It is hoped by the officials that the result of the use of the serum will be as gratifying as the introduction of the anti-typhoid serum of Colonel Russell, who was the first to bring it to America.

Precedents Followed

In the Spanish-American War, with an army of 200,000 men, there were 6,000 cases of typhoid, resulting in 2,4000 deaths. In the first year of the present war, with 1,000,000 in camp, all of whom have been vaccinated, there have only been nine cases of typhoid and one death. Eight of these cases, however, were contracted before the men entered the army.

It is on account of the success of the anti-typhoid and the fact that some of the same bacteriologists are working on the pneumonia serum that army heads are confident we may see the end of pneumonia in army camps and later in all walks of life, and that the deadly disease which is cynically known as "the friend of the old" because it kills them quickly will become a thing of the past.

~~~~

ATLANTA LIFTS BAN

ATLANTA, Ga. (Oct. 27, 1918) – The influenza ban on theaters and public gatherings has been raised here. Owing to the power shortage, theaters will only be permitted to operate six hours per day.

29 DEATHS SHOW PLAGUE ON WANE

THE WASHINGTON TIMES

Washington, D.C. (Oct. 27, 1918) – Influenza continued to decrease in Washington yesterday, with but twenty-nine deaths reported to health officials during the twenty-four-hour period ending at 9 o'clock last night.

Dr. William O. Fowler, District health officer, and Dr. H. S. Mustard, or the public health service, were agreed in the belief that the end of the epidemic is in sight.

District Commissioners yesterday refused to lift the ban on today's church services.

"No action to open churches and theaters will be taken until the feasibility of the move Is absolutely certain," said Dr. Fowler.

Automobile owners in Washington are appealed to by the public health service to offer their cars to Influenza relief workers to aid in the fight against the epidemic. Motorists willing to donate the services of their cars should call Dr. Herdliska or Lieutenant Fisk, Main 5520, or go to the Webster school, Tenth and H Streets northwest.

DEATHS IN D. C. FROM INFLUENZA

THE WASHINGTON TIMES

Washington, D.C. (Oct. 27, 1918) – These twenty-nine deaths were reported to the District Health Department during the twenty-four hours ending at 9 o'clock last night:

Elma Smith, 26, 3312 Sherman Avenue northwest.

Mary Camington,2T, 2524 Mozart Street northwest.

Nina Thomas, 25, 2720 N Street northwest.

Merina Johnson, 31, 1505 Fourth, Street northwest.

Marie Thomas, 11, 38 Rock Creek Church Road,

Patrick J. Dougherty, 48, St. Elizabeth's Hospital. ,

Evelyn M. Bailey, 2720 N Street northwest.

Elizabeth Smallwood, 3, 1933 Eleventh Street northwest.

Agnes Howell, 9. Freedman's Hospital

Ella B. Hyde, 33, Providence Hospital.

Sarah Cleveland, 28. U. S. Public Health Hospital No. 2.

Triphon Provest, 30, U. S. Public Health Hospital No. 2.

Nellie Freeborn, 28. U. S. Public Health Hospital, No. 2.

Charles J. Shields. 47, St. Elizabeth's Hospital.

Abraham Doebler, 75, St. Elizabeth Hospital.

Elizabeth Mulligan; 25. SL Elizabeth Hospital.

Mary Emma Combs, 47, 1350 Brentwood Road northeast.

Geraldine L. Callan, 1, 4004 Illinois Avenue.

Ethel Osborne, 30, Garfield Hospital.

Christina Green. 35, U. S. P. H. S. Hospital.

Mary Fletcher, 28, 9 Crays Street southwest.

Francis Nelson Dixon, two months, 442 N Street northwest.

William Green, 68, U.S. Soldiers Home.

Benjamin L. Posey, 38, Providence Hospital.

Lavinia A. Obrene, 28, 540 Fifteenth Street northeast.

William Farhood, 33, 3125 Fourteenth Street northwest.

Ella Flags Young, 73, Chatham Courts.

Clarence W. Horner, 61, 4600 Fourteenth Street northwest.

Josephine Hesslinger, 44, St. Elizabeth's Hospital.

"FLU" SILENCES PHONES

PINEVILLE, Ky, (Oct. 27,1918) Telephone exchanges of Harlan, Middleboro, Corbin, and this town are closed because all the operators are stricken with Spanish influenza.

New cases of the disease are being reported daily in this section. Operations In the coalfields are tied up by the epidemic.

"FLU" ORDER LIFTED

PHILADELPHIA. (Oct. 27, 1918) – The Spanish influenza order closing theaters, motion picture houses, and saloons his been canceled, effective Wednesday.

T. R. IS SIXTY TODAY

OYSTER BAY, Long Island (Oct. 27, 1918) – Col. Theodore Roosevelt is spending his sixtieth birthday anniversary quietly with his wife at his home at Sagamore Hill today. No celebration of the day was planned.

The colonel, having reached the Osler age, is hale and hearty and is enjoying the best of health.

Flu Beats Foe Bullets In Killing U.S. Soldiers, Senate Committee Informed

THE WASHINGTON TIMES

Washington, D.C. (Oct. 27, 1918) – The epidemic of Spanish Influenza has been checked in army camps, but while it was in progress more deaths were caused by the disease than were killed by German bullets in the same period, the Senate Military Affairs Committee was informed at the War Council this afternoon.

BOOTLEG AUTOS ARE CONFISCATED

NASHVILLE, Tenn. (Oct. 27, 1918) – Fifty thousand dollars' worth of 'booze' carrying automobiles and $15,000 worth of liquor is stored in the Federal building here. Federal authorities in the past few weeks have enacted a heavy toll on the confiscation of liquor stocks and automobiles.

As a result, the operation of high-powered 'booze' cars between Hopkinsville, Ky., and Nashville has been practically suspended.

The suitcase system is again growing popular with the bootleggers, it is stated.

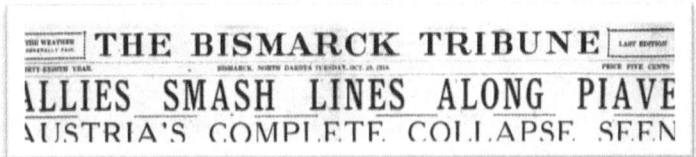

FLU MAY CUT DOWN VOTE ON ELECTION DAY

Estimated That 15,000 Cases Now
Are Prevalent in North Dakota.
REGISTRATION IS SMALL

THE BISMARCK TRIBUNE

Bismarck, N.D. (Oct. 29, 1918) – North Dakota voters not previously registered today had their last opportunity to sign up for next Tuesday's ballot bee. So general is the effects of Spanish influenza that a large registration today is not believed possible and the illness of scores of electors who are required by law to register, because of having changed their residence, or for other reasons, will necessitate swearing in their votes next Tuesday.

Campaign managers are already beginning to speculate as to the effect of Spanish flu on next Tuesday's election. There are not less than 15,000 "active" cases of influenza in North Dakota today. The lighter attacks will have their course by the end of the week, but there is no guaranty that there will not be as many, if not more new cases to take their place.

The flu bug has been no respecter of parties but has attacked Nonpartisans and partisans alike. At the present moment, the country districts seem the hardest hit, a fact, which may seriously affect the Nonpartisan vote.

President Townley of the National Nonpartisan league is said to have admitted that an estimated "floating" vote of 10,000 will turn the tide one way or the other. How many of these "floaters" will be too ill next Tuesday to go to the polls is a question which- not even Mr. Townley can answer. If the epidemic grows much more severe, health authorities may even consider the heretofore unheard of the possibility of postponing the general election.

Country towns, with few or no doctors, without hospitals and1 with no trained nurses, are reporting very heavy mortality from flu. One town in the southwestern part of the state with a population of but 300 has fifty, percent of its people ill, and nine deaths already have occurred. Some of the smaller villages are almost deserted, and business of all kinds is practically suspended. Bismarck, while it has had in all 750 cases of flu in a population of 9,.000, has had comparatively light mortality, and its total number of deaths is less than a dozen. There have, however, been more than a score of deaths in the city's two large hospitals, which have been filled from the beginning of the epidemic with patients brought in from surrounding towns.

DEATH STEAMER
HAS 192 BODIES
OF WRECK VICTIMS

THE BISMARCK TRIBUNE

Juneau, Alaska, (Oct. 29, 1918) —Loaded with bodies of the dead of the lost steamer *Princess Sofia*, the steamer *Princess Alice*, a sister ship, will leave here for Vancouver, B. C., in a day or two. She will carry the 192 bodies already found, and others may be found before she sails.

Coffins were being rushed here today from Seattle and Alaska points. Rescue workers expect to recover 90 percent of the bodies of the 343 lost.

LARGEST CARRIER
IS LAUNCHED

Philadelphia, Oct. 29—The steamship South Bend, said to be the largest cargo carrier ever built in the country, was launched today at the Delaware Yard of the Sun Shipbuilding Co., at Westchester.

The ship originally intended for a commercial company Was taken over by the government soon after the work was started on it. It is 475 1-2 feet long and 60 feet wide, it is the fifth ship launched by the Sun Shipbuilding Co. in the last few months.

EXTRA SUGAR
PERMITS FOR
FLU VICTIMS

Individuals or families suffering from influenza will be allowed an extra allotment of sugar by O. W. Roberts, Burleigh county food commissioner. Under directions received today from Dr. E. Ladd, federal food administrator for North Dakota. Mr. Roberts wired yesterday for permission to grant additional sugar to those who require it for the manufacture of hot lemonade and other flu cures, and grocers have been instructed to honor requisitions from flu sufferers.

NINE DEATHS!
LAST 24 HOURS
FROMINFLUENZA

Dread Epidemic Continues to Take
Heavy Toll From Smaller Towns.

Nine deaths, one of them from Bismarck, have occurred at Bismarck two large hospitals during the last 24 hours. All of the deceased were victims of Spanish influenza. Today's death list is as follows.

Joseph Rodek, Menoken farmer, aged 28

Mrs. C. I. Dunahey, Mandan

Iona Woods, Hazelton, aged 12

Russell Pogue, Moffit, aged 26

Mrs. Joseph Daugherty, Wing, aged 30

Walter W. Small, Fort Lincoln, aged 24

David A. Olson, Menoken, aged 20.

Mrs. Anna Neubauer, Steele, aged 26

John Pixatonis, Bismarck, aged 30.

Coroner A. E. Shipp was called today to Sterling to investigate the death of William Schafer, a young farmer residing near that place, who died from Spanish influenza, leaving a young widow and several children. The coroner is called; it is understood because the deceased had no medical attendance.

Walter W. Small, son of Mr. and Mrs. Irvin Small of Fort Lincoln, was one of Burleigh county's best-known young farmers, and his death is a bitter blow to his scores of friends. Funeral services will be held Thursday afternoon at the Lucas undertaking rooms.

The remains of Mrs. Anna Neubauer of Steele were taken this morning on train No. 4 enroute to her former home at Niles, Ill. The funeral of John Pixatonis, a member of the Bismarck Greek colony, was held from the Lucas undertaking rooms this afternoon.

The body of Mrs. Dunahey has been removed to Mandan, and the remains of Mrs. Daugherty will be taken to Wing for interment.

TWO BROTHERS DIE.

As she was about to leave for her home at Clyde Park, Mont., Miss Madeline McMurda, a form-probationer at St. Alexius hospital, today received notice that the bodies of two brothers who had died at Fortress Monroe, Va., from Spanish influenza, would pass through the city today.

Miss McMurda had expected that the bodies would be on train No. 3, upon which she proceeded to Miles City, but upon the train's arrival, she learned that the remains of her brothers would go through tonight on the North Coast Limited.

Mr. and Mrs. R. K. Batzer III.

Mrs. R. K. Batzer, of Hazelton, was brought to St. Alexius hospital last night, ill from Spanish influenza. Her husband, suffering from the same malady, and in a serious condition, came in today—Mrs. Batzer, who has been at. St. Alexius, for several days, is improving.

Little Girl Dies.

Iona, the twelve-year-old daughter of Mr. and Mrs. L. H. Woods of Hazelton, passed away at a local hospital last night as a result of Spanish influenza.

From Hazelton.

W. Burkholz, manager of the Hazelton elevator and Bert Hartman of the Wonder Store, were brought into St. Alexius hospital yesterday in a very serious condition as a result of Spanish influenza.

In Bismarck Hospital,

Dr. and Mrs. H. E. Winchester of Hazelton are both in the Bismarck hospital with Spanish influenza. Dr. Winchester is making a satisfactory recovery, but Mrs. Winchester's condition is still grave.

Whole Family in Hospital.

Mrs. E. M. Serr and four children have been transferred within the last few days from their home on Fourth

OLDER MEN TO BE TRAINED BY EASY DEGREES

THE BISMARCK TRIBUNE

Washington, D.C., (Oct. 29, 1918) —Older drafted men are to be put into shape for service through modified physical training less arduous than the program arranged for the younger draftees.

Camp commanders were instructed today to train the older men gradually.

BISMARCK NIGHT SCHOOL TO OPEN AFTER FLU QUITS

The Bismarck board of education announces that as- soon as the present epidemic of influenza subsides, a night school for the benefit of those who are not eligible to attend the regular day school will be opened in the high school building. English, civics, manual training, domestic science, including cooking and sewing, and commercial Subjects will be taught by competent instructors in the pay of and under the direction of the board of education. There will be no volunteer teaching, doing away with a situation that grew out of a former night school experiment, which resulted in some criticism.

CASHIER OF WISHEK BANK TILTED THE LID

Ashley, N. D. (Oct. 29, 1918) – W. L. Johnson, cashier of the Ashley State Bank of which John H. Wishek is president, has been arrested by federal authorities on a charge of violating the North Dakota Bone Dry Act, and the federal statutes which support it. He has furnished $500 cash bail for his appearance in U. S. District Court.

FLU EPIDEMIC
IS ON WANE

Washington, D. C. (Oct. 20, 1918) — The United States Surgeon General announced today that the epidemic has passed in ten naval districts and is on the wane in all other districts except in South Carolina and California.

LISBON WOMAN EDITOR
VICTIM OF INFLUENZA

Lisbon, N. D., (Oct. 29, 1918) – Holding the fort alone, so that her husband, William M. Jones Jr. might accompany the Fighting First regiment band to France, his wife, while acting as editor of the Lisbon Gazette, contracted Spanish influenza and died within three days. Mrs. Jones had been publishing the Gazette for more than a year and had proven a thoroughly capable newspaperwoman.

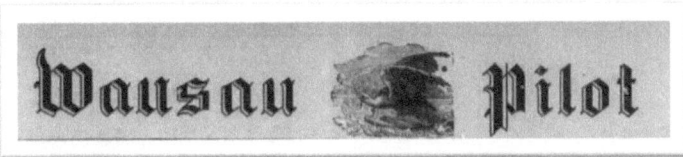

WAUSAU STILL IN ITS GRIP
Influenza Cases Number Fully a Thousand in Wausau

—

Many Deaths

THE WAUSAU PILOT

Wausau, Wis. (Oct. 29, 1918) – "Can I help? What can I do?" Thus, she spoke a young miss as she stepped into the Health Office at the city hall. It was a surprise to those who heard her. She was so young and apparently carefree. But she had uttered the word that was the keynote of the work now going on—helpfulness.

It is a peculiar truth that the people who make up a community and have a casual acquaintance with each other, are practically strangers in some respects, and it takes some big situation to bring them to really know each other. The fact has been and is being practically demonstrated in Wausau during the present epidemic.

Wausau citizens are united in one big family, or army, whose slogan is, "Fight the Flu." Men and women from every profession, business, and calling are putting their best and earnest efforts foremost in the work.

Doctors and nurses are working day and night, as are also volunteer workers who go into the homes. The members of the Motor corps have worked tirelessly, one of their chief duties being the carrying of food to some of the homes of those who are ill.

And this food has been just as tirelessly prepared by experienced cooks at the High school, Training school and in private homes.

The hospital forces have segregated a part of their buildings to influenza and pneumonia patients, and pending operations have been postponed that the greatest possible care might be given those afflicted with the diseases. Perhaps those who are really the heroes and heroines of the work and deserving of the greatest commendation are the volunteer workers. Among them are men, women who are wives, teachers, and girls who are employed and unemployed, who have voluntarily given their services to go into homes and care for the sick, cook and clean for the family and have not shrunk from any menial task whereby they might be of help.

A man who stands high in the community has done just this thing. Also, his wife, both working in an undemonstrative and unobtrusive way in different homes where sickness surrounded them, and death often hovered near. Another woman entered a home of people unknown to her, where both parents lay ill and held a little dying baby in her arms until it breathed its last, her daughter doing the housework for the rest of the children. Teachers have washed dishes, swept, and mopped, and still found time to bathe the children. There are many such cases, and we who help from the safe seclusion of our homes are moved to lift our hats to the brave workers in the volunteer force. Everyone is doing his or her utmost to help; the fountains of deep feeling have been touched, and through it all, we are learning something of the real sympathy which lies in hearts where one would least suspect it. And each one is working in unity and harmony with his neighbor. A spirit of helpfulness permeates the air. The alleviation of suffering is a big idea now, and working closely together through it all, we observe the tender hidden springs in our fellow men and find the milk of human kindness in the breasts of those whom we have considered worldly frivolous or thoughtless. Life is a wonderful thing, but life lived in appreciation of the good in those about us, is glorious.

Meals are being furnished about one hundred people on the west side. These meals are taken around by the motor squad in cans; cooked in the Agricultural schoolroom. On the East Side, more than that number are being fed, in the same manner, the meals being cooked at the High school. The cans are afterward collected and sterilized.

John Dern, who has been at home for the past two weeks, ill with influenza, is now convalescing and will soon be about. Mrs. Dern and son, John, Jr., have also been very sick with the disease, but are now much improved. Mark Bellis and family have been on the sick list with influenza, but all are now "out of the woods" and improving.

In many of the establishments in our city, masks are being worn by all employees.

W. J. Webster, the general agent for the Central Life Assurance society, has been extremely ill with influenza. He was taken to St. Mary's hospital at the outset. Three days afterward, pneumonia developed. He is an extremely sick man but is improving with hopes of recovery.

The schools, churches, Sunday schools, moving picture houses, all lodges, etc., remain closed going on for the third week. Wausau is simply trying to keep the disease from spreading. It included all mercantile establishments, saloons, and general places of gathering. It was ordered that only as many passengers as could be seated be allowed on streetcars.

Dr. L. E. Spencer is aiding the health department, and many good suggestions of the department are being put into practice with the result that now the number of cases is being lessened.

Businesses ordered closed with exceptions

B. L. Schuster, health officer, issued an order Friday to close all places of business Saturday evening at six o'clock, except for drug stores, hotels, and such places as must be open for the public.

Pray for Pastor

Rev. Fr. E. P. O'Toole, pastor of St. James' Church, is at St. Mary's Hospital experiencing an attack of influenza. The latest reports find him improving.

1000 Cases in Marshfield, Wisconsin

Perhaps the city which has been the hardest hit by influenza near

Wausa is Marshfield. Over 1,000 cases were reported there last week.

L. E. Blackmer of the University Extension has arranged a card index system for tabulating cases, which will be a great help.

Patients Kept in High School Gym

The infirmary has been opened, and a number of patients are being cared for there as well as in the gymnasium of the High school.

VACCINE FROM MAYO CLINIC

ADMINISTERED TO 100 IN 4 HOURS

Green Bay physicians injected one hundred doses of anti-flu vaccine within four hours after its receipt from Rochester, Minn.

Undertaker down with flu

A. M. Petersen, the undertaker, is going through a siege o influenza at his home on Maple street, being attacked Friday.

William Hussong, Albert Wendorf, Anton Goetzman all of the fire department, are ill with influenza.

Mrs. Elmer Lucas is in St. Mary's hospital with influenza. She is improving.

Help is badly needed, and all who can give their assistance are implored to do so.

Joseph Mayer was laid up last week with a touch of the prevailing illness.

Miss Irene Strupp has been ill since Friday. She is improving.

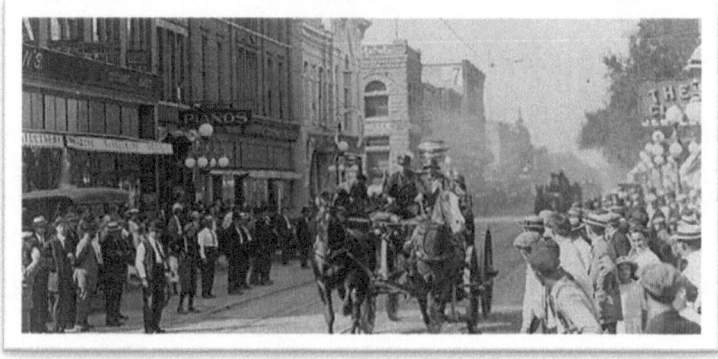

Crowds watch a horse-drawn firewagon down the main street of Wausau, Wisconsin, in 1913. Photo by J. M. Colby, Library of Congress.

SUCCUMBS TO MALADY

George Sutter, Jr. Dies of influenza
While on His Way to France

THE WAUSAU PILOT

Wausau, Wisconsin (Oct. 29, 1918) – George Sutter, Jr., son of Mrs. George Sutter, of Athens, died of influenza, on the 4th of October 1918, on shipboard while on his way to France. He went into the service in August, leaving Wausau with about sixty others. He was well known in Wausau, having come to this city often and had many friends here. His loss was an awfully hard blow to his widowed mother. He was thirty years old and is survived by his mother, one sister, Mrs. Wm. Langsdorf, of Athens, and two brothers, Clarence, who resides at home in Athens and Andrew, who is in the U. S. service in France. The remains were taken to the home of his mother in Athens, from which place the funeral will take place.

NOW LOCATED IN CALIFORNIA

Word has been received from Mrs. A. H. Grout that she arrived safe and well in California and is now pleasantly located in the same apartments with her sister. Miss Lillian Rounds, in Redlands. She reports the weather there as being delightful and warm and the flowers beautiful.

She was met at San Bernardino by her daughter. Miss Edith and her sister by auto and the ride from there to Redlands was very enjoyable. Influenza in California is about the same as in Wisconsin. In Los Angeles, there is a great deal of illness, and public places are closed. While the epidemic is not as great in Redlands, all schools, churches, and public places are closed.

Letter of condolence from Superintendent of the Yakima Indian Agency, Washington, Bureau of Indian Affairs.

October 29, 1918

Mrs. Grace Nye

Toppenish, Washington

My Dear Mrs. Nye.

During the scourge of Spanish Influenza from which your daughter Cecilia died, I was so extremely busy that it was impossible for me to tell you the particulars in connection with the death of Cecilia.

This plague attacked this school on the 13th of October. It was brought here at first by new students coming in, and it spread rapidly until we had about 250 cases. The entire school stopped its regular activities and devoted itself to absolutely to the care and nursing of the sick. Out of the 250 cases, we lost comparatively few. Among that number was your daughter. Absolutely everything possible was done in the way of medical care and nursing. The sick was never left alone for one minute, someone was administering to their needs and looking after them, and I want you to feel that in this sickness that your daughter had had as good attention as she possibly could have had in any hospital or home. I have spared neither expense nor time nor trouble. Altogether I feel that we have done just as well as could be done. This disease, which has taken thousands upon thousands throughout the country, was no worse here than elsewhere. It was no due to Chama or its location. It was a general disease everywhere.

Now that the plague is over, we have resumed our regular schoolwork. All of the students we have now are well and strong and getting along all right.

Trusting that Cecilia's body reached you in good shape and sympathizing with you, I am

Sincerely your friend,

Harwood Hall

Superintendent

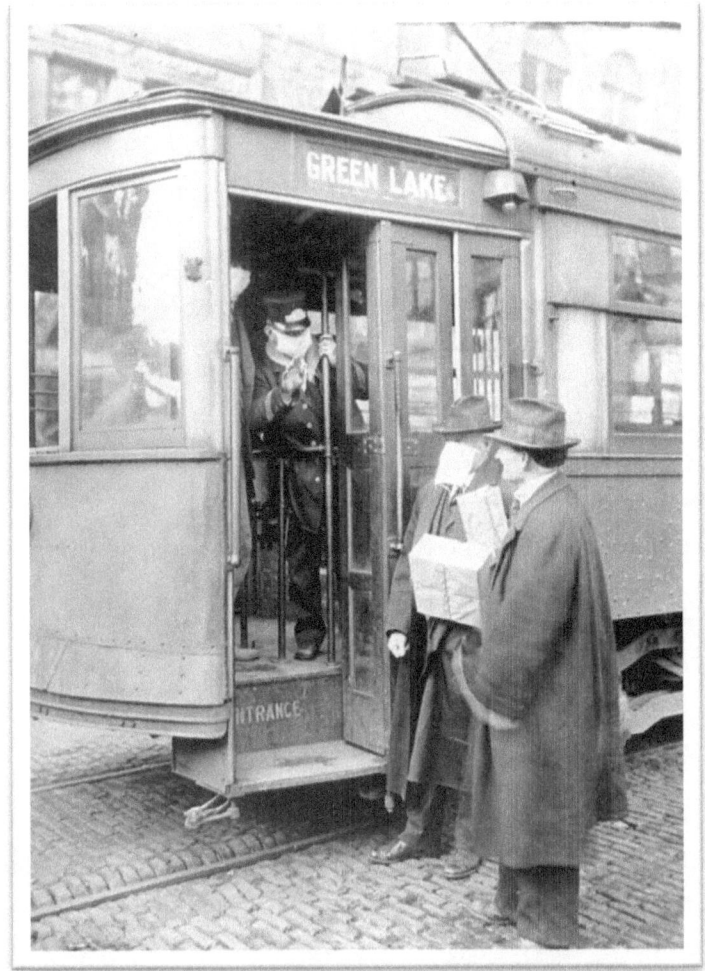

Streetcar conductor in Seattle, Washington, prevents rider without a mask from boarding in this 1918 photo. – *National Archives*

ARMY SURGEONS HAVE CURE FOR PNEUMONIA

Rogue River Courier – Grants Pass, Oregon

San Jose, Cal. (Oct. 31, 1918) – Headquarters at the base hospital Camp Fremont, today announced the discovery of a cure for pneumonia, which follows Spanish Influenza, and which has always been the fatal stage of the disease. The treatment consists of intravenous injections of coagulate and has been found, it was announced, to prevent hemorrhages of the lungs which characterize this new type of pneumonia.

INFLUENZA VACCINE READY FOR ALL U.S. SOLDIERS

Rogue River Courier

Washington, (Oct. 31, 1918) – The Surgeon General of the Army announced today that vaccination against pneumonia is available now for every officer, enlisted man, and civilian employee of the Army. The vaccine is said to have been proved to prevent pneumonia following influenza.

INFLUENZA CASES DECLINE
Pilot Boat Capt. Harry Shute Dead of Flu
THE REPUBLICAN JOURNAL

Belfast, Maine (Oct. 31, 1918)- Mrs. Carrie A. Gardner is recovering from an attack of influenza. Mrs. Ramsdall is with her at present, having been called here by the illness of Mr. Ramsdall, who was stricken with the prevailing distemper.

There are numerous cases of influenza in the outlying portions of the town, but in the village, it seems to be abating, though the newest victims are Mr. and Mrs. Pinkham and Mr. and Mrs. William Smith and Mrs. Ernest McLaughlin.

 Mr. John McLaughlin has recently purchased the house formerly owned by Capt. Isaac Lanpher, and will put it in thorough repair for the occupancy of his son Archie and family. This is a fine old place beautifully located on high ground with a fine view of the river.

We are fortunate to have a district nurse, Miss Towle of Augusta, in our village at present, sent by the State, who is doing effective work. There is also a special nurse attending to the needs of those connected with the Sandy Point shipyard, many of whom are ill.

Charles Foster arrived home on Thursday of last week, having been absent four months. He has been doing farm work in several towns, but for the past two weeks has been a victim of influenza in a hospital at Presque Isle. He expresses himself as having liked his work — "doing his bit."

Mrs. Alvah Treat of this place and her sister, Mrs. James Freeman of Winter port, returned to their respective homes on Thursday of last week, after having spent some time in the home of their sister, Mrs. J. F. Gerrity, in Bangor, where they were called by the illness and death of their beloved niece, Miss Helen Gerrity.

Mr. and Mrs. Eugene Shute of Boston and Mr. and Mrs. Elden Shute of Sagamore, Mass., arrived Monday to be present at the funeral services of their brother, **Capt. Harry D. Shute**, Oct. 22nd. Eugene and wife left for home the following Wednesday, and Elden and wife left on Monday morning's train. The funeral of Capt. Harry D. Shute took place on October 22nd at the home of his wife's mother, Mrs. A. C. Colcord. His death at his home in Rockland, Maine, was a shock to our community among whom he was a great favorite because of his genial ways and general good comradeship.

He was born in this town, October 20, 1883, the eldest son of Capt. and Mrs. Elden S. Shute and like his father followed the sea. He was united in marriage on January 23, 1911, with Miss Evelyn A. Colcord of this place, and to the happy young couple was born a son, Harry D. Jr., while living in Rockland, Maine, where they have made their home for the past six years.

For several years he was quartermaster and pilot on the Rockland and

Bar Harbor boats, finally rising to the captaincy of the J. P. Morse, the Monhegan, and the Mineola.

Attacked by the dread influenza, followed by pneumonia, the heart gave way, and the bright young life so full of promise slipped from the scenes of earth, into the fuller life beyond, leaving behind him a void which nothing can fill. He was a member of the Masonic order, and his brethren attended the funeral services in a body.

Rev. Ashley A. Smith of Bangor, our former pastor, spoke words of sympathy and comfort. The interment was in our village cemetery, and the profusion of flowers, among them a Masonic pillow, spoke mutely of the love and esteem of friends. May the good Father comfort the sorrowing wife and the bereaved members of his immediate family, parents, brothers, and sisters, in their loneliness. He was ever a most exemplary son, thoughtful and affectionate, and a most devoted husband and father.

 Those who were privileged to see him, in his own home, will ever remember the picture of his bright, young manhood.

They are not lost;

They are but gone before!

And we shall find them,

Waiting at the door.

Our community was for a second time deeply shocked by the death of another of our young townsmen, Mr. Edric A. Coleman, on the 22nd of October from influenza, followed by pneumonia. His devoted wife and little daughter, Ada, were attacked by the dread disease on the morning of the day on which he died and were taken to the home of her parents,

Mr. and Mrs. Levi Griffin, where they were ill in bed at the time of the funeral and unable to be present at the services in their own home, an unusually hard and distressing circumstance.

Mr. Coleman was born in Medway, Mass., January 29, 1884, the son of Frederick E. and Jennie Cummings Coleman. His mother was dying when he was but two years old, he was carefully reared by his maternal aunt, Miss Ida Cummings, in Medway. He married Miss Amy G. Griffin of this town, March 9, 190C, in Medfield, Mass., and one little daughter, Ada, came to bless their union. The young couple lived in Milford, Mass., until four years ago when they moved to this place, where he has since been employed in the sardine factory.

He was of a very home-loving nature, always giving closest attention to the needs of his family—a devoted husband and father. The loss to his wife is irreparable, and his genial smile and cordial and cheery words will long be missed by all his associates. He was a constant reader and always well informed upon topics of the day.

The funeral services were held at his late home on the afternoon of Oct. 24th, Rev. Harry Hully officiating. The beautiful flowers testified to the loving thought of family and friends. He leaves a bereaved widow and daughter and one sister, Mrs. Edgar Walton of Needham Heights, Mass., and one brother, Warren Coleman of Norwood, Mass., beside his aunt, Miss Ida Cummings, who through illness was prevented from being present for the funeral services.

"There is no Death!

What seems so is Transition!

The portal we call Death,

Is but the doorway to the Life Elysian!"

****

Mrs. Wallace F. Sprague has been assisting at the Waldo County Hospital during the rush occasioned by the influenza epidemic.

Sam Alexander of Camden, very well known in this city as the young Syrian lace vender, was one of the recent victims of influenza and died of pneumonia, which followed.

****

Murder Trial Canceled: Roy L. Pease Dead.
THE REPUBLICAN JOURNAL

Belfast, Maine (Oct. 31, 1918)

Last Thursday morning, a rumor reached Belfast that Roy L. Pease of Appleton had died in the Bangor Insane Hospital Wednesday night.

Sheriff Frank A. Cushman was not notified officially but called the hospital and learned that the young man had died of pneumonia following influenza. He was 28 years old and is survived by his two little sons, Maurice and Lloyd of North Searsmont. Pease had been in custody since May 11th as the alleged slayer of his wife, Ellen Cooper Pease of North Searsmont. He was indicted at the September term of the S. J. Court for Waldo County. Still, his trial was postponed to the January term at the request of Dr. Pearl T. Haskell of the hospital, who was not ready to report regarding his condition.

POOR'S MILLS.

The school commenced Monday again, but some of the children still have bad colds.

Mrs. Richard Merriam, who was a nurse in the Waldo County hospital and came home on account of sickness, is still quite poorly.

Mrs. Lester Wilson is at Dr. Wilson's taking care of her daughter Hazel, who is just recovering from pneumonia.

It has come to the knowledge of the Public Safety Organization that, even though the epidemic of Spanish influenza is on the wane here in Belfast, there is a lot of sickness throughout the county. In many places, nurses are needed very much. If all those in the county who are willing to volunteer as nurses will kindly send their names to the Public Safety office, we will register their names, and have them registered with the Public Safety office at Augusta. If those who require nurses will communicate with us, we will endeavor from our list to furnish nurses that are registered with the Augusta office.

The nurses are entitled to have their traveling expenses paid and will be paid the regular trained nurses' wages.

It is the desire of the Public Safety Organization to cooperate with the people, and by this arrangement, we believe we can be of very material assistance.

The influenza epidemic has rapidly decreased in town, and we are glad to see those who have been seriously ill able to be out of doors again.

NEW ENGLAND NEWS IN TABLOID FORM
Items of interest from all Sections of Yankeeland

FORMER CONGRESSMAN DEAD OF FLU
THE OXFORD DEMOCRAT

Paris, Maine - (Oct. 31,1918) – **Postmaster William Murray** died at the Boston City Hospital of pneumonia Saturday night, the result of an attack of the grippe. He was one of the youngest men ever elected to Congress and one of the youngest postmasters Boston ever had. He was scarcely 30 years of age when he entered Congress and but turning 36 when he died. His views on National problems were eagerly sought by leaders in National affairs.

Dr. H. A. Hands of, North Cambridge, was stricken ill and died before medical attendance could reach him while administering to a patient In West Somerville.

Patrick J. Griffin, a centenarian on March 18, the oldest resident of Burlington, Vt, was found dead in his bed at the home of his son, John S. Griffin. He formerly resided in Hartford, Conn

Arrest Made for Defaming President, Old Glory and the USA

Peter Rugis was arrested In Lawrence and held for the federal authorities on a charge of making remarks defaming President Wilson, the American flag, and the United States government.

Jobs Moved Due to Labor Strife

It is reported that the Rockville, Ct. branch of the Daniels Manufacturing Company has been closed. Labor difficulties are said to have arisen, which have forced the management to move the machinery to the plant in East Brookfield, Mass.

Disloyal Charges against Minister Dropped

The Rev. John Steik, the former pastor of the Lettish Lutheran Church in Roxbury, who was arrested a few weeks ago on the charge of making disloyal remarks, was discharged from custody by United States Commissioner Hayes for lack of evidence.

Big Haul of Moonshiners

Sixteen men, arrested in Fall River and Dighton by federal officers in the biggest haul of men alleged to have been in the business of manufacturing whiskey in this section of the country, were arraigned before U.S. Commissioner A. McF. Goodspeed. All were held on $1,000 bonds.

Mr. and Mrs. E. N. Anderson received word last Monday afternoon that their son, Harold C. Anderson, and daughter were sick with Spanish influenza. They left on the early train Tuesday, arriving in Wollaston a little past one o'clock. The disease developed double pneumonia. He has passed the crisis and is improving. Little Helen bad a light attack and is improving though still confined to her bed. Everything is closed there, even the churches.

Mrs. Hannah Whitney of Concord, Vt., came on Wednesday, Sept. 18, to visit her brother, J. B. Barnett of Hill Street. At noon on Thursday, she suffered a stroke of apoplexy and died the following day. The remains were taken to Concord, where she had made her home with her daughter. Mrs. Whitney was a few days less than 82 years of age. She was the widow of Frank Whitney; she leaves two daughters. She was the oldest of a family of nine children, of whom only two remain, J. B. Barnett of this place and another brother who lives in South Dakota.

The streetcar of the Norway and Paris railway is not yet out of commission, nor will it be on Tuesday as had been expected. According to the latest in instructions from headquarters, it will run at least until Thursday, possibly longer.

When its service la discontinued, a passenger service will be started by the Norway and Paris Transfer Co., in which Carl P. Dunham and Alton C. Maxim are associated. They expect to run their truck hourly trip·, probably leaving South Paris at a quarter before the hour and Norway on the hour, though the schedule is not definitely fixed set yet.

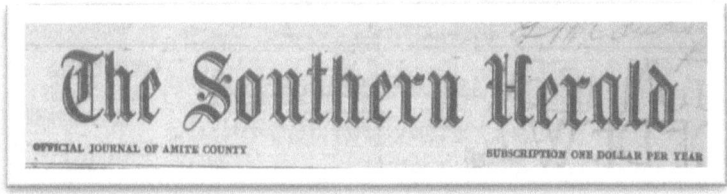

THE SOUTHERN HERALD

Liberty, Mississippi (Nov. 1, 1918) – For three weeks, this town and Bolivar county have been in the throes of the worst epidemic that ever visited the county. Thousands of people have been attacked by the malady, and many have died, while others have been left weakened and physically u fit for work for some time to come.

Jackson. Glass containers for soda fountain beverages are doomed in Mississippi. The executive committee of the state board of health passed an order placing these containers under the ban, the ruling to go into effect within 30 days. Paper containers are suggested. A temporary rule to this effect Is at present being enforced all over the state to aid In checking the Influenza epidemic. The board further ruled that where coffee or other hot drinks were served by soda fountains, all vessels used must be thoroughly sterilized, and silverware gave the same treatment—failure to meet these requirements subject one to fine or Imprisonment.

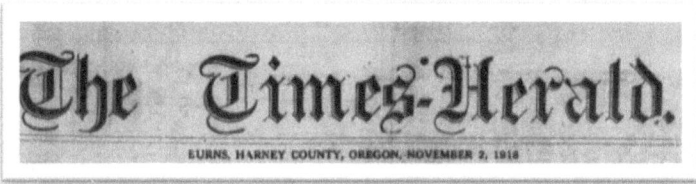

The Times-Herald.

BURNS, HARNEY COUNTY, OREGON, NOVEMBER 2, 1918

QUARANTINE RAISED ON ADVICE HEALTH DOCTOR

~~~

Representative of State Health Board Finds Cases of Spanish Influenza in City and Confers With Doctors and Authorities.

Burns, Harney County, Oregon (Nov. 2, 1918) – On the advice of medical men, the city dads of Bums placed a strict quarantine in effect last Tuesday against the outside because of the epidemic of influenza. This worked quite a hardship on the people of the community who were inside the city as well as those outsides. It took the time of the City Marshal McDonald with several helpers to guard the entrances to town and see the people of the country were supplied with what they wanted from the business houses of this city.

The action of the authorities had the approval of the citizens with, but few exceptions and each one tried to aid in every way possible. At the time the quarantine went into effect, it was not known that Burns had a case of Spanish Influenza, and It was the hope that It might be kept out until the epidemic had subsided and the danger of its spread less.

Yesterday Mayor Mothershead telephoned to the representative of the State Board of Health, Dr. Douglass, who was at Crane, asking that he come to Burns and consult with local physicians in the matter and observe some suspected cases.

Accordingly, Dr. Douglass came up and in company with Dr. Smith visited one or more cases and, at a meeting with the city council, later announced that there were cases of influenza in Burns and advised that since the epidemic was already here, the quarantine was of little avail.

He advised that it be raised but to keep patients and Inmates of the homes where influenza has already appeared. Consequently, this was followed by the city dads after consulting with Dr. Douglass, who has had experience with the epidemic.

Dr. Douglass thought that this section would witness an epidemic as it now had such a hold and was in several places, and under the circumstances, he suggested that we prepare to combat the disease.

The Times Herald has had no opportunity to Interview Dr. Smith since the state man was here as he is about the busiest man in all of this part of the country. Therefore It does not really know how many cases have been reported definitely. Dr. Douglass strongly recommended vaccination and sent up 500 doses from Crane this morning and wired for 1500 more to follow. As a consequence, Dr. Smith's office resembles the front of a popular theatre just at opening time, as his front yard and the street in front of his office, is filled with people waiting to "get scratched."

Three more deaths have occurred at Crane since our last Issue from Influenza and other cases have developed, but according to information, the situation there Is much Improved. Dr. J. W. Geary has been constantly on the job at Crane since early in the week and has had the assistance of the State Health Doctor and a Red Cross nurse.

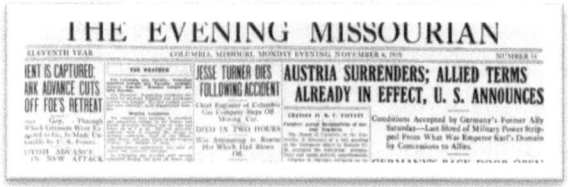

TWO MORE DEATHS
Influenza Takes James H. Chick
And Miss Mary Ellen Prather.

THE EVENING MISSOURIAN

Columbian, Missouri (Nov. 4, 1918) – James H. Chick, 60 years old, died of Spanish influenza on his farm about six miles northwest of Columbia yesterday and was buried today at Providence cemetery.

Miss Mary Ellen Prather, 70 years old, died of Spanish influenza this morning at the county infirmary.

Since last Friday, 47 new cases of Spanish influenza and five new cases of pneumonia were reported by physicians for Columbia and vicinity.

Three influenza patients were admitted at the City Emergency Hospital yesterday, all members of the same family. One patient was discharged.

INFLUENZA BAN LIFTS
TOMORROW AFTER 5 WEEKS
Local Situation is Reported
Much Improved Over the Weekend

HARRISBURG TELEGRAPH

Harrisburg, Penn. (Nov. 4, 1918) – All restrictions in force In Harrisburg for the last month as quarantine measures by the State Department of Health and City Health Bureau to check the influenza epidemic will be lifted at noon tomorrow. The local authorities were announcing today that the local situation has improved greatly over the weekend and that from present indications, there will be no danger in raising the ban.

Saloons, however, will not be permitted to open as tomorrow is election day, and state law requires them to remain close then. All other business places, including theaters, soda fountains, poolrooms, will reopen, and some of the private schools also will resume sessions.

The public schools will reopen next Monday and the Harrisburg Academy on Wednesday morning of this week.

Dr. J. M. J. Raunick, City health Officer, said today he was well pleased with the local situation and appreciated the continued cooperation of the public until the ban is lifted.

"Tell the people that afternoon tomorrow there will be absolutely no restrictions on anything in the city. Every place of business and all schools may open, and public meetings or gatherings of any nature will be permitted. There Is no need to communicate with health authorities about anything which is planned for any time afternoon tomorrow.

"At the emergency hospital, Fifth and Seneca streets, there are twenty-six patients yet, and with the city school teachers leaving today for a week's rest, there is an urgent need for assistants until the place is closed. The. teachers who came to the hospital and volunteered their services have been a great help."

Samuel Adley, aged 46, Grantville, R. D. 2, died at the hospital last night. He was brought there a few days ago from his home In Fishing Greek Valley. Two of his children died at home, and two more are in the hospital in a serious condition.

Five deaths from influenza were reported today by the local bureau of vital statistics, and five more from the disease yesterday. There have been no deaths from pneumonia reported.

On Saturday evening, merchants and other businessmen in the city cooperated with the health bureau and closed promptly at 6.30 o'clock. It was the fourth Saturday night that the stores were closed, only druggists and restaurant proprietors being permitted to remain open. Churches and Sunday schools also were not permitted to bold services. They will resume next Sunday again, after being closed for five weeks.

Reports from the Lykens Valley, Hershey, and other sections of Dauphin County not Included in the order raising the ban in Dauphin. York, Lancaster, and other counties tomorrow are so encouraging that the State Department of Health will likely issue an order very soon freeing those districts. The Emergency Hospital in the Lykens Valley mining region is being closed.

State Policemen, reserve Militiamen, doctors, and nurses have been dispatched to the Farview state institution where reports show 126 persons sick with Influenza, Including a number of the guards.

A well-defined case of smallpox at Grantville, Dauphin County, has been reported to the State Department of Health.

The case Is that of Fay E. Shertzer, eleven years old, who has been ill since October 23, 1918. The case traces back to three other cases in the house of Harry Hedrich, a farmer residing near Grantville, Penn. Dr. C. R. Phillips made a careful investigation of the case yesterday and vaccinated a large number of persons in that vicinity of Dauphin County. It is possible that cases may have extended into Lebanon County.

The Manchester Journal.

VACCINE PROVED EFFECTIVE IN LARGE TEST
THE MANCHESTER JOURNAL

Manchester, Vermont (Nov. 14, 1918) – Pneumonia preventing serum has been adopted by the army surgeons after experiments conducted in the Army medical school in Washington.

The first of the new serum has been received by the Boston army medical department. It is being administered to volunteers by Maj. Arthur E. Austin, attending surgeon at the Northeastern department headquarters. Experiments were made a short time ago to test the merits of the new serum. Two detachments of 10,000 soldiers were selected. One detachment was inoculated, and the other was not. The subsequent developments showed that in the detachment where the men had been given the vaccine, not a single case of pneumonia developed. At the same time, in the other division, there were numerous cases of the disease.

NEW TRIAL GRANTED KILLER DUE TO JURY BET

Manchester, Vermont (Nov. 14, 1918) – Because a wager was placed on the outcome of a murder trial by a member of the Jury before he was drawn on the panel, the Vermont Supreme Court has awarded a new trial to Robert Warren of St. Albans, found guilty last year of the murder of Jennie Hemingway. Warren was a soldier at Fort Ethan Allen at the time of his arrest and was tried in Franklin County.

FLU OVER, PRAISE THE DOCTORS
ST. MARY'S BEACON

Leonardtown, Md. (Nov. 14, 1918) – At last, the county has been freed from the epidemic of influenza. All praise to the doctors, to whose unceasing labors so many of our people owe their lives.

Joseph Xavier Thompson Dies at Camp Meade
ST. MARY'S BEACON

LEONARDTOWN, MD. (Nov. 14, 1918) – Joseph Xavier Thompson, son of Mr. and Mrs. John L. Thompson, of near Laurel Grove, died at Camp Meade of pneumonia on Sunday, October 20, 1918, in the 22nd year of his age.

His remains were brought to St. Mary's and laid to rest beneath the grand old Stars and Stripes in St. Joseph's New Cemetery, Thursday, October 24th.

Warren Ellis Died of Flu
Word was received on Sunday of the death of Warren Ellis of St. Patrick's Creek. Influenza, followed by pneumonia, was the cause of death.

Gave Up His Life for Liberty
Leonardtown, Md. (Nov. 14, 1918) – In the casualty list of Aug. 26, 2018, under the caption, "Died of Wound," is the name of **James Archibald Pilkerton**, of Mechanicsville, this county, the first St. Mary's Countian to make the supreme sacrifice "somewhere in France, on account of wounds received in the line of duty.

James Archibald Pilkerton was born at Mechanicsville on November 19th, 1895, and was in his twenty-third year, the son of Mr. and Mrs. James R. Pilkerton. He was a most dutiful and devoted home-loving son. Promptly answering the call of his country, he presented himself for registration on June 5, 1917, and just four months later, on October 5, he was inducted into the military service. Reporting at Camp Meade, he was assigned to Battery E 310th Field Artillery. After spending the winter training, he was sent to France early in the spring of this year.

His death is a great shock not only to his family and personal friends but to every loyal citizen of this country. We cannot help feeling a deeper and closer interest in the war when we realize that the life of one of our most exemplary young me has been sacrificed to the greed of Prussianism.

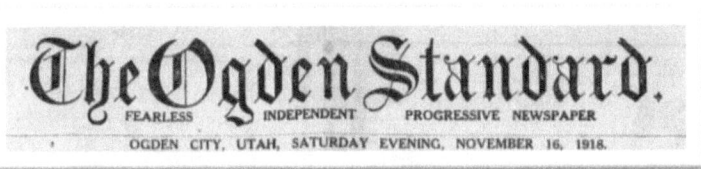

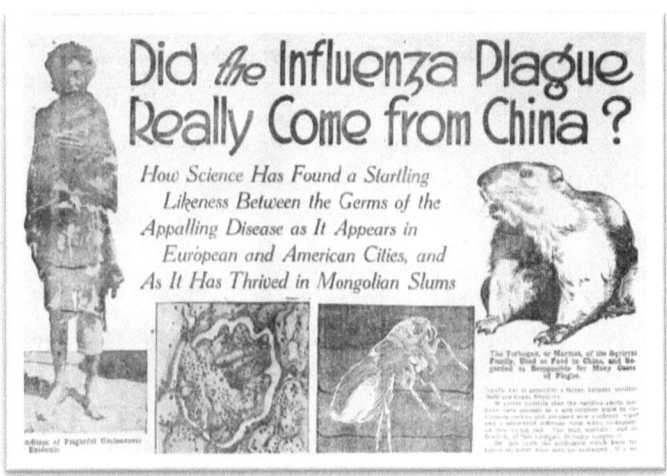

HOW SCIENCE HAS FOUND A STARTLING LIKENESS BETWEEN THE GERMS OF THE APPALLING DISEASE AS IT APPEARS IN EUROPEAN AND AMERICAN CITIES, AND AS IT HAS THRIVED IN MONGOLIAN SLUMS

BY JAMES JOSEPH KING, A. B., M.D
Captain, U. S. Army Medical Corps

THE OGDEN STANDARD

Ogden City, Utah (Nov. 16, 1918) – A COMPARISON of the epidemic of the disease known "Spanish Influenza," with the epidemic of pneumonic plague that broke out in Harbin, China, in October 1910, and spread continuously throughout northern China at the time, reveals so many points of similarity as strongly to suggest that the disease which became epidemic this fall may be the same malady, but modified by racial and topographical differences that ravaged northern China eight years ago. The origin of the influenza plague was suggested to the writer soon after its outbreak in our camps, by Mr. Guy M. Walker, an eminent American authority on Chinese affairs. This suggestion led to an investigation of the reports of the pneumonic plague in China, and there is sufficient likeness of that disease to the so-called Spanish Influenza as to warrant consideration of it.

Pneumonia in Harbin

The pneumonic plague first appeared in Harbin, a town in Manchuria under Chinese control.

Harbin is on the Trans-Siberian Railroad and was the original hotbed of the disease. The plague had prevailed in Russia, previous to November 1910, but the Russians, alert to Its danger, took immediate action and stamped it out. It was believed that the Plague was carried into Harbin by the fur dealers, the furs themselves, and by Chinese laborers returning to their homes to celebrate New Year's Day, a custom universally observed In China. From Harbin, the plague rapidly spread in all directions, usually following the lines of traffic along the railroads.

It spread as far south as Chelu, a seaport town, probably having been carried there by Chinese coolies returning from the north.

By Jan. 24, 1911, 1500 Chinese and 27 Europeans, two of whom were physicians, and an assistant had died of it; in fact, nearly all who had the disease perished of it.

The Spread in China

The plague had been profoundly serious, the mortality being fearfully high. This malady has spread throughout China. Wherever Chinese coolies from the north have traveled, they have carried this disease. From 1910 up to 1917, China has not been free from it. The writer heard of several cases being present in Peking last year.

 In the early part of 1917, about 200,000 Chinese coolies collected from the northern part of China, where the pneumonic plague has raged at intervals since 1910, were sent to France as laborers. Part of them was sent around through the Mediterranean; some, and perhaps the majority, were sent across the Pacific and then through Canada and America to be transported across the Atlantic to France. Entire trainloads of these coolies were carried across the United States to the port of New York and thence to France.

The photograph showing the boatloads of the coolies at Weiheiwei ready for embarkation to France via Pacific, Canada, America, and Atlantic were taken by Mr. L. P. Frieder.

Coolies Carrying the Plague

The coolies made splendid laborers in France and were in the back of the lines during the German drive of March 1918. No doubt, many of them were captured by the Germans at that time. Hence the outbreak of the disease In the German army and its rapid spread to Spain.

So far as medical science knows today, this disease first broke out last spring in the German army, where it was said to have been very serious. Next, it was heard of in Spain, hence the name Spanish Influenza. The name is really a misnomer, but it has stuck, probably because it was the first epidemic of influenza that Spain ever had.

Since our soldiers and sailors have been returning from the battlefields of France, it has become very prevalent and serious in our camps and cities all over the country.

After this brief review of the pneumonic plague and the narration of its possible connection with the present epidemic, it is of interest to compare the clinical and bacteriological malady.

The Symptoms in China

It is not necessary here to go into concerning the clinical data except in a very general way. In the Chinese epidemic, there were few definite symptoms at the outset of the disease except the general malaise, prostration, loss of appetite, often soon to be followed by the pneumonic process and death. So, it is in the present epidemic. There have been indefinite symptoms with great prostration rapidly followed by pneumonia and death in the most virulent forms. The outstanding features of the Chinese pneumonic plague were its high inactivity and high mortality. So, this so-called influenza epidemic, which is more contagious, is followed more frequently by pneumonia and attended with higher mortality than in any previous influenza epidemic.

In the pneumonic plague epidemic of China, the bacillus pestis was almost constantly found associated with the pneumococcus and the streptococcus. These organisms were found in different localities where the plague was prevalent.

The virulence of the disease likewise varied. For instance, Dr. Shibayama made a report on eight different strains of pneumonic plague organisms before the International Plague Conference held in Mukden in April 1911.

The bacteria found in patients in the influenza epidemic have been the Influenza bacillus associated with the four groups of pneumococci, the streptococcus hemolyticus, and the micrococcus cararralo. For instance, in one camp the organisms found wore, the influenza bacillus associated with group 1 pneumococcus in another it was the influenza bacillus associated with group 3 pneumococci in another influenza and streptococcus

We see, therefore, how different strains of pneumococcus and strep associated with a bacillus were the exciting cause of the epidemic in different localities. Likewise, the mortally and virulence of the has varied in different localities.

The similarity in the Two Plagues

Thus, we have shown a striking similarity between the pneumonic plague of north China and the so-called Spanish influenza epidemic. It is not unreasonable to believe that the two diseases may be the same. The influenza bacillus and the bacillus pestis in atypical forms may simulate each other. We know that organisms may assume different forms and have different cultural characteristics under different conditions.

The ordinary influenza bacillus is a short slender bacillus. The bacillus pestis is about the same length but Is generally a fatter, broader bacillus. Both are Gram-Negative.

It seems possible that the bacillus pestis may have been present in a non-virulent state in the Chinese coolies and assumed new virulence, vigor, and a somewhat different form when transplanted into virgin soil. The high mortality and infectivity of this epidemic strongly suggest it.

On this basis, the epidemics which have followed all great wars may be explained. If a nation or tribe can survive any disease long enough, it will acquire immunity to that disease. When, however, foreign people comingle freely and intimately as in war, the epidemic will break out. The inactive, non-virulent organisms in one race will become virulent in some other race, which has not acquired Immunity to that specific organism.

~~~~

Vaccine for the Plague
By Dr. Leonard Keene Hirshberg
THE OGDEN STANDARD

Ogden, Utah (Nov. 16, 1918) – The successful work of American physicians in applying preventive measures against the plague gives great interest to the following statement by Dr. Leonard Keene Hirshberg:

Once the germ was brought to light, isolated, and cultivated by itself, the doctors in several American army camps at once set to work to boil and bottle the dead microbes as a vaccine.

The new vaccine – sometimes absurdly called a serum – is nearly a complete and positive preventive of Spanish influenza and its complications.

So successful has its use as a preventive inoculation been proved that since the first day it was introduced on a large-scale Sept. 28, 1918, when 51,117 new victims were reported, there has been a steady decline in the number of soldiers and civilians affected.

The use of the vaccine will be widely extended since Congress appropriated 1 million dollars to be used by the public health service in fighting this communicable disease.

The public health service, aided by the medical forces of the army and navy, took steps to render effective aid to all districts in which influenza made its appearance.

The vaccine has been used in several camps, but no announcement had been made of its discovery pending the results of widespread tests. Physicians connected with the army medical school developed the vaccine, which was manufactured in quantities sufficient to provide for the treatment of 50,000 persons daily. The vaccine is designed primarily for pneumonia, which often follows attacks of influenza and which is the cause of practically all the deaths attributed to influenza.

One treatment with the vaccine only is needed, although, in the early stages of its development, three vaccinations were found necessary.

There are a number of vaccines now employed successfully in army and navy cantonments. It is a pathetic reflection upon so-called "human intelligence" that is necessary to have the military discipline to prevent people from getting typhoid, dysentery, meningitis, influenza, and pneumonia.

COURT ADJOURNED UNTIL MARCH 17

Jurors Notified Not to Appear for the Fall Term Next Week

WARREN SHEAF

Warren, Minnesota (Nov. 20, 1918) – Owing to the prevalence of Spanish Influenza in many localities throughout the county, Judge Grindeland has found it advisable to adjourn the fall term of the district court, which should have convened here last week, until March 17, 1919. Both grand and petit jurors have been notified not to appear next week. In view of the further fact, also, that there is no pressing litigation that requires immediate attention, the adjournment is a wise move for the safeguarding of the public health.

INFLUENZA CASES CONTINUE TO DECREASE AND PEOPLE ARE RUSHING TO GET MASKS

THE OGDEN STANDARD

Ogden, Utah (Nov. 30, 1918) – The doctors report for Thursday and Friday of this week made to the city health board, respecting the epidemic of Influenza, Is to the effect that on two days there was a total of 103 new cases. This shows a decrease from 64 reported on Wednesday, proving, says Mr. Shorten, that the rigid quarantine, the wearing of masks, the avoidance of crowds, and that the health rules generally are being well obeyed by the people at large.

"We shall have to remind one or two people that we mean business in this matter, though. There is a notion that the rules and regulations may still be regarded as a joke, but surely when people read of the decrease in the number of cases, they will be bound to admit that the experiment is well worthwhile."

The long looked for vaccine arrived from Salt Lake this morning just in time to save Mr. Shorten a journey to the capital city in quest of it. Dr. Brown, the city health physician, will administer the vaccine to any who cares to have it. His hours will be from 10 a. m. to 4 p. m. The treatment calls for three applications at an Interval of forty-eight hours. The vaccine is highly spoken of by medical authorities.

The difficulty of procuring enough masks to satisfy the public demand was again evident this morning. Although ladies of the Red Cross turned over to the city board another four hundred masks Friday afternoon, the masks were quickly called for. Every energy Is being turned on to meet the demand.

Inspector Shorten expressed himself as bitterly disappointed with the action of the school board, who last night, at their joint meeting with the new emergency hospital committee, turned down the proposal made to the afternoon meeting in their name by Henry C. Johnson, superintendent of public schools.

"The high school would have been an ideal place," says Mr. Shorten, "for the kind of hospital we need and which, in the opinion of Dr. Harrison and Dr. McGuilicudy, would have aided us in downing the epidemic. We will have to look round again to find another place, though."

Since *The Standard* went to press yesterday, there have been reported the following deaths:

Rebecca Matthews, who died at 8:40 this morning; Albert Scowcroft, who died at 11:15 last night.

~~~~

REBECCA MATTHEWS IS A VICTIM OF INFLUENZA

Ogden, Utah (Nov. 30, 1918) – Rebecca Matthews, 20, wife of Charles Matthews and daughter of Mr. and Mrs. Alexander C. Yarrington of 516 Twenty-first street, died this morning at 8:40 of influenza-pneumonia.

She is survived by her parents and one brother, Herbert, who is with the U. S. forces in France, one sister, Mrs. Ruth Greenwell who lives in Wyoming, and the following uncles: R. W. Yarrington, Robert T. Yarrington, David C. Yarrington all of Ogden and employed with her father in the S. P. shops, and Guy Yarrington who Is a machinist on the Southern Pacific system in California,

The husband Is now down with influenza. The funeral arrangements will be announced later.

SERGEANT O'BRIEN

W. S. O'Brien, Sr., manager of the Postal Telegraph Company, received advice today from his son William S. O'Brien, Jr., a member of Battery E,146th field artillery, announcing he had been promoted to sergeant. Sergeant O'Brien is one of the authors of the book of Camp Kearny poems, which are highly prized by the members of the families of the boys in the Utah organization.

OGDEN CAN KEEP DOWN INFLUENZA

Dr. W. S. Harrison, assistant surgeon U. S. Public Health Service, will leave Ogden for his home in San Francisco at 2 p. m. today. The doctor said:

"If Ogden will only go whole-heartedly into the matter of another well-equipped and fairly large emergency hospital, there is no doubt that, with the rigid quarantine and wearing of masks that have already been put into effect, the city will make a record in the combatting of the epidemic. No city of its size in the United States has a better opportunity or greater power to put it into effect."

Dr. Harrison said he had enjoyed his stay here, and that nothing but his own poor health would have caused him to go home so soon.

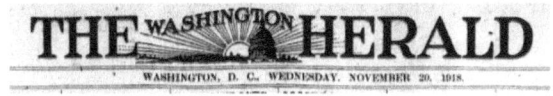

WASHINGTON, D. C., WEDNESDAY, NOVEMBER 20, 1918.

By Nov. 20, 1918, the Armistice had been declared ending the World War. The front page of the Washington Herald did not have a single news story about the Spanish Influenza. The following article was a paid opinion piece published by the *Herald* on page three:

INFLUENZA, EPIDEMICS, AND VACCINATION

THE WASHINGTON HERALD
Washington, D.C. (Nov. 20, 1918)

By Chas. M. Higgins, Brooklyn, New York

Vaccination a proven cause of epidemic and a possible or partial cause of the present epidemic of influenza and pneumonia.

Request to the U.S. War Department to suspend all army vaccination during the epidemics and to make all vaccinations wholly voluntary, as is now the case in the English army.

Congress and the Government should investigate all vaccine factories as a possible and proved source of epidemics.

HON. NEWTON D. BAKER, SECRETARY OF WAR, WAR DEPARTMENT, WASHINGTON, D.C.

Dear Sir: As a lifelong student of the nature and effects of vaccination and its relation to public health, and as an American citizen interested in the best welfare of our soldiers and citizens, please permit me to suggest that your department might now very properly direct that all army vaccination should be suspended during the present epidemic of

355

influenza and pneumonia which is now prevailing in a different part of the country causing many deaths.

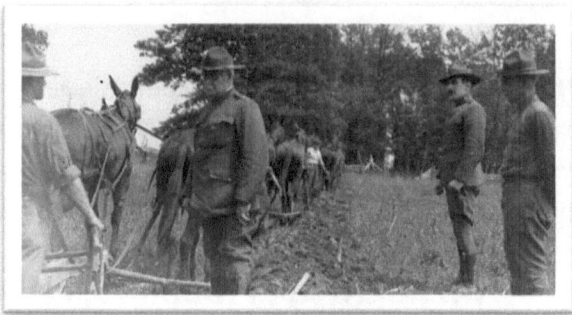

Gen. Hugh L. Scott at Camp Dix in 1918. Harris & Ewing

Medical Authority Forbids Vaccination During Epidemics and Opposes Compulsion.

The highest medical authorities, even the strongest pro-vaccinators, advise the suspension of all vaccination during epidemics of contagious diseases.

See Osler's Modern Medicine, edition of 1913, Vol. 1, pages 847 and 848.

This recent work of high authority also condemns all compulsory vaccination and admits its dangers as follows: After advising against all vaccination during epidemics of dangerous diseases, it states:

"With the greatest care, however, certain risks are present, and so it is unwise for the physician to force the operation on those who are unwilling or to give assurance of absolute harmlessness."

There is some suspicion now existing that the multiple and widespread vaccinations of different kinds to which the soldiers have been subjected for some time past in the several camps throughout the country may be a cause, or at least a condition of the present epidemic, which may favor its spread, for, as a matter of fact, it has spread more severely in these camps, particularly in New England and more especially in Massachusetts, where the epidemic seems to be the most fatal. The great number of cases occurring in the Massachusetts camps and at Camp Dix, in New Jersey, with the big mortality 25 percent, seems to show that whatever the disease truly is – it is surely, in its worst types a very dangerous and fatal Infection and calls for the most serious and careful precautions, one of these being the suspension of all infecting operations, like vaccination, while such a dangerous epidemic exists.

Grave Nature of Present Epidemic

From the rapidity, severity, and mortality of the disease it would seem not to be true influenza, as heretofore known, and as its worst cases are characterized by a rapid and fatal ending, sometimes with a few days sicknesses, in malignant or septic pneumonia, with abscesses in the lungs. It seems more related to the very fatal "Pneumonic plague," which raged in Manchuria after the Japanese war. This suspicion is strengthened by the fact, just reported in the newspapers, that the chief germ found in the fatal cases is the "streptococcus" which is found in the worst forms of "blood poisoning" or "septicemia" and also in vaccination. Now the act of ordinary vaccination is, in itself, an act of blood poisoning, pure and simple, and It is so classed in medical and statistical works as a form of "septicemia." and one disease germ commonly found, with many others, in vaccine virus is the streptococcus, which is the chief germ found in all bad pus infections and abscess formations.

See Manual of Causes of Death. U. S. Census Bureau. 1913, page 56. No. 20.

Therefore, as the act of vaccination simply the impregnation of the body and blood with a pus infection identical with "septicemia" or "pyemia," and as this infecting process is repeated at wholesale in the bodies of thousands and tens of thousands of men closely massed in camps, should it be any wonder if an epidemic of some sort of "septicemia" should crop out at some time under such conditions?

Possible Relation of Vaccination to Present Epidemic.

In leading medical and statistical works both influenza and Pneumonia and typhoid fever and vaccination are all classed as a different form of "septicemia," and while I do not of course know, and do not say, that the present epidemic of influenza and pneumonia is actually caused by vaccination, yet, I repeat that when the body and blood of millions of men all over this country.

Europe is deliberately impregnated with various septic diseases or septicemic infections, can any reasonable person, whether doctor or layman, be surprised if such world-wide. Million times repeated, acts of septicemic infection should ultimately be proved to have some causative or conditional relation to the present world-wide epidemic of septicemic disease?

Is it physically or medically possible to go on sowing and to spread some multi-diseases, at wholesale, within human bodies, without reaping some wild diseases at retail?

It has been suggested that this epidemic originated in the multi-vaccinated and diseased or impoverished German army and has traveled one quarter around the earth from that focus of infection.

Great Danger of Vaccination During Epidemics.

It is, of course, very difficult to prove or determine the real cause or origin of any epidemic disease, and aa a matter of fact, with few exceptions, these diseases are a mystery to the medical profession, and very little is as yet known about them. It Is known, however, that ordinary vaccination is very dangerous during epidemics and should be stopped. In contrast, the epidemic exists because what is called double or "mixed" infections are very dangerous and very likely to be fatal in the final effect.

> *See Osier's Modern Medicine. Vol. 1. pages 32 and 33.*

For example. If the infection of pneumonia entered the system at the same time when it was struggling with the vaccine infection, it would be almost sure to kill, particularly the severe type of septic poisoning now prevailing.

Hence the medical and hygienic wisdom of suspending all septic infecting operations, like vaccination, while any epidemic condition exists and also the wisdom of now making all vaccination voluntary, instead of compulsory, as advised by the high medical authority quoted and by the present example of the English army.

Logical aid Medical Relation Between Influenza and Vaccination.

Another Interesting: point in this connection is the actual relation between influenza and the two closely related diseases of vaccination and smallpox. Of course, you know that vaccination and smallpox are simply varieties of the same disease and that modern vaccine virus originates directly from human smallpox, which is transplanted to the cow and thence used from the cow on the human body, instead of being taken directly from some natural or inoculated disease of the cow, called "cowpox" as in the original vaccination of Jenner, which was taken from the cow directly to the human arm and thence from arm to arm – a form of vaccination which was long ago given up and prohibited as most dangerous to human health and life.

You must also know that smallpox is a very "various" disease and that this is the probable reason for its Latin name, "Variola," because it exists in so many forms of "variations." One of these varieties is a puzzling and misleading form, without eruption, which is almost identical with influenza, so that one disease can be, and often is, mistaken for the other. In fact, true smallpox might be described simply as influenza with the eruption and mild smallpox or vaccination as influenza without eruption!

This, you will see, establishes a logical and medical relation between vaccination and influenza and further strengthens the suspicions stated that the present epidemic of influenza and septicemia or septic pneumonia may have some causative relation to the extensive wholesale and repeated vaccinations in the military camps throughout the world and would indicate that this vaccine infection was now escaping from and overflowing its usual bounds and running wild as a world-wide epidemic infection; and hence the positive and compelling reasons for now checking this overflowing infection by suspending all further vaccination while this epidemic and infecting condition exist.

Influenza Vaccination and Smallpox on the USS Ohio.

To show that the relation above outlined, between influenza, variola land vaccination, is no mere fancy, let me cite the instance of influenza and smallpox epidemics in the vaccinated crew of the U. S. Battleship *Ohio* in December 1913, as taken from the U. S. Naval Medical Bulletin of October 1914. Here I think you will find a most interesting confirmation of this point, as follows:

"Coincident with the outbreak of smallpox on the *Ohio,* an epidemic of influenza was present and had been for several days. The Initial symptoms of both diseases are so similar that until the eruption appears in smallpox, it is impossible always to differentiate between the two, and, indeed, it is possible that some of the cases classed as influenza may have been smallpox without eruption."

In this epidemic of influenza and smallpox in the generally vaccinated crew of the battleship, there were twenty-nine cases of smallpox and five deaths, which is rather high mortality of nearly twenty percent and shows that general vaccination, to say the least, is not such a very infallible preventive of smallpox as vaccinators claim it to be, and this is another very good reason why compulsory vaccination should not be forced on any person.

Epidemic Actually Caused by Vaccination.

That the hypothetical condition suggested in a preceding paragraph that the wholesale and worldwide vaccine Infection going on for the past few years has possibly now escaped from its usual bounds and is now overflowing and running wild and thus causing epidemics in mankind or animals: that this, I say maybe no mere hypothesis or theory, but rather a hard fact, is proved by the frightful epidemics of "foot and mouth disease" In the United States in 1902, 1908 and 1914, which originated from two of the largest vaccine factories in this country – one in Philadelphia and the other In Detroit – and was widely distributed to cattle and mankind in several of our States.

> *See reports of U. S. Bureau of Animal Industry. 1903 and 1908.*
> *Also, Yearbook of U.S. Dept. of Agriculture, 1914, page 30*

It is clearly shown in these reports that vaccine infection was the direct cause of these epidemics 1902 and 1908. Still, the cause of the epidemic of 1914 and 1915 is not so clearly proven, although there is a strong suspicion that it was caused by vaccine infection like the two others. As a matter of fact, it originated in the same state – Michigan – where the epidemic of 1908 originated and where the largest vaccine factory in the country is located.

These vaccine epidemics caused the destruction of hundreds of thousands of cattle and other domestic animals in over a score of States, at a loss of many millions of dollars to the Government and people of this country.

KEN ROSSIGNOL

Surely any medical operation so inherently dangerous and capable of inflicting such injury on animals or man should not be forced on any person against conscientious objection or without free will and consent and should not be required by our enlightened domestic government in our army in any form except purely voluntary like all other medical remedies and operations.

 There is an attempt made in some of the official reports to deny that these epidemics of "foot and mouth" disease caused by vaccination could be or were transmitted to mankind in virus and were limited to domestic animals. Still, this I believe to be a grave mistake, as I have the most convincing evidence that this disease was so transmitted to many human victims, both child and adult, with the awful effects in 1902 and 1908 and is frequently transmitted to mankind in vaccine virus.

Vaccine Factories at Possible and Proved Source of Epidemics and Should be Investigated by Congress and the Government

This foot and mouth disease Is a horrible eruptive fever, a kind of "cowpox" or something like a mongrel smallpox and diphtheria combined or also like very bad chickenpox with successive crops of blisters or blotches, something like cold sores, large and small, breaking out all over the body, but chiefly on the hoofs or hands and feet, lips, and nostrils, also inside the mouth and throat.

Sometimes these blotches become confluent and pustular and continue for months but, usually, the eruption ends in a few weeks in recovery or death. In the worst cases, with internal eruptions and pus infection affecting vital nerve centers. The end comes in a few days by the victim choking to death from paralysis of the heart and breathing organs like what happens in infant paralysis, rabies, and lockjaw.

Now here we see that at least two and probably three, great epidemics of the fatal disease have originated from vaccine factories and this raises the serious question as to how far other epidemics, or even the present epidemic, may have originated from some vaccine factory or from some of their products extensively or carelessly used. Surely, the places where dangerous infectious diseases are constantly propagated on a gigantic scale and disseminated from that place into the bodies of millions of animals and mankind should be the very possible or probable source of epidemic disease. Obviously, therefore, this entire subject of the present extensive manufacture and distribution of diseases or disease cultures or products and its relation to epidemics and public health should be thoroughly investigated by Congress and the Government at an early date.

To show you what a gigantic and dangerous medical interest this vaccine manufacture has now become, it may be sufficient to state that there are now about 150 concerns licensed by the U. S. Government to manufacture vaccines and serums for animal or veterinary use, and about fifty concerns licensed to make vaccines and serums for human use with a capital of about fifty million!

This is one of the great medical interests supporting compulsory vaccination, which is a grave medical malpractice, which should be abolished wherever it exists and be **replaced by wholly voluntary vaccination** as already shown.

Data Proving Danger and Fatality of Vaccination and Its Needlessness Where Sanitation and Hygiene Are Used

With this letter, I send you three pamphlets containing facts which will verify some of the statements herein made—first, my pamphlet. *"Open Your Eyes,"* which on pages 21 to 31 will show how vaccine virus is made and how diseases are transmitted by it to animals and mankind, including the serious epidemics of 1902 and 1908. In pages 32 to 35 you will find data from the Registrar General of England, one of the highest statistical authorities In the world, showing yearly mortality from vaccination which is often greater than that from smallpox, particularly in little children, where it is frequently many times more than that from smallpox. We have a similar or even greater mortality from vaccination in this country. Still, it is most shamefully denied and concealed by that part of the medical profession, which is fanatical on compulsory vaccination and which now controls most of our Departments of Health and Vital Statistics.

This serious charge I am prepared to legally prove when necessary. On page 48 of the pamphlet you will find testimony from the English Minister of Health that the partial repeal and the consequent decline in vaccination and increase in sanitation have not increased smallpox but greatly reduced it and that actually, is his own words – "as exemptions from vaccination have gone up from four percent to thirty percent, so deaths from smallpox have declined."

It is estimated that over fifty percent of the children and from five to ten percent of the army In England are not vaccinated.

Second: In Mr. Loyster's pamphlet entitled "Vaccination Results in New York State in 1914," you will find a record of about thirty deaths of little children, including the author's own son, which were caused by vaccination. They were ending fatally in lockjaw, paralysis, or septicemia. Photographs and particulars of these cases are given, which makes a most shocking record of the dangers of vaccination to health and life and the shameful efforts of a dominating part of the medical profession to constantly deny, minimize and conceal this very grave fact.

Third: In my latest pamphlet, "Vaccination and Lockjaw," you will find an exhaustive explanation of the true relation of vaccination to lockjaw and how it causes many deaths from lockjaw in little children. And the falsity of the apologies and arguments by which some doctors try to deny and conceal this fatal responsibility of vaccination for such deaths, which should be now unquestionable to any honest or competent doctor.

Wonderful Work of the War Department and Army Acknowledged

Before closing, please permit me to express my full appreciation of the wonderful work done by your department and our army officials in raising, encamping and equipping our present great army and putting it into the fighting field so quickly and potently, with the result your department and our army officers most fully deserve, as they undoubtedly have, the unstinted thanks and congratulations of our whole citizenry, civil and military, man and woman.

No army in the field or camp has ever been taken better care of in a general sanitary, hygiene, and medical sense than our army during this grueling war. The able and liberal way in which the physical, moral, mental, religious, and recreational needs of the men have been covered by various bodies, military, medical, civic and religious, is the wonder of all our citizens who have visited our camps. And to this undoubtedly is due to the cheerful and high spirits, the wonderful morale and fighting power of our brave soldiers that has made itself instantly felt on the battlefields of Europe and has already brought the barbarous enemy to his knees and will undoubtedly soon result In a complete victory for basic American principles of democratic government for the whole world – Equality – Consent of the governed and rational liberty for all citizens in their inherent rights.

Compulsory Vaccination Condemned as Un-American

I feel, therefore, that the only blot on this glorious record of our army is the dangerous medical practice, or rather malpractice of compulsory vaccination. which clearly violates fundamental American principles and also violates the oath which the soldier takes as to "Liberty and Justice for all."

In compulsory vaccination, there is obviously neither "liberty" nor "justice," and it is utterly opposed to the fundamental American principle of the inherent human right to medical liberty and choice and to the sanctity of the body. It, therefore, fits property only with some code of Prussianism from which It has been, in fact, copied. And I believe, further, that with the excellent sanitary and hygienic conditions now used in our army this medieval medical barbarism of compulsory disease inoculation, ostensibly to produce health, is, to say the least, neither necessary nor ultimately useful but probably produces far more disease than it prevents.

For example: for one death that naturally occurs from smallpox or typhoid fever, ten to one hundred occur from the far more frequent and fatal diseases of tuberculosis, pneumonia, and meningitis. And let us here ask what the use is of having the soldiers forced to submit to a whole series of disease infections, if these infections, at best, only give Immunity for a little while from such diseases as typhoid and smallpox and make the system more susceptible to greater mortality from the far worse diseases of pneumonia and meningitis, which actually seems to be a possible effect of vaccinations from the recurring epidemics of these dangerous diseases in our heavily vaccinated camps.

Proved Value of English System of Non-Compulsion

I feel sure, therefore, that this now well-tested English reform of abolishing compulsory vaccination and making all vaccination voluntary will prove equally successful with us as in England, in the increase of general health and reduction of disease as is clearly stated in the quota already given from the English Minister of Health.
See also the recent English work, *"The Vaccination Question."* London. 1914. by Dr. Millard, a pro-vaccinator, health officer of the unvaccinated city of Leicester, who gives similar testimony. After many years' experience condemning compulsory vaccination and showing its needlessness for public health and its great dangers to human life.

Conclusion

In conclusion, I hope, therefore, that your Department will see the truth and wisdom of the suggestions here offered and will do what seems best to you to have these suggestions adopted in the army, to suspend all vaccination during epidemic conditions and make all vaccination voluntary as it now in the English army. This reform will I am sure to conduce to the best health and welfare of the whole army and particularly to the newest or youngest part of it. The boys under 21, now called into military service, and which is one of the most precious possessions of the nation to be most carefully conserved in every way we can.

Petition for Redress of Grievances
a Constitutional Right

I also wish to here finally remind you that in laying this important matter or "grievance" before you I am exercising an essential constitutional right of the citizen as expressed in Article 1 of the First Amendment, vis: the right "to petition the government for a redress of grievances.," which right the article states cannot be abridged or denied.

Respectfully submitted.

CHARLES M. HIGGINS

271 Ninth Street, Brooklyn, N. Y.

Oct. 14, 1918

(The above letter was carried in THE WASHINGTON HERALD as a paid advertisement in the Nov. 20, 1918 edition.)

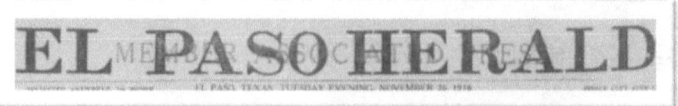

EL PASO DOCTORS GET
ROSENOWS "FLU" VACCINE

EL PASO HERALD

El Paso, Texas (Nov. 26, 1918) – El Paso doctors have recently received consignments of Dr. E. C. Rosenow's influenza vaccine for a trial here. The vaccine has been tried out in several places, but as local physicians say, It Is yet an experiment; they are not urging It upon their patients. For those who have heard of it and asked that it be given them as a possible preventive against the disease, local physicians have administered it.

Considerable is claimed for the vaccine. It is declared that in the city of Rochester, Minn., of the 15,000 people who were given this vaccine, not one has suffered from influenza nor pneumonia: that In one school, 356 children were vaccinated with It and returned to school and not one of them had the disease. Also, 14 nurses of St. Mary's hospital, Rochester, had influenza before the vaccine was given, but that after the staff had been given the treatment, not another case occurred.

Another hospital in Rochester reports that not a case of pneumonia nor influenza occurred among the 1600 people vaccinated with this serum.

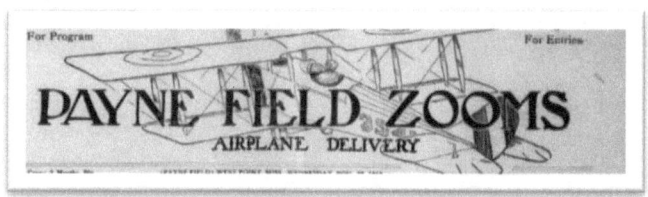

CONSIGNMENT OF FLU VACCINE ARRIVES

PAYNE FIELD

West Point, Miss. (Nov. 27, 1918) – Along with all the other recruit horrors, which include pneumonia vaccine, typhoid vaccine, paratyphoid vaccine, and smallpox vaccine, somebody off in the wilds of the army medical research for something or other, has found another vaccine.

A consignment of vaccine for the prevention of the contraction of influenza or something is the official title of the fluid, and the Post Hospital at Payne Field is now prepared to inject this bit of liquid into anyone who so desires it.

The authorities of the hospital recently announced the receipt of some pneumonia vaccine for the purpose of injection, as a preventive.

PART FOUR

NO CHANGE HERE
IN FLU SITUATION

THE MEDINA SENTINEL
Medina, Ohio (Dec. 6, 1918)

The flu situation in Medina and vicinity has not improved any since last week and if anything is not so well. There are innumerable cases, the but few serious ones reported.

While many are recovering from recent attacks, others are coming down with it," and it is impossible to tell just what the situation is.

The ban on all public gatherings, of course, still obtains and will continue so long as there is any apparent danger. Judging from present conditions, then it is probable that the schools will remain closed the balance of the year, as well as the churches and all other places of public gathering.

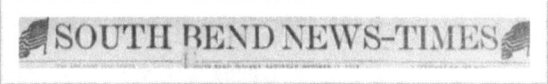

INFLUENZA CLAIMS
LAPORTE EDITOR

E. J. Widdell of the Herald Dies
Friday After Brief Illness.

News-Times Special Service

LAPORTE, Ind., (Dec. 7, 1918) E. J. Waddell, 42 years old, managing editor of the LaPorte Herald, died at the Richter hotel here at 4:10 o'clock Friday afternoon, following a week's Illness of influenza which developed into pneumonia. He is survived by his mother, Mrs. Louise Widdell of Mishawaka; two sisters, Mrs. J. M. DeLap of Mishawaka, and Mrs. C. N. Dolk of South Bend; four nieces and four nephews.

Mr. Widdell had been employed by the Herald since he was 12 years old, starting as a carrier boy.

Private funeral services will be held on Monday afternoon, and burial will be in St. John's Lutheran cemetery.

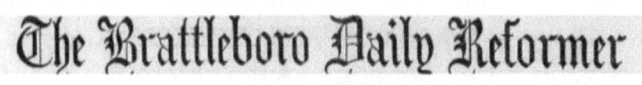

NINETY PERCENT OF
FLU DEATHS ARE PREVENTABLE

Influenza Cases Can be Cured, Dr. Rosenow Says

THE BRATTLEBORO DAILY REFORMER

Brattleboro, Vermont (Dec. 10, 1918)

CHICAGO, Ninety percent of the deaths from influenza and pneumonia are preventable when a properly prepared vaccine is used, according to an address by Dr. E. C. Rosenow of Rochester, Minn., before the annual meeting of the American Public Health Association today.

FLU AGAIN INCREASING IN LOS ANGELES AND FRISCO IN LATE FIGURES; CONDEMNS BANS

By Associated Press to THE SUN
LOS ANGELES, CALIF. Dec. 10, 1918

Eight hundred five new cases of influenza were reported today to the board of health here. This represented an Increase oi 110 over new cases reported yesterday. Health authorities said the increase was accounted for in part by the compliance of physicians with a request of the board that they are more prompt in reporting new cases.

IN FRISCO ALSO

SAN FRANCISCO. Dec. 10, 1918 – An increase in the number of new cases of influenza but a decrease in the number of deaths was announced tonight by Dr. William C. Hassler, city health officer. For the 24 hours ending at 5'clock, 244 new cases and three deaths had been reported. Yesterday's record was 115 new cases and five deaths. Dr. Hassler said he would appear before the board of supervisors Thursday with a request that the mask-wearing ordinance is reinvoked. He said the pressure of official business made impossible his earlier appearance before the board.

ONLY SECONDARY WAVE

SACRAMENTO, Dec 10, 1918 – The flareup of Spanish influenza in various parts of California was described today as "a slight secondary wave, common to practically all cases of contagious diseases," by Guy P. Jones, assistant secretary of the state board of health. Reports received by the board show there have been about 184,000 cases to date of Influenza and pneumonia since the beginning of the epidemic.

ARMY CAMPS RESULTS

WASHINGTON, Dec. 10, 1918 – An official summary of the results of the influenza epidemic in army camps and military centers in the United States, made public by the War Department today, shows there were 338,257 cases of the disease up to December 1, with approximately 17,000 deaths.

IS MORE VIRULENT

CHICAGO, Dec. 10, 1918 – The influenza epidemics which many health officials believe came to this country from the battlefronts in Europe are returning in the more virulent form now, declared Dr. Woods Hutchinson, of New York, at the annual meeting of the American Public Health Association today.

England and Italy are experiencing epidemics now, he said, and by royal proclamation, masks are worn by everyone In Italy. It may have been carried across by our latest troop shipments, he said. Dr. Hutchinson said he had communicated to Sir Arthur Newsholme, Chief health commissioner of Great Britain, the result of his investigations in various parts of this country concerning the use of gauze masks and vaccines.

A combination of these two was virtually the only successful method of fighting the epidemics. Dr. Hutchinson said, and he declared quarantine and the closing of all public meeting places "a relic of barbarism," with no value whatever.

"To pull the people from one public meeting merely drives them into another, where they talk to each other and exchange influenza germs if they carry the infection." he declared.

Col. V. C. Vaughn of the army medical corps advocated federal control of a part of the school program regarding school hygiene and education of the large percentage of foreign-born in our armies under federal direction.

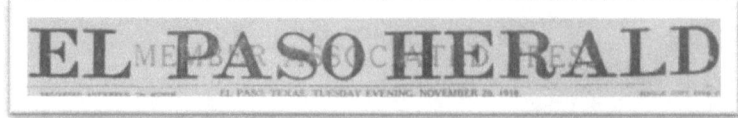

COMPULSORY VACCINATION IN TEXAS UPHELD BY TEXAS SUPREME COURT

EL PASO HERALD

Austin, Texas (Dec. 12, 1918) – Cities and towns in Texas have a legal right to pass an ordinance requiring compulsory it was held by the Texas Supreme Court yesterday in the case of the City of New Braunfels. et al., against Fritz Waldschmidt et al., from Comal County. The judgment of the District Court is affirmed, and that of the Third Court of Civil Appeals reversed.

New Braunfels passed an ordinance requiring compulsory vaccination of pupils before attending the schools there. Waldschmidt et al. attacked Its validity on the ground that it was unconstitutional. The district court refused to enjoin the enforcement of the ordinance, and this action was sustained by the Supreme Court. This decision also upholds an act of the legislature requiring vaccination as one of the conditions of the privilege of attending public schools.

THE RULING OF THE TEXAS SUPREME COURT

We cannot assent to the proposition that with smallpox still in New Braunfels, and in other nearby communities with which commercial and social intercourse was continuous, the trial court would have been warranted in declaring the ordinance unreasonable, having for its object to protect as far as practicable, by means of vaccination, the health and lives of the children and all the people of that community. As declared in Blue v. Beach, 155 Ind. 136: "It is a well-recognized fact that our public schools in the past have been the means of spreading contagious diseases throughout an entire community. They have been the source from which diphtheria, scarlet fever, and other contagious diseases have carried distress and death into many families. Surely there can be no substantial argument advanced adverse to the reasonableness of a rule or order of health officials which is intended and calculated to protect, in a time of danger, all school children, and the families of which they form a part, from smallpox or other infectious diseases."

Enough has been said to show that the rule laid down in Houston T.C. Ry. Co. v. City of Dallas, 98 Tex. 417, 418, precludes our sustaining the decision of the Court of Civil Appeals that this ordinance is invalid as lacking in reasonableness or want of necessity. This court announced in that case: "As was said by the Supreme Court of Minnesota, in the Evison case, supra: 'Much must be left to the judgment and discretion of the city council, and when they have exercised their judgment and discretion in passing an ordinance it is prima facie valid, and, to justify a court in setting aside their action, its unreasonableness, and the want of necessity for it as a measure for the protection of life and property, must be clear, manifest and undoubted, to amount, not to a fair exercise, but abuse of discretion, or a mere arbitrary exercise of the power of the council.'" *Evison v. Railway Co., 11 Law Rep. Ann., 436.*

There is no conflict between this ordinance and our law for compulsory education. For that law expressly exempts from its requirements "any child who's bodily . . . condition is such as to render attendance inadvisable." Certainly, an unvaccinated child would come within that classification when those charged with the duty to protect the public health in his community had declared that before he could be considered bodily fit to attend the school, he must be vaccinated.

The effect of our conclusions is not to impose compulsory vaccination on the minor defendants in error nor to subject their parent to prosecution if he withdraws them from school, because of his

375

opposition to vaccination. It is simply to deny these minors the privileges of the schools until they comply with the ordinance passed for their own protection and for the protection of their families, along with all others residing in the community, as has been pointed out by the New York Court of Appeals. Viemeister v. White, 179 N.Y. 235, 1 Ann. Cas.. 334.

The judgment of the Court of Civil Appeals is reversed, and the judgment of the District Court is affirmed.

City of New Braunfels v. Waldschmidt, 109 Tex. 302, 310-11 (Tex. 1918)

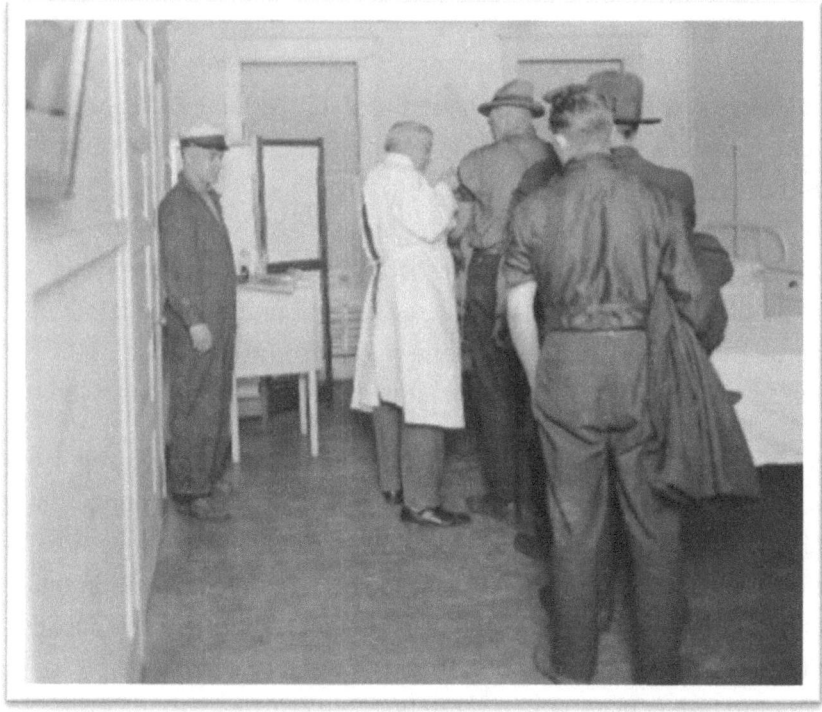

Citizens in Seattle line up for injections for the Spanish Influenza in 1918. *National Archives*

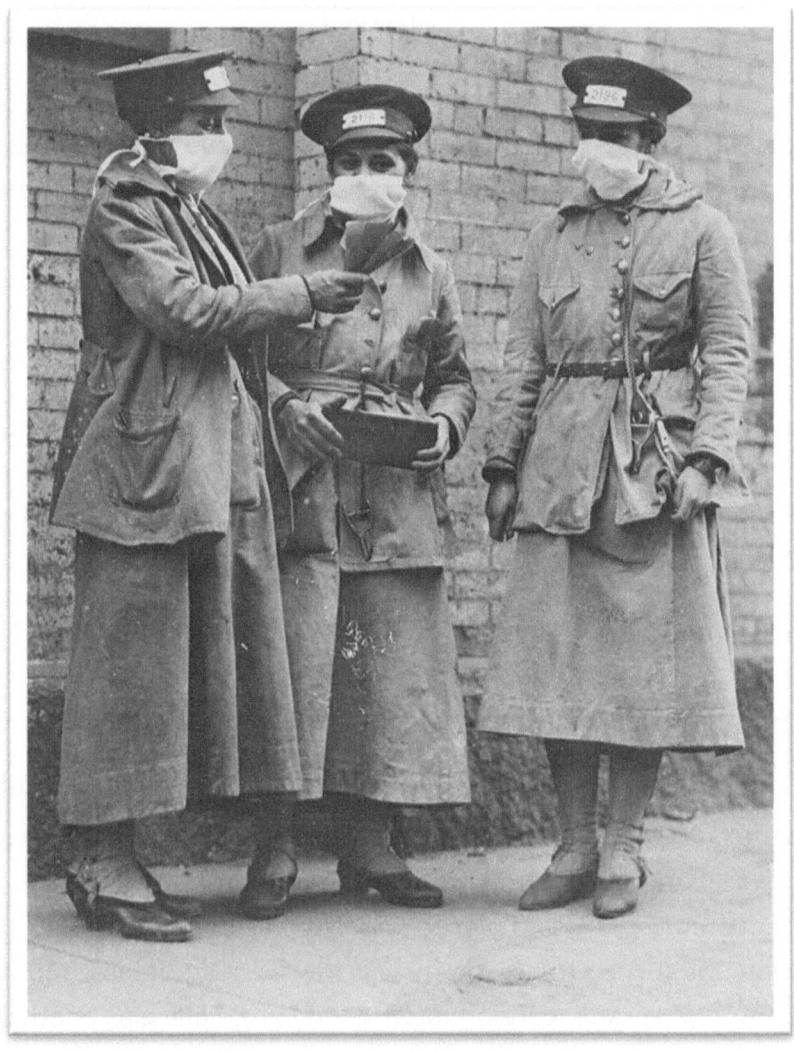

New York City female conductors on trains don their gear for work. *National Archives*

THE FLU

THE OXFORD EAGLE

Oxford, Mississippi (Dec. 12, 1918) – One of the old fabulists tells of a man who was trudging along the highway leading into a great city when he met a pestilence coming out.

After the usual greetings, the man marked: "You certainly have done your work well; you have killed most of the inhabitants of the city which you have just left."

"You were wrong, friend," said the pestilence, "I did kill some people, but most of them killed themselves by yielding to fear and panic.

Many scourges have done the same thing. The present epidemic of influenza is an exception. There has been no panic, although the disease carries off its victims as fast as any of its predecessors, some of them not lasting 24 hours after being attacked.

But people do not fear it as they did yellow fever or cholera. No effort was made to run away from it. One potent reason for this was because there was no place to go. No matter in what direction one turned to go, the flu was there ahead of him, and his chances of escape were about as good in one place as another. In the Delta below us this scourge is carrying off a great many people, and among the number are a large number of colored people, who usually enjoy immunity from other visitations. But little noise is being made, and we hear no outcry made, which is good because when people are alarmed and frightened, they fancy they are attacked, and they die from symptoms without actually ever having the disease.

People who compose themselves and who do not give way to alarm may be taken sick, but their chances of escape art much enhance. So long as they keep up courage, they seldom fall victim, and this courage wards off the disease, even from those who have exposed themselves to the contagion. On the other hand, fear invites the attack and lessens the power to resist its destructive force.

Prudence in avoiding exposure, and courage to meet the evil if it comes, save many lives, and minimizes the work of the scourge. The doctors have given liberal and lucid instructions to the public, and if these are followed, the disease can be stamped out in a short time. The flu has done much damage more than is apparent – but the people have acted wisely, and while it is not past, its ravages are being controlled by the medical men, and we will soon be free of it.

News Scimitar.

FLU TAKES TOLL OF MILLIONS BY RECENT EPIDEMIC

New York, (Dec. 11, 1918) —The Spanish influenza epidemic which swept this country during the autumn "stole" millions of the best years of life from American manhood and womanhood, Henry Moir, an insurance authority of this city, declared here.

The average economic loss of active life in each case of death from the malady of its aftermath was at least 25 years, said Mr. Moir, emphasizing the peculiarity of the epidemic, which found most of its victims under 30 years of age, as compared with the average life of 55 and 60 years of persons insured in well-established companies.

Addressing the Association of Life Insurance President, Mr. Moir, who is president of the Actuarial Society of America, described how the epidemic had dislocated the standard mortality experience of the insurance companies in the past 15 years.

With no pestilence taking toll of lives in the United States and Canada during that period, he said, the standards of health of persons under 50 were found to be much better than at any recorded time in the past.

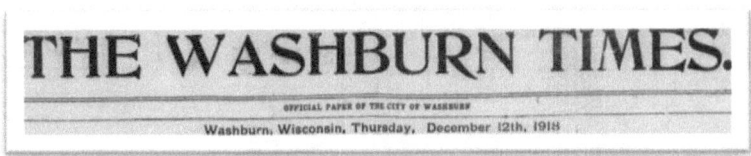

HOLDING COURT AT COURTHOUSE

Jury Cases Will Not Be Held Until Influenza Ban Has Been Lifted.

Washburn, Wisconsin (December 12, 1918) – Circuit Judge G. N. Rigjord has been hearing fact for court cases at the Court House in this city this week, and this part of the fall calendar will be cleaned up during the remainder of the week when the court will again adjourn until some future date.

The regular term of Circuit Court for Bayfield County was not held this year as per dates on account of the influenza epidemic in this city and cases demanding jury trial and numbers of witnesses will not be called until the ban has been lifted.

The adjournment of the court was deemed necessary by Judge Risjord after a conference with physicians in this city in order to prevent a spread of the epidemic to the rural sections of the county.

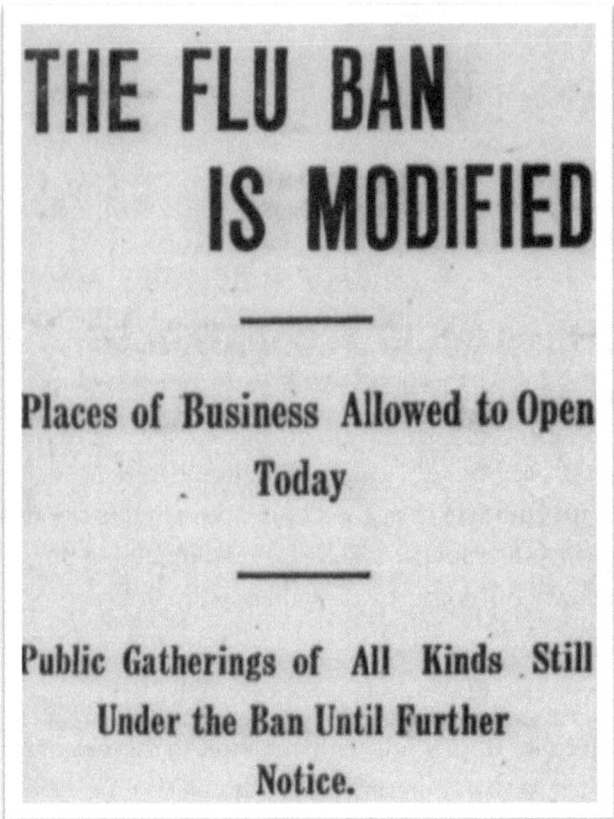

THE FLU BAN IS MODIFIED

Places of Business Allowed to Open Today Public Gatherings of All Kinds Still Under the Ban Until Further Notice. A notice of the Health Department was issued today, allowing a partial lifting of the influenza ban, which has been rigidly enforced in the city during the past two weeks.

The Health Department will now permit places of business to remain open during the day and evening, but the proprietors are cautioned not to permit crowds to congregate and to take all other precautions to prevent a spread of the epidemic. Pool rooms that are now allowed to open will not be permitted to let crowds congregate in their places of business, and any person going contrary to the order will have his place of business closed by the Department.

All public gatherings of all kinds are still under the ban.

This includes churches, lodges, skating rinks, picture shows, entertainments, and all places where crowds might congregate.

According to doctors of the city, there seems to be an improvement of the influenza situation during the week, but everyone is urged to use due precautions that a further spread of the disease may be averted.

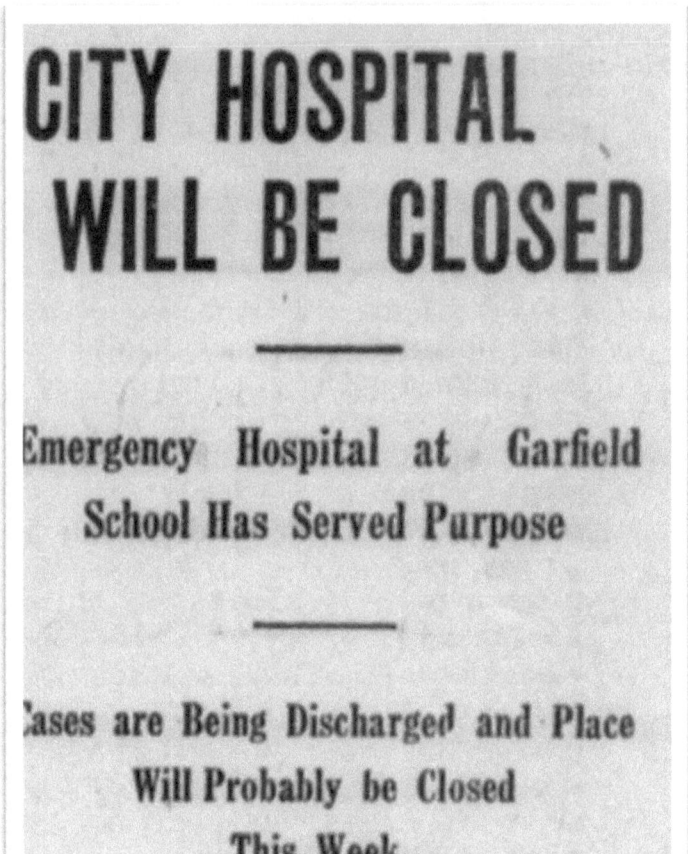

CITY HOSPITAL WILL BE CLOSED

Emergency Hospital at Garfield School Has Served Purpose

Cases are Being Discharged and Place Will Probably be Closed This Week.

Washburn, Wisc. (Dec. 12, 1918) – Emergency Hospital at Garfield Has Served Purpose

The Emergency Hospital, which was established in the Garfield school building about seven weeks ago to care for cases of influenza where the persons do not otherwise get the proper care at home, will probably be closed sometime this week, according to City Health authorities.

The maintaining of the hospital has largely been done by volunteer help with the valued assistance of Visiting Nurse Mrs. Bertha Olson and has been a big undertaking. Still, without it, many cases that were treated at the institution might have resulted seriously. The hospital was established for persons having no place where they could be treated, and for cases where the entire family was ill with the disease and in caring for these persons, it has served its purpose.

The epidemic seems to be holding its own at this time, and because of the large amount of work in keeping the Emergency hospital open, it has been decided to close the institution this week. The building is now being cleaned and will be thoroughly fumigated.

The ladies and the men who have volunteered their time and services in hospital work are entitled to a great deal of credit from the community. They have risked their health in order to relieve the suffering of others. At the hospital, many cases were treated, there being as many as twenty-seven patients in the institution at one time, and because of these being kept all at one place, the spread of the disease was curtailed in large measure.

The patients at the institution were given the very best of care and treatment, and all have the greatest praise for the volunteers and others in charge.

The Emergency hospital has demonstrated the need for a hospital for this city. Some such hospital should be established., It need not be a large one to answer the purposes of the people of the city.

Died at Hospital

Mrs. Minnie Bushey, the wife of Arthur Bushey, died Monday morning from pneumonia and influenza at the Emergency hospital after a few days' illness with the disease. Mrs. Bushey was in a serious condition when taken to the hospital, and despite the efforts of nurses and physicians, her life could not be saved.

The funeral was held Tuesday afternoon from the late residence on Bayfield street, and interment was in Woodland cemetery. Mrs. Bushey is survived by a husband and three children, besides a number of other relatives. They have the sympathy of friends in their bereavement.

FLU BAN IS TO BE LIFTED THIS WEEK
Churches and Lodges to be Allowed to Open
Picture Shows Will Open Next Monday
Evening According to Health Officers.

THE WASHBURN TIMES, Washburn, Wisc. (Dec. 19, 2018) – The influenza ban, which has been on in the city since the second week in October, is to be raised this week, and churches will be allowed to open next Sunday morning for regular church services. Still, children will not be permitted to attend, and there will be no Sunday school allowed. The picture shows, which have also been closed for the same period, will reopen next Monday evening, but children under 18 years of age will not be permitted at the show.

This was the decision reached by health authorities today. There has been an improvement in the influenza situation, but there are still several active cases in the city, and people are urged to use due precautions to prevent the spread of the disease.

Schools in the city will open again on December 31st.

SCHOOLS OPEN NEXT MONDAY

Influenza Has Been Raised on Educational Institutions Courses Being Arranged to Make up for Lost Time

THE WASHBURN TIMES

Washburn, Wisc. (Dec. 19, 1918) – The Board of Education of the City of Washburn has decided to open the public schools of the city next Monday, the influenza ban having been raised by the health authorities to permit the opening of the schools.

The schools of the city have been closed since the second week of October, and to make up for the lost time, the courses of study are being rearranged somewhat, and only the essential studies will be taken up by the children in order to catch up.

The schools in the city will not open at the same time. This is being done to give Visiting Nurse Mrs. Bertha Olson time to examine the children. The Walker school will open Monday morning, the Lincoln school Monday noon, the Garfield school Tuesday morning, and the Pioneer school Tuesday afternoon.

Pupils who show the least sign of being ill will be sent home with instructions to see a physician. Any child sent home from school or absent for a day must present a written certificate signed by the Health Nurse before being admitted to school again.

Influenza at the University of Maine

THE REPUBLICAN JOURNAL

Belfast, Maine (December 12, 1918) – Owing to a new outbreak of influenza in Orono, the town board of health has again forbidden public assemblage and the schools, churches, and places of amusement were closed Dec. 4. Over 100 cases of influenza were reported in town, and two of the public-school teachers have died within a few days.

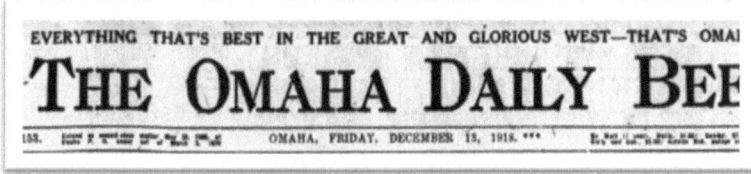

MUST EDUCATE PUBLIC TO FIGHT FLU EPIDEMIC

Manning Says Little Good Would Result from Closing Town Unless Others Do Likewise.

The quickest and most effectual method of ridding Omaha of influenzas is to inaugurate a campaign of education.

OMAHA DAILY BEE

Omaha, Nebraska, (Dec. 13, 1918) – This is what Health Commissioner Manning told the Associated Retailers of the city at a meeting Thursday afternoon in the rooms of Secretary J. W. Metcalfe.

Health Commissioner Manning told the retailers it would do little permanent good to put on the lid and close up the town. This, he said, would be beneficial if every city, town, and community would adopt the tight closing plan. However, so long as such a rule was not applied elsewhere, the disease could not be kept out of Omaha.

"There must be co-operation among the merchants," asserted the health commissioner, "and if the disease is to be eradicated, they must all work together." He urged that they impress upon their patrons the idea of early shopping and see to it that as much as possible of the trading is done during the morning hours.

Urges Early Opening.

Opening the stores early in the morning and spreading the trade over the entire day, the commissioner believes, would prevent large crowds at any one time and consequently would materially help to prevent the spreading of the disease. It was recommended that there be a limit placed on the number of persons riding on elevators, and it was urged that people be encouraged to walk downstairs instead of riding the cars.

The matter of the best method of encouraging early shopping was referred to as the dry goods committee. It will meet in the office of Secretary Metcalfe, room 733 Brandeis building, this morning and submit its report.

The Associated Retailers resolved that beginning Monday, December 16, and continuing to and including December 24, stores of members will be kept open until 9 o'clock each night.

DOCTORS FAIL TO AGREE ON MEANS TO PREVENT FLU

Wearing of Mask and Ban on Public Gatherings Ridiculed by Detroit Health Commissioner. 400,000 Flu Victims in Three Months – Mostly men between 20 and 40

OMAHA DAILY BEE

Chicago, (Dec. 12, 1918) – Instead of a definite program for fighting influenza outbreaks, the American Public Health association adjourned late today, giving copies to each of the health officers attending the annual meeting of all the medical and scientific data presented during four days and nights of discussion.

"The various communities for which we are working will know that we have at hand the best available information science has yet discovered concerning the disease," said Dr. Charles J. Hastings, of Toronto, Canada, the retiring president, "but we cannot expect to draw up a definite program for combatting influenza epidemics when we see so wide a divergence of opinion among medical authorities as has been shown here."

The organization of a federal department of health and the combining of various semi-public and private associations interested in various phases of public health movements were urged in an address by Dr. George E. Vincent, head of the Rockefeller Foundation.

Health Commissioner Dr. J. W. Inches of Detroit led the argument against closed public meetings, schools, theaters, and stores. He ridiculed the use of the mask as not a feasible measure in large cities.

On the other hand, Dr. J. A. Heyne of Charleston, S. C; Dr. M. T. Flannigan of Richmond. Va.: Dr. W. R. Stokes of Baltimore and Dr. W. E. Moore of Sioux Falls, S. D., held that closing public meetings in rural districts is efficacious.

Dr. W. H. Park of the committee on vaccines said the disease was due to an undetermined organism, and the dominating variety of the organism differs according to various localities. His report condemned the indiscriminate use of "stock vaccine" and held that the vaccine should be used only in controlled cases until its efficacy could be established. He admitted that the most generally used form of vaccine offered some protection against the secondary stages of influenza, but little against the mild form of the disease, and added that the vaccine generally had not been used until the peak of the disease, thus proving little.

Frederick L. Hoffman of Newark, N. J., reporting for the committee on vital statistics, said nearly 400,000 had died in this country the last three months and that they were chiefly men between 20 and 40 years old.

Omaha Doctors Coining Money Off People's Misery

City Health Commissioner Manning is aroused against exorbitant charges being made by some Omaha doctors for services in the influenza epidemic. A woman called him up Thursday morning and said she was anxious to have the vaccine treatment for prevention of pneumonia, but the doctor was going to charge her $10.

"Some of the doctors, who are getting plenty of practice for the first time in their lives in the present Spanish influenza crisis, are proving themselves nothing but human vultures," he declared.

"Now here's a fellow trying to charge $10 for the vaccine treatment. We give them this vaccine for nothing. We made it and did so to try to do something to curb the epidemic, and then they try to profiteer off of it. Think of doing a thing like that at a time like the present, coining the miseries of the people into money.

"I'm going after those fellows if they don't stop it. They are a disgrace to the profession. I might even publish their names if it goes any farther."

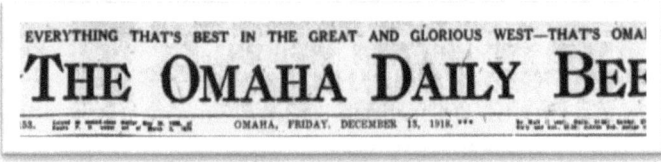

Mother, Daughter and Son Die of Flu, Father and Two Sons Are Idle

OMAHA DAILY BEE

Omaha, Nebraska (Dec. 13, 1918) – John Bugher, 4612 South Thirty-fifth street, is ill in the home of a neighbor with tuberculosis of the throat, his son George, ten years of age, is ill with influenza and his daughter Clara, five years of age, is in the Nicholas Senn hospital with the same disease. Early Thursday morning, Mrs. Bugher died of Spanish influenza, and funeral arrangements are pending the arrival of Mrs. Bugher s relatives from Staple ton, Neb.

The Bughers' stroke of hard luck began Thanksgiving when the entire family was stricken with influenza. Mr. Bugher recovered sufficiently to care for his family and was obliged to remain at home to nurse them instead of going to his work at the packing house. December 5, Bertha, the oldest daughter, died of influenza, and two days later, Earl, the youngest son, died of the same disease. Mr. Bugher has only recently regained the use of his voice.

South Side Brevities

The funeral of Mrs. A. C. Carlson will be held Sunday afternoon at 1:30 o'clock In Brewer's chapel, with Interment in Graceland Park cemetery. The Rev. R. L. Wheeler will have charge of the service.

Martin Cunningham and his son, Leonard of Colome, S. D. are ill with Influenza at the home of Police Sergeant J. H. Carey, 4542 South Seventeenth street, whom they stopped to visit for a few days on their way to Mission, Tex.

Mrs. Emma Collins, with her two children, who formerly lived at 3018 W street, left Wednesday for Los Angeles, where they will make their future home. Mrs. Collins is a sister-in-law of Justice-elect, George Collins.

Mrs. Augusta Schulz, 73 years of age, died in her home, 3952 Q street, Tuesday evening. The funeral will be held Saturday afternoon at 1:30 o'clock in the German Lutheran church, with interment in Graceland Park cemetery. Mrs. Schulz is survived by three sons, Hall, Theodore, and Carl.

NEW FLU VACCINE PRODUCED AT UNIVERSITY OF MISSOURI

OMAHA DAILY BEE

Columbia, Mo. (Dec. 13, 1918) – An influenza vaccine said to differ from any other hitherto offered the medical profession has been produced and is now being manufactured for free distribution to registered physicians' by the public health laboratory of the School of Medicine of the University of Missouri.

While it has not been tried on a large number of cases, tests conducted by the university medical authorities are said to have been sufficient to convince them of its efficacy.

NO ABATEMENT IN FLU SITUATION
MANY CASES REPORTED BUT FEW SERIOUS ONES
State Department of Health Advises Against Quarantining Patients
THE MEDINA SENTINEL Dec. 13, 1918

The epidemic of influenza that has pervaded Medina and Medina County for several weeks does not appear to be abating to any perceptible extent. However, the situation is not regarded as any more acute than it has been during any of the time. Local physicians report no diminution of cases, but no noticeable increase in virulence.

Health Officer Harding states that many think that closer restrictions should be made on even informs assemblages of a half dozen or more persons and complain that no quarantine order has been issued.

A closer restriction, says Mr. Harding, would prevent the congregating of any large number of persons in the stores while shopping, to be consistent.

And so far as the question of quarantine is concerned, the State Health Board has advised against it. The general belief seems to be that as the disease is not gaining any, it is probable that it will subside soon.

The general recurrence of influenza, which Ohio is experiencing, the percentage of fatal cases is running only about one-half as great as in the earlier outbreak. Despite all precautions that can be taken, says the State Health Department, the epidemic may be expected to continue until at least 40 percent of the people of the State have had the disease. The longer the time over which this number of cases can be distributed, the less will be the demoralization caused by the outbreak. Enforcement of regulations against public gatherings in places where the disease is prevalent will achieve this 'slowing up' and is therefore desirable even though it is not likely to reduce the total number of cases.

The recurrence of the influenza outbreak is being noted in other states as well as in Ohio, according to the health department. Experience indicates, it is held, that Ohio has followed the proper course in refraining from the quarantine of individual cases and in checking the spread of the disease by restricting public gatherings.

Influenza is so highly contagious during the preliminary stage, before the infected person knows he has the disease, that quarantine after the case is diagnosed fails to prevent a large number of exposures, health officers say. Regulations for placarding of houses for influenza, it has been observed, often lead patients to fail to call a physician.

From the standpoint of deaths, the health department points out, and the epidemic is much-less serious than formerly. Many communities are reporting large numbers of cases with few or no deaths. This condition is attributed partly to decreased virulence of the disease, partly to the better facilities now available for the care of patients and partly to the more widespread knowledge of the disease among the public.

Fear of Flu Gets Best of Juryman
Teeple as He Serves in District Court

Elmer Teeple, 2304 Vinton street, fainted Thursday afternoon while serving as a juryman in district court. Fear of the "flu" and some medicine he had taken got the best of Teeple. Dr. Charles Rosewater was called to attend him.

Judge Estelle excused Teeple from further service in the trial.

FT. OMAHA MAN GIVEN MILITARY FUNERAL HERE

Services Over Body of Lieutenant Horning Held with Honors; Body Sent to Phoenix, New York.

The military funeral of Lieut. D. A. Horning, who died Tuesday night at Fort Omaha of pneumonia following influenza, was held Thursday afternoon at 3 o'clock in the Cole & McKay undertaking parlors.

The Rev. Father James W. Stinson, the pastor of the Saint Philomena Church, performed the absolution service of the Catholic Church.

At the close of the service, the casket was draped in a large American flag, and while it was being borne from the chapel to the caisson, the Fort Omaha band played "Nearer My God to Thee."

Body to Union Station.

The funeral cortege formed and slowly moved to Union Station, where the body was taken to Phoenix, New York.

The following is the order of formation and movement of the funeral procession as it passed to the depot: The Fort Omaha band, with muffled drums, played a dirge almost the entire distance, followed by an escort of flying cadets, 32 in number. Immediately behind the escort came the caisson bearing, the casket accompanied by the following lieutenants who acted as pallbearers: H. E. McNeill, T. H. Lewis, R. E. Thompson, T. E. Nelson, W. H. Collins "and W. E. Connolly. Following immediately behind the caisson came a riderless horse, symbolic that the deceased was a mounted officer. Next in order came the officers of the command followed by 500 of the enlisted men from the fort.

Lieutenant Horning entered the service as private and was sent to the Hawaiian Islands. While there, he became a company clerk, and in November 1917, he was ordered to Fort Omaha by official wire from

Washington.

Praised by Comrade.

Captain Alexander, in speaking of his friend and companion, said: "He was an excellent soldier in every respect; careful and attentive to every detail of his work. He was an expert rifleman, pistol-man and swordsman, and always regretted that he did not get an opportunity to give service across the seas."

Lieutenant Horning leaves a father, mother, and four brothers, all of whom live at Phoenix, N. Y, where the body will be accompanied by Lieut. Roy Perkins.

Thomas Kerl, Wealthy Farmer, Is Guilty of Seditious Utterances

Thomas Kerl, wealthy lawyer farmer of Oakland, Neb., and Coeur d'Alene, Idaho, was found guilty yesterday before a federal jury on the charge of sedition. Judge Woodrough granted Kerl ten days for filing an appeal for a new trial. The jury was out just ten minutes.

Kerl was accused of saying that the American soldiers are a bloodthirsty bunch and should be killing hogs the South Omaha packing houses. Most of the morning session was passed in presenting evidence to uphold this charge.

R. E. McFarland, a lawyer from Coeur d' Alene, Idaho, where Kerl owns extensive interests, and Senator Norris Brown and Irving F. Baxter of Omaha, represented the defendant in the trial. United States District Attorney Allen and his assistant, Howard Saxton, conducted the trial tor the government.

Kerl is a scientific farmer and rancher. He is said to be enormously wealthy.

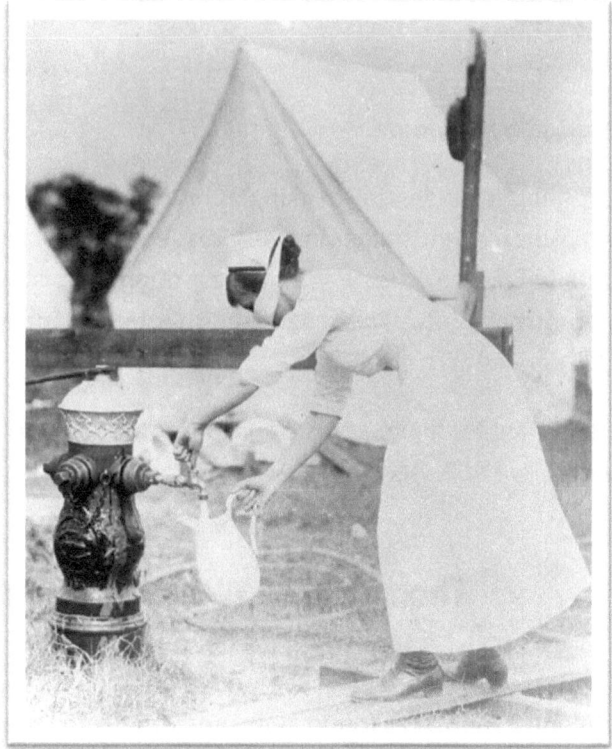

RED CROSS REPORTS
SCARCITY OF NURSES

Because of the great demand for nurses in caring for Cleveland's own influenza nurses, the Red Cross has not been able to secure additional nurses. Nurses have been doing valiant service but are far too few. Neighbors and friends must, in many cases, lend the necessary helping hand. It is urged that the following precautions are observed. Fresh air, cleanliness, and masks of cheesecloth over the nose and mouth will help to ward off the contagion.

Families in great need of help in nursing may inquire concerning nurses of Mrs. J. R. Kennan; also, nurses in taking or leaving cases will please report to her.

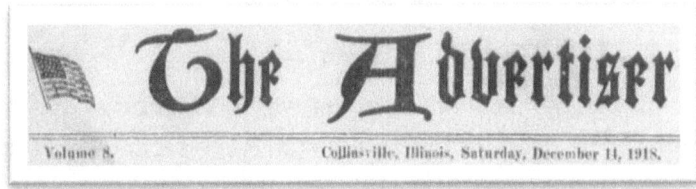

"FLU" BAN LIFTED; SCHOOL OPENS MONDAY.

THE ADVERTISER

Collinsville, Illinois - (Dec. 14, 1918) – The "flu" ban was lifted Wednesday night, and it is announced that school will resume Monday. The churches will resume their regular services Sunday, and other activities about the city are taking on their usual life. It was stated last night that there were only thirty-eight influenza cases in the city.

Chief of Police Joe Needles and Patrolman Mike Dobner are experiencing a siege of the "flu" this week.

SEVERAL DEATHS OCCUR DURING PAST WEEK.
Snadden Family Doubly Bereaved
During Little More Than a Month

Leo Ignatius Snadden, aged 22 years, son of John and the late Hannah Snadden, died at the family residence at 207 North Hesperia street on Friday evening of last week after a short illness of pneumonia.

Young Snadden was born and raised in this city and received his early education in the Saints Peter and Paul's Catholic schools and afterward attending the Collinsville Township High School, graduating with the class of 1916. His late employment was with the Consolidated Coal Company at mine No. 17, where he served in the capacity of a clerk for the past six months. He was a member of the Knights of Columbus Council 1712 of this city.

Deceased is survived by the father, one brother, Joseph, and seven sisters as follows: Margaret, Jennie, Mary, Elizabeth, Rose Ellen, Agnes, and Ruth, all residing at the family home.

Funeral services were conducted Monday afternoon at 3 o'clock from the family residence, and interment was in SS. Peter and Paul's Catholic cemetery. The death of this young man is the second bereavement that has come to this family in a very short time. Another son, John Snadden, who was with the American Expeditionary Forces in France, died on October 22, 1918, and friends and acquaintances mourn with the bereaved in the double affliction which they have been called on to bear in so short a time.

SUPERINTENDENT ADVISES TEACHERS
Asks That More Important Work
Be Given Especial Attention.

THE ADVERTISER

Collinsville, Illinois (Oct. 14, 1918) County Superintendent of Schools H. T. McCrea has sent out a circular to school officers and teachers in which he takes up many points concerning the present state of school affairs resulting from the loss of work as a result of the closing by the influenza epidemic.

He suggests that instead of endeavoring to complete the whole course as laid out for the year's schoolwork, that the more important subjects be taken up and given thorough attention for the remainder of the term.

Superintendent McCrea has ruled that it is not advisable to cancel the Saturday holiday or other holidays to make up for lost time, stating that in both city and country, the services of the school children were valuable to the parents in many ways on Saturdays.

State Superintendent of Public Instruction F. G. Blair has ruled against holding school on Saturdays. Superintendent McCrea's letter follows:

To Teachers and School Officers: A readjustment of the plans outlined for the present school year has been made necessary by the epidemic of influenza, which has been so widespread throughout the county. Two months of the regular schoolwork have been lost by several schools. It is impossible- to fully make up for a time, thus lost. We suggest that teachers devote as much time as possible, during the remaining part of the school term, to the more essential subjects of the course of study. They should exercise their best judgment in selecting the studies to be emphasized.

Examinations – While the plans previously suggested for holding the bi-monthly central and final examinations will be carried out, yet, we shall endeavor to take into consideration the many interruptions in the school work caused by the epidemic when the questions for the examinations are prepared. It is better to do thoroughly that which is attempted than to cover superficially a much wider field.

Teachers Institute – No attempt will be made this year to conduct an institute such as has been held in the past few years. Owing to the many breaks in the continuity of the schools, it has been thought wise to annul the call for a regular institute. In lieu thereof, the following will be considered institute days: Saturday, February 1, 1919. Saturday, March 1, 1919. Friday, April 11, 1919. Saturday, April 12, 1919, Saturday, May 3, 1919.

The meetings for February and May are the dates set for the quarterly meetings of the Madison County Teachers Association. The meeting for March is on the date set for the meeting of the School Officers Association. On this day, a joint session of the Institute and School Officers Association will be held. These three institute sessions will be held at the Wildey Theatre in Edwardsville. The meetings in April are on the dates set for the sessions of the Southwestern Division of the State

Teachers Association and will be held at the High School building in East St. Louis. Teachers must hold themselves in readiness to attend each of these meetings and arrange their plans accordingly.

Spelling Contest – For reasons previously given, the call for the spelling contest has been canceled. No effort will be made to take part in the state spelling contest this year. We regret this very much, as the prospect of making a good showing was excellent until influenza interfered with our plans.

Emergency Certificates – Teachers holding emergency certificates expiring on November 30, who expected to write in the examination December 5 and 6, and who are now teaching, may by making personal application at the office of the county superintendent, obtain a certificate to cover the full term of school. This concession is granted as a special privilege but will not excuse the holder from writing in the examination when one is called.

Announcements – Programs of the meetings on institute days will be mailed to teachers at the proper time, but we suggest that you make a note of the dates set so that they may not come upon you unprepared. Requests to be excused from attendance at any of these meetings must be of a very urgent nature to receive any consideration at this office.

Sincerely yours,

HUGH T. McCREA,

County Superintendent of Schools.

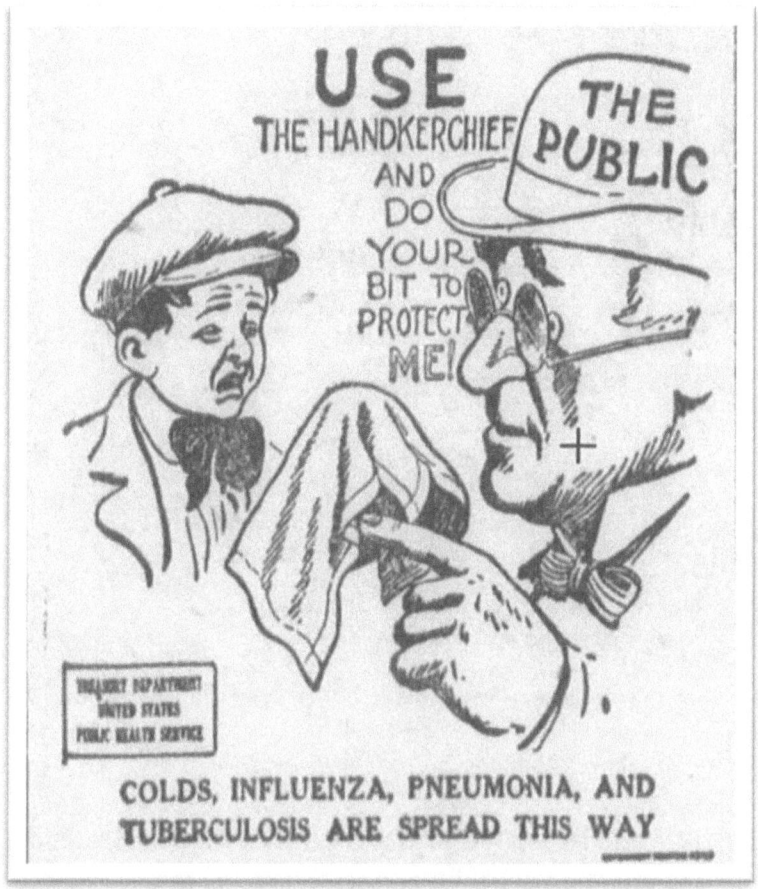

This poster was contributed by Evening Star cartoonist Jim Berryman for the Public Health Service in 1918

U. S. HEALTH SERVICE ISSUES WARNING

Increase in All Respiratory Diseases After the Influenza Epidemic Probable.

Influenza Expected to Lurk for Months. How to Guard Against Pneumonia. Common Colds Highly Catching—Importance of Suitable Clothing—Could Save 100,000 Lives.

THE ADVERTISER – Collinsville, Illinois

(Dec. 14, 1918) Washington, D. C With the subsidence of the epidemic of Influenza, the attention of health officers Is directed to pneumonia, bronchitis, and other diseases of the respiratory system, which regularly cause a large number of deaths, especially during the winter season.

According to Rupert Blue, Surgeon General of the United States Public Health Service, these diseases will be especially prevalent this winter unless the people are particularly careful to obey health instructions.

"The present epidemic," said Surgeon General Blue, "has taught by bitter experience how readily a condition beginning apparently as a slight cold may go on to pneumonia and death. Although the worst of the epidemic is over, there will continue to be a large number of scattered cases, many of them mild and unrecognized, which will be dangerous spots to be guarded against."

The Surgeon General likened the present situation to that after a great fire, saying, "No fire chief who understands his business stops playing the hose on the charred debris as soon as the flames and visible fire have disappeared. On the contrary, he continues the water for hours and even days, for he knows that there is a danger of the fire rekindling from smoldering embers."

"Then you fear another outbreak of Influenza?" he was asked. "Not necessarily another large epidemic," said the Surgeon General, "but unless the people learn to realize the seriousness of the danger, they will be compelled to pay a heavy death toll from pneumonia and other respiratory diseases.

Common Colds Highly Catching.

"It Is encouraging to observe that people are beginning to learn that ordinary coughs and colds are highly catching and are spread from person to person by means of droplets of germ-laden mucus. Such droplets are sprayed into the air when careless or ignorant people cough or sneeze without covering their mouth and nose. It is also good to know that people have learned something about the value of fresh air. In summer, when people are largely out of doors, the respiratory diseases (coughs, colds, pneumonia, etc.) are Infrequent; in the fall, as people begin to remain indoors, the respiratory diseases increase; In the winter, when people are prone to stay In badly ventilated, overheated rooms, the respiratory diseases become very prevalent

Suitable Clothing Important.

"Still another factor in the production of colds, pneumonia and other respiratory diseases is carelessness or Ignorance of the people regarding suitable clothing during the seasons when the weather suddenly changes seasons."

FLU VACCINES ARE IN EXPERIMENTAL STAGE, SAYS DR. PIKE

HEALTH OFFICERS ANNOUNCES DISEASE VARIES IN DIFFERENT LOCALITIES ATTENDS CHICAGO HEALTH CONFERENCE.

FREE TRADER-JOURNAL

Ottawa, Ill. (Dec. 17, 1918) – Many Ottawans have considered taking serum inoculations for the prevention of influenza and are interested In knowing just whether it is effective as a preventative or not, the city health officer, Dr. W. A. Pike, has Just returned home after spending several days at the health conference in Chicago, and today issued the following statement regarding the vaccine treatment:

"Many inquiries are being made relative to the value of vaccines and serums to be used for the prevention and treatment of influenza. In this regard, I wish to state that I attended the meeting of the American Public Health Association held last week in Chicago at which there were gathered together health authorities from all parts of the United States and Canada. Reports there presented showed that the type of the disease differed in different localities and a vaccine in order to be of value must necessarily be adapted to the type of the disease prevalent In the community in which it is to be used. This, of course, can only be determined by bacteriological analysis."

"The same holds true with regard to serum to lie used for treatment. Serums are made from the blood of convalescent patients.

"Cases must be typed individually, and the serum to be of value must be made from the blood of patients convalescent from the same type of the disease as that from which the patient is suffering.

"The public must understand that as yet the matter of vaccines and serums is still in the experimental stage and that the results so far reported following their use, are so conflicting that their indiscriminate use is to be deplored."

W. A. PIKE

Health Officer

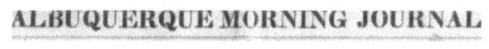

ATTORNEY KILLED WHEN
KNOCKED DOWN IN FIGHT

By Morning Journal Special Leased Wires

LIVINGSTON, MONT. Dec. 23, 1918 – O. M. Harvey, Republican State Chairman and one of the most prominent attorneys in Montana, died at 6 o'clock tonight from a fractured skull sustained in a fall to the sidewalk during a fistfight on the streets her half an hour earlier, with Postmaster J. Swindlehurst. Swindlehurst gave himself up to the Sheriff and is in the county jail.

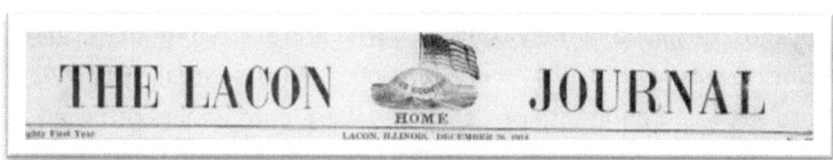

TEXAS ST. CLAIR KILLED

Notorious Marshall County Bandit Slain in Des Moines
After Killing Chief of Police of That City

THE LACON HOME JOURNAL

Lacon, Illinois, (Dec. 26, 1918) – Word comes from Des Moines, Iowa, that Texas St. Clair, alias "Dutch" Cross, a former resident of Marshall

County and notorious in half a dozen states as an all-round bad man, was recently shot and killed in that city after he had mortally wounded C. C. Jackson, chief of police, who is also dead as the result of a revolver duel with the bandit.

For some time, St. Clair had been a prisoner in the jail at Newton, Iowa, awaiting trial for a crime committed in that county. He recently escaped from the Newton jail and a few days ago was located in Des Moines by the police of that city which surrounded the house in which he was known to be hiding and demanded his surrender. St. Clair refused to come out of the house, and Chief Jackson and two officers started to enter, when the bandit opened fire on them, the chief falling at the first shot.

St. Clair ran to the rear of the house, pursued by bullets from the guns in the hands of the other two officers who, with the chief, had entered the house. As he rushed out through the rear door, his body was riddled with bullets from revolvers in the hands of three officers who had been on guard outside, and he fell dead.

Thus, ended the career of a man whose entire life was one long record of crime. Most of the readers of the Journal are more or less familiar with the life history of the St. Clair brothers Frank and Texas.

Years ago, they lived in the vicinity of Varna and started on their career of crime in this county. They were convicted of horse stealing and were sent to the Joliet penitentiary. Later they were paroled and returned to this county, one of them being paroled to a gentleman in Henry and the other to a gentleman near Varna.

Within a year after their return to Marshall county, several horses were stolen hereabouts, and they were at once suspected of the crime. A little later, Frank broke into a freight car near Varna and stole some hides, which he sold in Henry.

He was arrested and bound over to the grand jury. At about the same time, the brother, Texas, was arrested on the charge of being implicated in horse stealing, and he, too, was bound over to the grand jury. Both were indicted and were placed in the county jail to await the convening of the Circuit Court.

This was about two years ago. They remained in jail only a short time after their indictment, not because they were released by not by the process of law but rather because someone smuggled a saw to them, and one night, they sawed the bars and escaped from jail.

They were next heard from in Iowa when a raid was made on their home near Newton by the Jasper county officials, and great quantities of plunder were found. Texas succeeded in getting away, but Frank was caught and locked up in the county jail. Later he was returned to the Joliet penitentiary for violation of his parole and, as far as is known, he is still there. He is under indictment in this county on the charge of burglary and larceny and State's Attorney Black has arranged for his arrest upon the completion of his term at Joliet and his return to this county to stand trial under the indictment that has been brought against him.

Marshall County is not proud of her former residents, and no one hereabouts is mourning because of the death of Texas St. Clair. He was a bad actor and was wanted in Peoria and a dozen other places to answer criminal charges.

Rep. Mudd Has the Flu
St. Mary's Beacon Dec. 19, 1918

Leonardtown, Md. – The Baltimore Sun of Tuesday, Dec. 17, 1918, states that Rep. Sydney E. Mudd is very ill with influenza at Providence Hospital, Washington, where he was removed on Saturday, after having been sick for two weeks. His condition is not considered serious, and his physician believes he will soon resume his duties in Congress.

Calvert County Courts Closed

The November term of Court for Calvert County was only in session for two days, as most of the cases being continued. As none of them were of vital importance, this action was taken to guard against spreading influenza, which has again made its appearance in that county.

In the Casualty List

Wm. G. Hayden, son of Mr. and Mrs. Theo. Hayden, of Hermanville, Md., was reported in the casualty list of Thursday Dec. 12, 1918, as having been wounded, degree undetermined.

The list of Dec. 14 contained the name of Johnson M. Gatton, of Hollywood, Md., as missing in action.

Full Casualty List by Dec. 27

General Pershing has cabled the War Department that on Dec. 14, there remained 40,440 casualties in the process of verification, of which 1,069 were deaths and 39,371 severely wounded. His cable stated that the complete report of those killed would be received in the U. S. by Dec. 20 and the wounded by Dec. 27.

Many Indians Are Victims of the Spanish Influenza

By Associated Press to THE SUN

SAN FRANCISCO, Dec. 21,1918 – Spanish influenza, among; Indians at Manchester, California, brought today an appeal from the Indians to the Indian board of control in this city. There have been three deaths. Rev.

Frederick O. Collett, field secretary, has gone to Manchester to take charge of the situation.

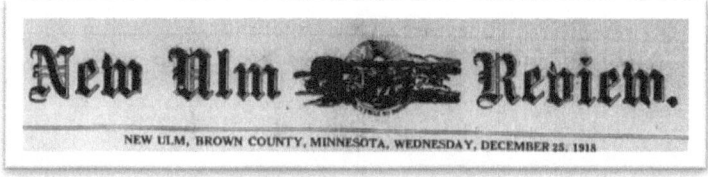

NEW ULM, BROWN COUNTY, MINNESOTA, WEDNESDAY, DECEMBER 25, 1918

FLU VACCINATION ADVISED FOR ALL
INSURANCE COMPANIES OFFER SUGGESTIONS TO THEIR POLICYHOLDERS
Epidemic Causes So Many Deaths That They Urge Prevention

NEW ULM REVIEW

New Ulm, Minnesota (Dec. 25, 1918) – Life insurance companies who keep accurate statistical records of life and death for human beings find their calculations somewhat upset by the influenza epidemic which has attacked chiefly those chances for many years of life were of the best, leaving the older and younger, the feebler members of the race untouched in the great majority of cases.

All this has had its effect on the business of the big insurance companies, and they have consequently been making a thorough investigation to see whether they can find some remedy to check the progress of the disease.

As a result of their investigations, they are advising their policyholders to be vaccinated. A part of one of the circulars sent out by a company represented here by J. R. Higgs says:

Get Vaccinated.

The epidemic of Spanish influenza has gone all over the United States, and not only that but to every part of the world. The disease has been very severe, and the fatalities have been enormous.

If this disease follows the course of the usual epidemics, we will have the return of the trouble at various times within the next few years, and with severity possibly diminished, but still sufficient to cause a great deal of trouble and a great deal of sorrow because of the number of deaths that will occur.

The medical profession is working hard to obtain some medication that will lessen the mortality in this disease, and to date, has obtained vaccines which, if properly given, seem to have a very marked effect in preventing infection.

Influenza in itself is not the most dangerous part of this trouble, but the various forms of pneumonia that seem to come with the disease have been the complications that have been responsible for most of the deaths.

The vaccines given at this time seem to vary materially lessen the probability of infection. We would advise our policyholders to see their family physicians and obtain this vaccine treatment without delay.

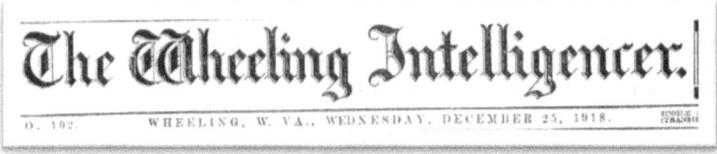

The Wheeling Intelligencer.

O. 102.   WHEELING, W. VA., WEDNESDAY, DECEMBER 25, 1918.

TWO CASES OF FLU REPORTED

THE WHEELING INTELLIGENCER

Wheeling, West Virginia (Dec. 26, 1918) – Two cases of influenza have reported to City Health Officer D. W. Boone, the first cases for several days.

Indications are that the disease is gradually stamped out here.

Special Dispatch to the Intelligencer

Steubenville, Ohio (Dec. 25, 1918) – The first application for a refund on a liquor license, because of being compelled to close by order of the hoard of health during the "flu" epidemic, has been file in common pleas court located here by H. M. Levinson, a local liquor dealer, who asks for a rebate of $71.7S. His place of business, along with all other local saloons, was closed 26 days during October and November. It is understood that all license holders here- and in the county who were forced to close, will apply for a refund. Under the law, it must be granted, and County Auditor Floyd is holding up the state tax settlement until the rebates are paid.

Refused to Confirm Effort to Oust
Health Officer for Shady Dealings

An effort on the part of Mayor O. Y. Crawford and Village Council of Toronto to oust Health Officer Dr. E. R. Giesey for alleged malfeasance in office has failed. Council at the request of the mayor suspended the doctor far fifteen days, pending an investigation into charges that he discriminated in favor of some business firms in enforcing the "flu" ban. James Shaw was appointed to succeed Dr. Giesey, but the state board of health has refused to confirm his appointment, holding that Dr. Giesey's dismissal at this time is "very unwise."

The doctor is still in power, and the "flu" ban, which has been in effect eleven weeks, still holds.

Good Health Record,

Bridgeport, West Virginia (Dec. 25, 1918) – This city still continues to maintain its good record so far as the health condition is concerned, and no new cases of influenza were reported to the health officer yesterday. There are still two cases of influenza and one of diphtheria.

Thirteen Cases in Police Court.

Mayor Junkins had thirteen offenders before him yesterday morning, and all were on charges of drunkenness. The mayor was a little lenient with the bunch yesterday, and all were let out with fines of one dollar and costs. Only one arrest had been made at a late hour last night.

.

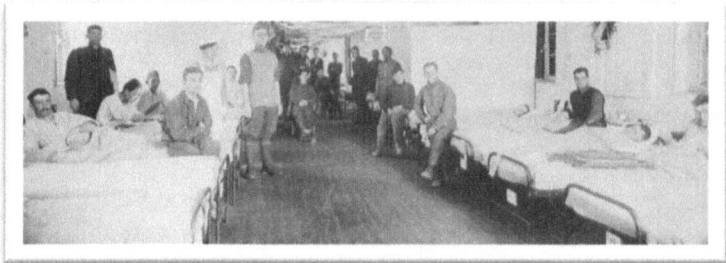

This influenza ward of an Army Hospital in France was taken on Dec. 28, 1918. *National Archives.*

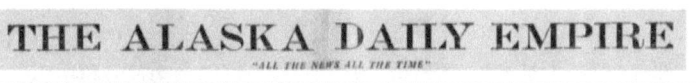

VACCINE LIKE GUM DROPS TO ESKIMOS
Krulish Expedition Doing Wonderful Work Among Indians of Alaska.

THE ALASKA DAILY EMPIRE

Juneau, Alaska (Dec. 31, 1918) – Alaska Indians take to the Influenza vaccine-like Eskimos to gumdrops, according to W. T. Lopp, chief of the Alaskan division of the United States Bureau of education, who has just returned after a five-week inspection of schools in the South Eastern district of Alaska, says the Post-Intelligencer.

"They like it," said Lopp in discussing the conditions of the Indians in connection with the Spanish influenza epidemic. "The Krulish expedition is doing wonderful work in Alaska. There is free use of the influenza vaccine, and it seems very successful as a preventive measure."

According to Mr. Lopp, conditions in the schools of Alaska are good at the present time, and the epidemic toll has been light. The maximum number of deaths reported in one village in the southeastern district was eleven, the casualties running between two and five deaths, and in some cases, entire villages escaped without a death. In the northern part of Alaska on the coast, Mr. Lopp says, the toll taken by influenza among the Eskimos was terrific. Cable dispatches received at the offices of the bureau headquarters here show that 200 natives have died and that there are only fifty adult survivors in a village on Cape Prince of Wales.

Numbered among these are three of the village's prominent men, James Keok, said to be the largest native reindeer stockman in Alaska, died from the disease. His reindeer number between 1,600 and 2,000 head. Warner Adlooat and Charles Kitook, two native instructors, were also claimed.

The influenza is gradually waning in the North country now, according to Mr. Lopp, and conditions are expected to be normal again soon.

UNITED STATES HAS MORE THAN ONE-THIRD OF GOLD

NEW YORK, Dec. 31. —Notwithstanding that the total supply of the gold in the world has increased $1,500,000,000 since the war began, the United States now has more than one-third of the total supply as against less than one-fourth of it before the war began.

GRANDVIEW STRICKEN WITH INFLUENZA IN WASHINGTON

YAKIMA (Dec. 31, 1918) – The town of Grandview, south of here, is in dire straits from influenza. One hundred cases developed in the past two days. Whole families are stricken. Doctors and nurses are being sent from here to establish an emergency hospital.

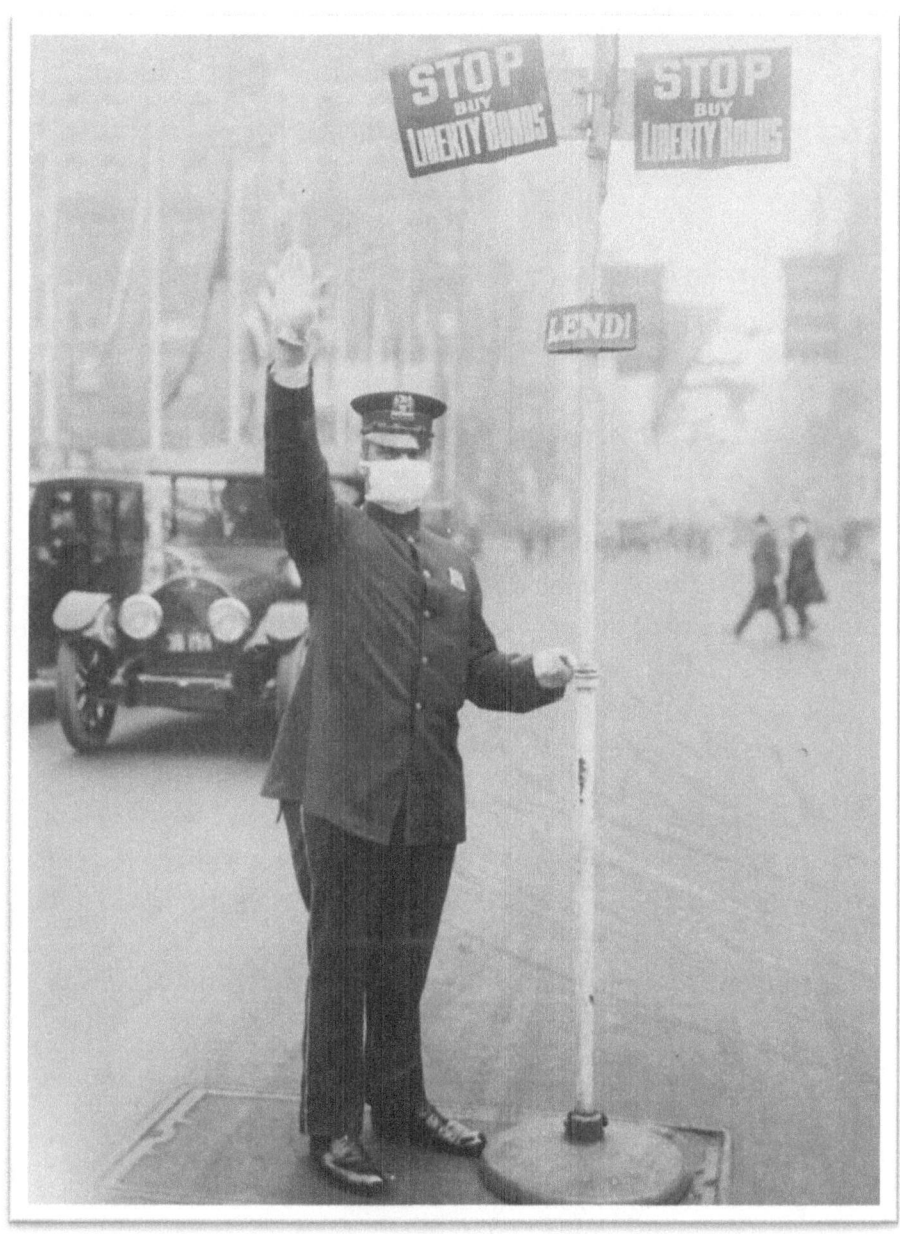

Traffic cop in New York City.

THE ARIZONA REPUBLICAN
AN INDEPENDENT PROGRESSIVE JOURNAL

INCREASE OF 98
FLU CASES FOR
PAST 24 HOURS

Total Cases In City Now 536 Within About 100 of Peak of First Wave of Epidemic Police Enforce Laws

ARIZONA REPUBLICAN

Phoenix, Arizona (Jan. 8, 1919) – Last night found Phoenix completely in the grin of its second influenza epidemic, with a second strict quarantine in force and the city virtually closed up. At the same time, the epidemic made heavy gains, new cases for the 24-hour period reaching 122. Cases in the city, releases, and deaths being substituted, showed a total of nearly 550, approaching to within a little less than 100 of the peak the disease reached in the initial wave.

Following closely the quarantine measures announced by the health board, the city police department made active preparations yesterday to rigidly enforce the new health regulations. During the day, 22 special officers were sworn into the police department as deputies and assigned stations to further ensure quarantine enforcements and to assist in handling the situation.

Soldier Deputies

The new officers are mostly soldiers and sailors back from camp and overseas service and will be uniformed as police reserves. They will be scattered through all parts of the city to prevent crowds from gathering to see that quarantine rules are obeyed and to keep school children off the streets. If the number of deputies sworn in yesterday is insufficient for the purpose, Chief of Police Brisbois is prepared to swear in an equal number of others.

Among those sworn in yesterday as special police were Brandon brothers, owners of the American theater, closed by the epidemic.

In obedience to the rules of the Health Department, as contained in notices from Dr. H. K. Beauchamp, city health officer, every motion-picture show in the city, every theater and every pool hall was closed yesterday. The public schools were already closed, although the high school made an attempt to continue its classes. Dr. Beauchamp also announced his rules would apply to churches, dances, and all other public gatherings.

Quarantine Is Strict

The health board yesterday also put into effect some of the strictest quarantine measures ever seen in the city.

All houses in which influenza is prevalent must be quarantined, as well as the occupants. Persons coming in contact with the disease must wear masks.

An exception is made in the quarantine regulations, however, in the case of the wage-earner of the quarantined family. Although the household must be segregated, the wage-earner is permitted under the rules to leave the premises to work, on condition that he does not come in contact with the sickroom and sick persons.

It is these regulations that the Police department will co-operate with the health department in enforcing, as well as the regulations in regard to the closing of the theaters and dance halls and the like.

Depends on People

Dr. Beauchamp and other health authorities yesterday reiterated statements that the speedy stamping out of the second influenza wave in this city depends largely on the hearty support and co-operation given officials who are fighting the disease by the general public. If the regulations are obeyed and care exercised by everyone, it is thought the epidemic can be checked in the course of two weeks.

While the fight against the epidemic was being organized and started yesterday, the epidemic itself showed no signs of abatement. During the day, 122 cases were reported, with two doctors not reporting, against 154 for the two days preceding Twenty-three releases and one death brought the net advance of the epidemic down to 98 cases, against 102 for the previous two days.

Last Night's Report

New cases in the city – 115

New cases in hospital – 7

Total new cases – 122

Releases in the city – 23

Releases from hospitals – none

Total releases – 22

Deaths in city – 1

Previously reported live cases – 438

Net advance in cases yesterday – 98

Total cases in city – 536

At the same time, yesterday's total approaches closely the greatest number of cases recorded in the city, 634, about two months ago.

As a further aid in fighting the epidemic, the city vaccine station at 134 North Central Avenue will remain open, and vaccines for influenza and other disease furnished the public free.

To discuss the question of closing the churches during the present second wave of the influenza epidemic, the ministers of Phoenix met yesterday afternoon at the Y. M. C. A.

Under the impression that the matter of closing the churches was to be left to the judgment of the church people themselves, it was learned at the meeting that the city health officer had intended to include the churches in his closing order. There was no decision made at yesterday's meeting.

A meeting of the health board will be held this morning, at which time the question of the closing of the churches will be decided.

The Maricopa County Health Board this morning issued a public notice to all county schools, churches, picture shows, dance hall, and all places of entertainment, ordering them to be closed and to remain closed until further notice. The order is also signed by Dr. A. B. Nichols, county health officer.

REGULATIONS TO CONTROL SPANISH INFLUENZA

THE GARDEN ISLAND

Lihue, Kauai, Hawaii Territory (January 28, 1919)

THE FOLLOWING REGULATIONS CONCERNING THE PREVENTION AND CONTROL OF THE DISEASE" KNOWN AS SPANISH INFLUENZA WERE DULY ADOPTED BY THE TERRITORIAL BOARD OR HEALTH AT A SPECIAL

MEETING HELD AT THE OFFICE OF THE BOARD OF HEALTH ON THIS 23rd DAY OF JANUARY, A. D. 1919.

REGULATION NO. 1. That the proprietors of all hotels, restaurants, clubs, and boarding houses within the Territory of Hawaii be and are hereby required to sterilize after each and every use thereof, dishes, glassware, cutlery, and table linen by boiling the same for a period of at least twenty (20) minutes.

REGULATION NO. 2. That the proprietors of soda water fountains, soft drink, and Ice-cream establishments, counters, and fountains within the Territory of Hawaii, be and are hereby required to sterilize after each and every use thereof, all drinking glasses, spoons, and other eating and drinking utensils by boiling the same for a period of not less than twenty (20) minutes, PROVIDED, HOWEVER, that where paper cups are used in such establishments, the drinking utensils need not be so sterilized.

REGULATION. NO. .3. That all theatres, and churches be and are hereby ordered closed, and all other public gatherings held within enclosed buildings, except public and private secular schools, bo and are hereby prohibited.

The foregoing regulations shall be in full force and effect from and after the 25th day of January, A. D. 1919, and until revoked by the Board of Health.

DATED at Honolulu, January 23rd, A. D. 1019.

TERRITORIAL BOARD OF HEALTH

By S. S. PAXSON,

Its. President.

ATTEST:

K. B. PORTER,

Secretary, Territorial Board of Health.

The foregoing regulations are hereby sanctioned and approved on the 23rd day of January, A. D. 1919. C. J. McCarthy, Governor of Hawaii.

THE OGLALA LIGHT

PINE RIDGE, S.D. (Feb. 1, 1919)

The many local friends of Paul Hagel were saddened to hear of his death in France from Pneumonia following Flu. This information was not received until late in January, notwithstanding the fact that his death occurred on December 21st. The sympathy of the entire community is extended to the surviving wife and relatives.

The following recapitulation shows the ravages of Spanish Influenza on the reservation. This occurred mostly in the fall, but there are still a few sporadic cases here.

Districts	Cases	Deaths
Oglala Boarding School	149	1
Wakpamni	524	37
White Clay	275	33
Wounded Knee	608	52
Porcupine	306	45
Medicine Root	740	38
Pass Creek	740	20
Eagle Nest	30	41

Total for reservation   3642   267

WHAT CHEMISTS HAVE TO SAY
On the Subject of the Rosenow Vaccine, Information Secured at the Request of the EDITOR OF THE TIMES

THE WILSON TIMES

Wilson, North Carolina (Feb. 4, 1919) – Always desirous of helping our people in every line of activity, and certainly to eliminate the dread scourge influenza which has taken so many from our midst, as soon as he heard df the Rosenow vaccine discovered by an eminent bacteriologist of the Mayo group, probably the most advanced physicians and surgeons in the world, we endeavored to give our people information regarding the vaccine and get them in touch with it. Being a layman as far as the practice of medicine is concerned, we could not understand why Dr. Rosenow would create a vaccine and allow its use in any particular whatsoever unless he believes it to be of great virtue

The recent controversy over the matter published in the Times, created so much of wonderment and interest in the mind of the editor, regarding what seemed to us, inexplicable situations surrounding the use and application of this vaccine that we invoked the aid of Mr. E. L. Tarkenton of the Patterson Drug Co. to help us out of the dilemma that personally at least, we could arrive at some understanding of a few things connected with the profession,

Mr. Tarkenton has very kindly obliged us. We are publishing today the letter of Parke, Davis ft Co, manufacturing chemists who are placing the Rosenow vaccine on the market, and we give the explanation to our people in order to let them Judge for themselves.

Editor Times.

Detroit, Mich., Jan. 29, 1919

Patterson Drug Company,

Wilson, N. C.

Attention If r. E. L. Tarkenton

Gentlemen:

Your communication of January 22nd addressed to our Baltimore Branch, and referring to the question of influenza vaccine, has been forwarded to us for a reply. We have read with a great deal of interest not only your letter but also the enclosed clippings from the Daily Times.

It is certainly a matter to be sincerely regretted that the influenza situation has been the source of numerous controversies, many of which have undoubtedly impeded the step being taken to control the spread and the mortality of the disease. The attitude of many physicians towards vaccines is particularly difficult to understand. It is true that the efficiency of vaccines as prophylactic or therapeutic agents is not universally accepted, even by those whose training is such as to warrant them in Intelligently drawing conclusions.

Diametrically opposed opinions were expressed at the last meeting of the American Public Health Association in Chicago. This was not especially surprising; however, every topic taken up at this meeting was a subject of more or less dispute; in fact, the sessions had the earmarks of a debating society rather than of a scientific gathering. The objection to the use of vaccines rested largely on a theoretical basis, and on the other hand, the application of vaccination found its chief advocates among those who had been extensively trying out their efficacy.

The statement made regarding the committee appointed by the American Public Health Association to report on vaccines might carry the impression that they had found vaccination to be of rid avail. Such is not the case, however. The attitude of this committee is that the efficacy remains to be proved. We believe we can do no better than to quote verbatim that section of the committee report, which has reference to the use of vaccines.

Assuming that the cause of the epidemic 1b an unknown virus, it does not seem possible at present to prevent the primary disease by vaccination "with known organisms.

Against the secondary infections, there would seem to be a theoretical basis for the use of vaccines, and especially for the use of vaccines prepared from organisms responsible for complications that may differ in various localities at various times. This variable bacterial flora may militate against the practical -application of vaccination on a large scale because it would seem to require frequently repeated vaccinations with the flora that may be met with. It is impossible at present to evaluate the reports from the use of these vaccines adjusted to meet local conditions—more data obtained under carefully controlled conditions needed.

"Stock vaccines made from the influenza bacillus alone or from other bacteria, have been used to a considerable extent The injections of stock vaccines have seemed to mitigate to some degree some outbreaks of influenza and also the severity of the complicating infections; but in those instances in which the results of the use of vaccine have been controlled, no appreciable results have been obtained. The fact that the vaccine Is usually employed after the epidemic has broken out and is perhaps on a decline, and the fact that an unknown number of people have been exposed, make it very difficult to draw a conclusion as to the efficacy.

Recommendations

"Your committee recommends that until such time as the efficacy, or the lack of efficacy, of prophylactic vaccination against influenza, is established, vaccine it used, should be employed in a controlled manner, under conditions that will allow a fair comparison of the number cases and of deaths among the vaccinated and non-vaccinated groups. Particular attention should be directed to securing data as to the period in the epidemic at which vaccinated and non-vaccinated persons developed the disease.

"Nothing in these recommendations should be interpreted as discouraging the use of pneumococcus stock vaccine against lobar pneumonia deaths.

"This epidemic emphasizes the importance of properly equipped laboratories."

We entirely concur in the above recommendation against the "indiscriminate" use of vaccines. There is no question but that a lot of mushroom vaccines have sprung up during this epidemic, which is quite worthless. It is difficult to see, however, that anyone conscientiously endeavors to impartially determine the efficacy of the influenza-pneumonia vaccine can fail to be impressed with the results which have been reported up to date. The few negative reports are, for the most part, based on limited application. Where vaccination has been used on a massive scale, and with adequate provisions for controlling the results, it has consistently reduced the incidence of influenza, decreased its severity, and restricted its complications.

We are enclosing a circular containing an abstract of the report of Dr. E. C. Rosenow in the January 4, 1919, issue of the Journal of the American Medical Association

No amount of theoretical speculation can offset the facts there set forth.

The Bamberg Herald

BAMBERG, S. C., THURSDAY, FEBRUARY 27, 1919.

INFLUENZA IS A MYSTERY
So Far It Has Defeated Medical Skill and Science.

(By Frederick J. Haskin.)

Bamberg, S.C. (Feb. 27, 1919) – An experiment that makes the transmission of influenza a more baffling mystery than ever, and which at the same time places on record an act of self-sacrificing heroism by about one-hundred naval volunteers, has just been completed by officers of the United States Public Health Service cooperating with medical officers of the United States Navy at Boston and San Francisco. As nearly everyone knows, scientists all over the world, in combating the spread of influenza, which is still going on, have proceeded on the assumption that it is transmitted chiefly by coughing and spitting. The theory has been that the diseased mucus thrown out by these acts is filled with the germs of influenza, which thus find lodgment in healthy tissue.

All the experiments heretofore made seem to indicate strongly that influenza is transmitted in this way, and it is well accepted that most other respiratory diseases are so carried.
The latest experiment consisted of submitting the one-hundred men who volunteered for the purpose of every possible method of infection with influenza germs through the nose and throat. These men risked their lives for the general good, and for the advancement of science. They went through a singular trying and repulsive ordeal. They, and

everyone else, believed that they were being Inoculated with the dread disease, which is destroying millions of lives all over the world. Their heroism is fully equal to that displayed some years ago by the men of the army medical army corps who exposed themselves in Cuba to the bites of mosquitoes to determine finally whether yellow fever was transmitted by that insect. The only difference between the two experiments was in the result. Some of the officers who exposed themselves to the bite of the mosquito contracted yellow fever, and one of them died, thereby establishing the soundness of their theory. The volunteers who submitted themselves to inoculation with the germs of influenza were fully expected to take the disease and were prepared to die. But not one of them developed any symptoms of influenza.

This astonishing negative result, which is the sensation of the day in scientific circles, should not tempt anyone to be careless in the matter of coughing and spitting or ill exposing himself to infection by those acts. As officials of the public health service point out, it may be that the germs of the disease disappear as soon as or immediately after the symptoms appear. Something like this is true of other diseases. In measles, for example, it has been found that the germs which cause the disease all gone within five or six days after the appearance of the rash, and the ease is no longer contagious.

The discovery of this fact, which was made by Anderson and Goldberger of the public health service only a few years ago, has led to shortening the quarantine for measles by more than half.

"These new experiments in the transmission of influenza," said Surgeon General Blue, "show how difficult is the influenza problem. They by no means indicate that we can afford to disregard coughing, sneezing, and spitting as common means of spreading diseased, and even in the case of influenza, this source of infection should always be borne in mind.

I believe, however, that we have not paid sufficient attention to other paths of infection, especially to the lips, mouth, and hands. The fact that the disease was much less common in army camps where the sterilization of all eating utensils and dishes was rigidly enforced shows the importance of the mouth as an avenue of infection."

There can be no doubt that these experiments at Boston and San Francisco were carried out with the utmost thoroughness. Lieutenant Commander Rosenau of the Navy Medical Corps and Surgeon Joseph Goldberger of the Public Health Service were the officers in charge of the Boston experiment, which was made at the quarantine station on Gallop Island. Forty-seven men were the subjects of this part of the experiment. All of them had been more or less exposed to the disease, and thirty-nine of them had never had any bronchial disease. This means that some of them may have been naturally immune to influenza, but it is not at all probable that all of them were. The first experiment consisted of thoroughly infecting the noses of about ten of the men with cultures of Pfeiffer's influenza bacillus, a virulent germ commonly found in influenza.

None of the men developed any symptoms. The next form of the experiment was to take the secretions from the noses and throats of influenza patients and place them in the noses and throats of the volunteers by means of swabs and sprays. The time occupied in removing the diseased mucus from a sick man and putting it into the nose and throat of a well man was reduced to as little as 30 seconds. Yet none of the men so infected developed any symptoms of the disease.

Determined that the test should be exhaustive, the doctors next submitted a group of volunteers to infection by actual coughing and spitting.

For this purpose, ten volunteers were selected, and ten-bed patients who had recently come down with severe attacks of influenza.

Each of the volunteers leaned over the bed of each of the sick men, conversed with him for a few minutes, and allowed the patient to cough directly in his face so that then should be no doubt of transmission of diseased tissue. Each volunteer was thus exposed to ten different cases of influenza and was in close proximity with them for not less than three-quarters of an hour. Yet not one of these volunteers developed any symptoms of influenza.

The experiments in San Francisco which were carried out under the direction of Surgeon G. W. McCoy ol the Public Health Service, and Lieut. De Wayne Richey of the United States Navy at the Angel Island quarantine station, were very similar in method and in the result. The men who volunteered for these experiments had been vaccinated with Pfeiffer's influenza bacilli and pneumonia germs. If, as European reports would indicate, influenza is caused by an ultra-microscopic germ, such vaccination would be without protection to those so vaccinated. None of these men had been exposed to the influenza epidemic.
In this experiment, there was no direct exposure to patients, but the additional methods of infection were tried to inject the blood of an influenza patient into that of a volunteer and of introducing the pure cultures of influenza bacilli into a volunteer's eye. No one of these men developed influenza.

The result of this experiment has left the medical world completely bewildered.

The theory which has apparently been upset by these experiments was originated by a famous French physician Nicolle, who claimed to have produced influenza with a material obtained from mucus excretions. He produced the disease with this material after filtering through a fine porcelain filter showing that a germ was present, which was not only too small to be detected with the microscope but too small even to be held back by the fine pores of unglazed porcelain. Foster, an American army surgeon, showed that common colds were produced by equally minute germs. The work of Foster bore so directly on the problems presented by influenza that it may be said to have led to the experiments there described.

The only thing which can be considered proved about influenza so far is that it is still a mystery both as the nature of its causative germ and as to its means of transmission, and therefore especially dangerous. Authorities, however, still consider influenza a crowd disease, and all unnecessary gatherings of people should be discouraged when influenza is prevalent.

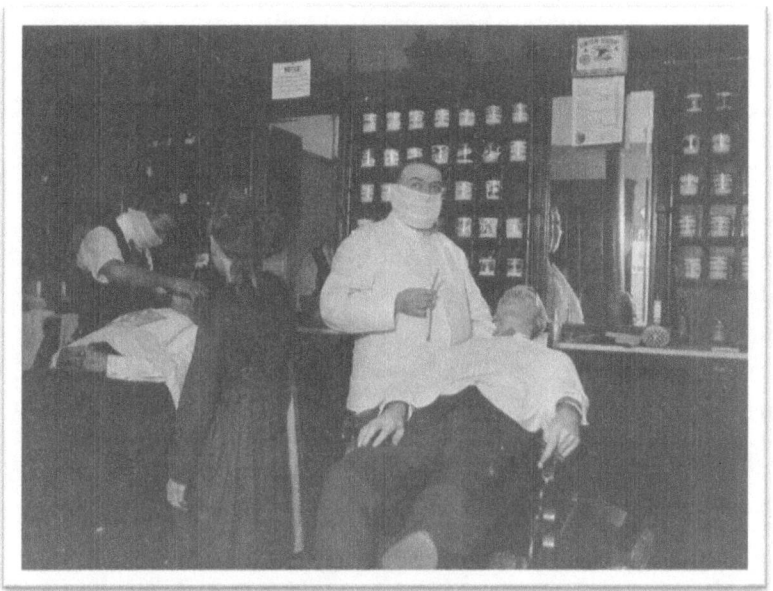

Barbers serve customers with masks in 1918. *National Archives*

INFLUENZA DOPE COSTS
DRUGGIST $100 FINE

THE WASHBURN TIMES
Washburn, Wisc. (February 13, 1919)

Ed Thoreson, a local druggist, was fined $100.00 and costs before Judge
H. P. Axelberg last Thursday afternoon when he appeared and entered a
plea of guilty to selling intoxicating liquors without a prescription.

Thoreson's arrest was caused by District Attorney Charles F. Morris and
was based on the information given by one Len Wilcox, who had been
arrested for breaking into the City Drug Store. Wilcox is a minor.

Druggist Thoreson claims that the liquor obtained by Wilcox was done
so upon Wilcox's presentation to him that he was suffering from an
attack of influenza and that the liquor was to be used strictly for
medicinal purposes. Thoreson claims this is the first and only time he
has ever sold liquor to any person without a prescription, and that had
Wilcox not claimed that he was suffering from the "flu" that he would
not have been in this predicament.

At any rate, it cost Thoreson $100.00 and costs for giving the "Flu"
medicine, which was probably many times more than the price paid by
Wilcox for the "medicine."

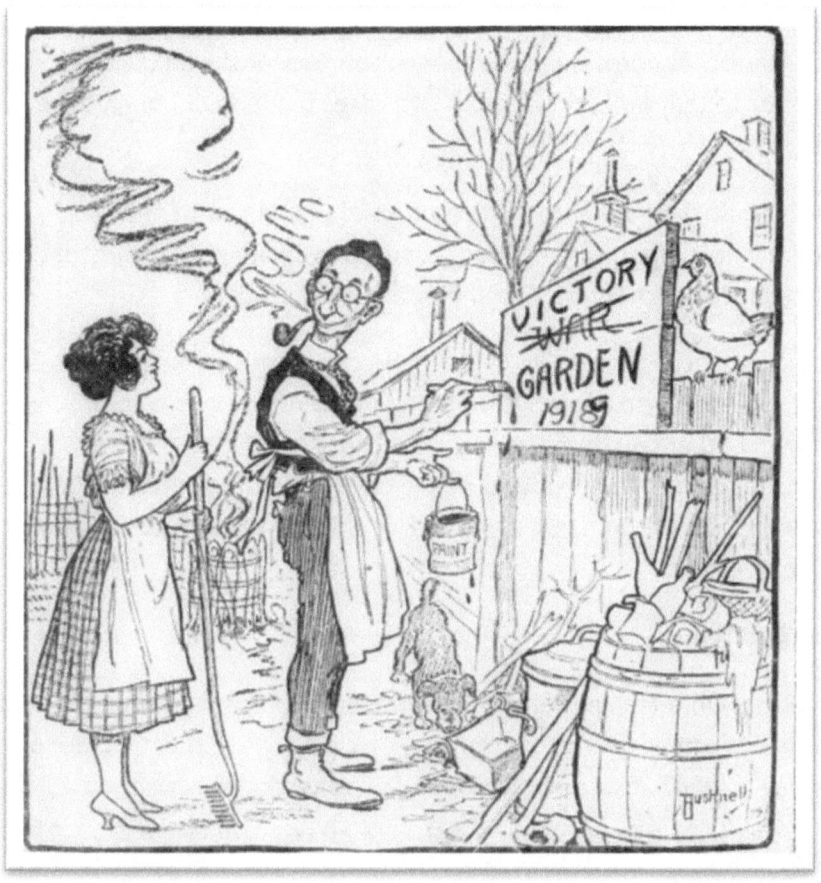

THE ROCK ISLAND ARGUS.

Rock Island Entirely Free of Disease That Resulted in
Numerous Untimely Deaths

IN DANGER OF THIRD WAVE

City More Susceptible if Another Epidemic Occurs,
Health Commissioner Says

ROCK ISLAND ARGUS

Rock Island, Illinois (March 12, 1919) – Spanish influenza is extinct in Rock Island, not one case having been reported for the last two weeks, and prior to that time, only one or two cases made their appearance daily.

However, Rock Island is not entirely free of the danger of another epidemic. It is reported by national and state health authorities that the United States is to experience a third influenza epidemic.

Rock Island, according to Dr. C. T. Foster, city health commissioner, is more susceptible to a third wave than any other city in this community and many other communities for the reason that during the first and second epidemics the residents of the city were not afflicted in such large numbers in comparison with other cities, leaving those unaffected still susceptible.

Has Third Wave

Cleveland, Ohio, is experiencing its third wave of Spanish influenza, and health authorities assert that the city is hit because of the mildness of the way in which it suffered from the first and second waves.

There is little indication that Rock Island is to suffer from a smallpox epidemic that is affecting other cities in the country. Only one case of smallpox exists in the city at present, and there is practically no other contagion.

Father Kelly Seriously Ill

ST. MARY'S BEACON

LEONARDTOWN, MD. (March 13, 1919) – Rev. Lawrence J. Kelly, S. J., formerly pastor of St. Aloysius Church, Leonardtown, is reported as dangerously ill of influenza at Yonkers, N. Y. This is sad news to his many friends in St. Mary's, who earnestly hope that he will speedily recover. Father Kelly is easily one of the ablest and most popular priests who have been stationed in this county, remarkable not only for his zeal for the spiritual welfare of his charge, but a man of broad learning and great public spirit.

Science's Latest on the Flu

OMAHA DAILY BEE

Omaha, Nebraska (April 3, 1919)

The London Times – The third wave of the influenza epidemic has now ended. The deaths from the disease recorded for the 96 great towns of England and Wales last week numbered 3,218, compared with 3,889 the previous week. In London, the deaths numbered 597, as against 808. What is more, it has ended to date? The mysterious periodicity which the mysterious disease seems to have established for itself has been maintained.

This periodicity is roughly 12 weeks. The first wave began .in July and died down about the end of August, a two months' course. Twelve weeks after the beginning of the first wave at the beginning of October, the second wave began to flow. The wave was spent by the middle of December. Again, 12 weeks after the beginning of the second wave, i. e., in January, the third wave appeared. It had begun to spend itself in the first days of March.

Meanwhile, the evidence that the causative organism of the epidemic is the filter-passing germ described by the late Major Graeme Gibson and also by Captain Wilson accumulates. It is a very strong body of evidence, and to a great extent, satisfies the requirements of proof laid down by Koch. That is to say, the germ can be recovered from patients affected by the disease; it can be cultivated outside the body; it can, when inoculated into animals, reproduce the phenomena of the disease, and it can be recovered again from the inoculated animals, and again grown.

It is just the failure to understand the necessity of proof of this sort, which has led so many observers to describe "germs of influenza" in these last weeks. This is, perhaps, especially true of the much-debated Pfeiffer's bacillus, which was originally discovered in the eighties, and has been discussed a hundred times since. The bacillus is one of the many which are very commonly present in the human nasopharynx.

(Other bacilli very frequently found in healthy throats and noses are the pneumonia bacillus, the streptococcus, and the staphylococcus.) This, by no means, establishes the Pfeiffer bacillus as the cause of a disease. Were such an argument admitted, there would be no limit to the number of things which might be suspected in the same connection, e. g., baldness, soft corns, all of which frequently occur in persons suffering from influenza. We should be back again in the dark ages.

We do not think that it has been established of the Pfeiffer bacillus or any other bacillus or coccus, except the one mentioned above, that it will produce influenza when inoculated into animals, or that it can be recovered from these animals after infection.

In the absence of proof of this kind, the statement that the bacillus is present in the throats of all influenza patients does not carry us much farther. It is in all probability. So are other bacilli. Admittedly these "residents" may and do afflict severe illness once the resistance which normally holds them at bay is broken down. It is exceedingly improbable that they are the agents that initiate the attack.

 This is the reason why vaccination against influenza is not generally advised. You cannot vaccinate against a disease the exact cause of which is in doubt (though now that Major Graeme Gibson's discovery has been announced, a vaccine of a new kind may possibly be available soon.) The best use that can be made of vaccination at present is to inoculate against the "residents," the germs which constantly lie in wait for their host, and visit pneumonia and blood-poisoning upon him when he is weak,

And there are, as has been pointed out before in these columns, objections even to this course.

Many announcements of "cures" of the disease have been made. The public should realize that probably upwards of 80 percent of all cases of uncomplicated influenza in this epidemic have got well by themselves when pneumonia has supervened it has, of course, been a different story. It is easy to see that an individual treating a limited number of cases in some particular way, by some particular serum or drug, might easily have recoveries in 100 percent of his patients. He would ascribe this good result to his drug or serum. In point of fact, his patients would have recovered in any case.

Rigid control of every new method is essential before it can be accepted; otherwise, vast disappointment must result. That means pitting a large number of treated cases against an equal number of untreated cases or cases treated by other methods. Only then can conclusions worth talking about being drawn. Bacteriologists and others who publish statements of results without having sufficiently controlled their work do no good service to science or to humanity.

A standardized vaccine is now available against the pneumonia complications, and the first authentic statistics are hopeful no more. Sera (a serum differs from a vaccine. It is an antidote; a vaccine if a "hair of the tail of the dog that bit you" or is likely to bite you) of all sorts have been tried during the pneumonia attacks. Good and bad results are spoken of, but perhaps, on the whole, the good outweighs the bad, especially as regards anti diphtheria serum, which does seem to exercise some beneficial effect in early cases.

COUNCIL TO PAY
'FLU' BILLS OUT
OF CITY FUNDS

Decides to Reject Alfred I. duPont's Offer
to Assume Expense
MOTHER ASKS MONEY TO
PAY FOR SON'S FUNERAL

THE EVENING JOURNAL

Wilmington, Del. (May 26, 1919) – Members of City Council last night decided to pay out of the city treasury all bills contracted by the public health committee of the State Council of Defense and the Board of Health of this city during the influenzas epidemic last fall, and thus ended a controversy which has been pending several months.

This decision was reached after the committee of three members appointed to confer with Alfred I duPont, who had offered to furnish the money to pay these bills, had submitted a report in which they recommended that the city should pay its own bills.

The attitude taken by Council was the same as that taken by John J. Raskob, chairman of the health committee of the State Defense Council, in a letter sent to President of the Council George T. Lyon several days ago. For some reason, Mr. Raskob's letter was not read at last night's session of Council. Councilman Mearns, in moving the adoption of the report of the special committee, read extracts of the letter of Mr. Raskob, which had been published in the newspapers. In on the subject, Mr. Mearns said that Mr. Raskob in appearing before the Board of Health during the 'flu' outbreak, when all hands were quibbling and offering to see that all bills were paid showed he had a big heart. "I thank God for what he did, and I thank him now," Mr. Mearns added. Mr. Mearns said that he did not think that the bills were handled In a business-like or man-fashion manner.

The action of Council In deciding to pay the hills, which amount to approximately about $30,000 caused little surprise, it being evident from the beginning that the city would have the bills to pay, as all other towns In the state took care of their own patients during the outbreak and paid their own bills.

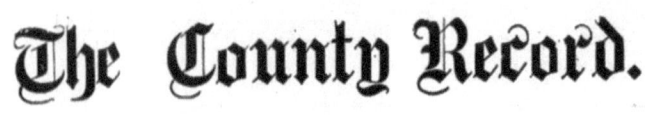

GOOD NEWS, IF TRUE
Pneumonia No More Than Boils
Of Neck says Dr. Duncan

THE COUNTY RECORD

Kingstree, S.C. (June 26, 1919) – Influenza and pneumonia are no more to be feared than a boil on the neck of the neck, according to Dr. Charles H. Duncan, one of the founders of the Volunteer Hospital, who, in an address in New York last week before the convention of the Allied Medical Association of America, described his method of combating Spanish influenza by means of "immunizing a patient to his own poison."

Upon 246 patients ill with pneumonia and influenza last winter. Dr. Duncan said he had used the treatment "without a single fatality or any complications."

"Briefly," the physician said, "I took one drachm of mucous from the infected area and pasteurized it in one ounce of filtered water where it remains several hours. One cubic centimeter of this toxin injected subcutaneously will effect a spontaneous cure of Spanish influenza, pneumonia, catarrh, or any similar localized infection. It will stop any cough except tuberculosis, inside of 24 hours."

Dr. Duncan declared that his discovery was based upon his observation of a dog licking a sore paw. He said the dog, by increasing germs of resistance at the place of infection, brought about a natural healing, and the method he employed was similar in that it increased the leucocytes or white corpuscles of the blood and these, in turn, carried the poisons out of the human system.

The doctor said that he had been using the method, which he calls "autotherapy" for about ten years and that it now was widely accepted by homeopaths and eclectic physicians, although it had not been endorsed by the American Medical Association.

Dr. Duncan said that by taking the poison from a boil and subjecting it to his process and injecting the sterilized product into a patient's body, he not only cured him of the boil but rendered him immune against a repetition of such afflictions. Similar results, he said, had been attained in cases of mastoiditis, ozoema, and certain types of local venereal diseases.

955 DIE BEFORE. RELIEF MISSION REACHES PORT

U. S. Cruiser Marblehead Returns From Relief Expedition to Bristol Bay

By Associated Press to THE SUN

SAN FRANCISCO July 12, 1919 – Confirmation of reports that the native Indian population of Bristol Bay, Alaska, virtually was wiped out by an epidemic of Influenza, was brought here today by the United States cruiser Marblehead, on its return from a relief expedition to the north.

According to Lieut. W. R. Leahy, senior medical officer of the expedition, 95 percent of a population of more than 900 persons, had died by the time the expedition reached Bristol Bay. Only approximately 50 of the influenza sufferers were alive when relief arrived, Lieutenant Leahy said, and half this number were saved.

He described finding babies and young children lying among the hundreds of dead, weak, and helpless from starvation.

The mortality, he said, almost was entirely confined to adults, the children apparently being immune to influenza. Lieutenant Leahy said the disease was a modified form of Spanish Influenza, but that the natives appeared to have no powers of resistance. He attributed this to other diseases prevalent among the population and the squalid conditions under which the natives lived. The first tasks of the relief party, according to Lieutenant Leahy, were to drive away dogs that were preying upon victims to conduct burials and care for the starving children.

Canneries operating on Bristol Bay supplied the coffins. Only a few cases of influenza were reported by the canneries, and the majority of these recovered. The Marblehead left here June 4 for Bristol Bay with doctors, nurses, and supplies.

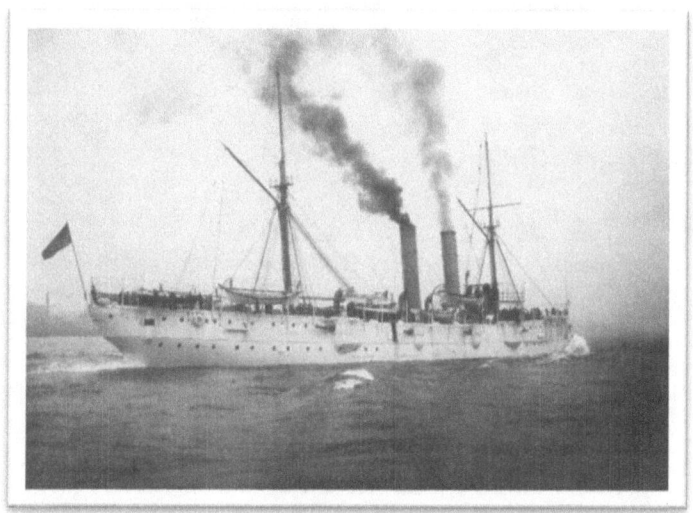

The Navy cruiser USS Marblehead.

PART FIVE

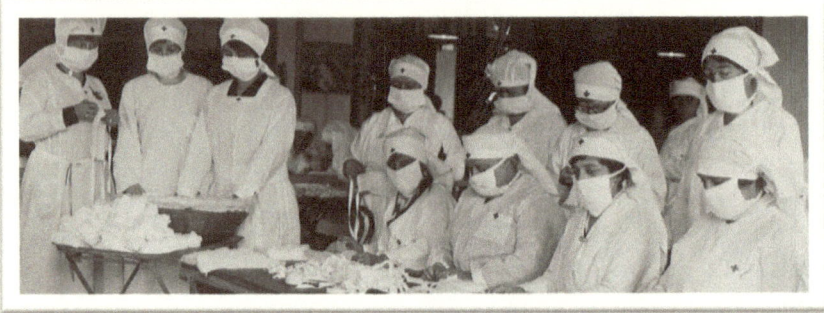

VACCINE DEVELOPMENT
Naval Hospital on League Island, Pennsylvania
(the Philadelphia Naval Shipyard)
Mayo Clinic Dr. Edward Carl Rosenow
Naval Training Station in San Francisco.
Puget Sound Navy Yard (Ely 1919).

The fate of Pfeiffer's bacillus as the probable cause of influenza is
reflected in the use of vaccines in the United States during the
pandemic of 1918–1919. By 1918, the successful use of some vaccines,
especially those against rabies, typhoid fever, and diphtheria, as well as

the use of diphtheria anti-toxin, had raised high expectations for a vaccine against influenza. Those who already had a vaccine in hand were quick off the mark to promote their vaccines as sure preventives or cures for influenza. Drug manufacturers aggressively promoted their stock vaccines for colds, grippe, and flu. These vaccines were of undisclosed composition. As public anxiety and demand swelled, there were complaints of price gouging and kickbacks. *– National Institutes of Health*

Philadelphia effort: "After the nature of a drowning person grasping at a straw, a stock influenza vaccine was used as a preventive in fifty individual cases and as a curative agent in fifty other uncomplicated cases" (Dever 1919). They made the vaccine made from B. influenza and strains of pneumococcus, streptococcus, staphylococcus, and Micrococcus catarrhalis (now Moraxella catarrhalis). Each dose contained between 100,000,000 and 200,000,000 bacteria per cubic centimeter, in a four-dose regimen. The investigators reported that no vaccinated individuals (who were hospital workers) became sick, but also noted that strict preventive measures were taken, such as the use of masks, gloves, and so on. In a group of ill patients treated therapeutically with the vaccine, none developed pneumonia, but one developed pleurisy (infection of the lining of the lungs). They noted, "The course of the disease (in those treated therapeutically) ...was definitely shortened, and prostration seemed less severe. The patients apparently not benefitted were those admitted from four to seven days after the onset of their illness. These were out of all proportion to the number of pneumonia that developed and the severity of the infection of the control cases. The effects were always more striking; the earlier the vaccine was administered." Finally, they concluded that "The number of patients treated with vaccines and the number immunized with it is entirely too small to allow of any certain deductions; but so far as no untoward results accompany their use, it would seem unquestionably safe and even advisable to recommend their employment."

San Francisco effort: In general, pneumococcus and streptococcus were seen as the cause of the most severe complications. Additionally, and amid dissent, they decided to obtain a culture of B. influenza from a fatal case at the Rockefeller Institute to include in the vaccine. In all, the vaccine contained B. influenza, 5 billion bacteria; pneumococcus Types I and II, 3 billion each; pneumococcus Type III, 1 billion; and Streptococcus hemolyticus (S. pyogenes), 100 million.

Guinea pigs were first injected with the vaccine to assess toxicity, and then five lab worker volunteers were inoculated. Lab tests determined that their white cell count increased, and their sera agglutinated B. influenza (meaning that they had antibodies in their blood that reacted to the bacteria). Side effects from the injection included local swelling and pain but no abscesses. Given permission to proceed, more vaccine was prepared, and 11,179 military and civilians were inoculated, including some at Mare Island (Vallejo, CA) and San Pedro as well as San Francisco civilians associated with the Naval Training station. In most experimental groups, the rate of influenza cases was lower than in the uninoculated groups (though no information is given on how the statistics for the uninoculated groups were gathered, nor is there information on how a case was defined). Moreover, people who were inoculated received the injections about three weeks after influenza appeared in California, so it's impossible to tell whether they had already been exposed and infected. The percent of influenza cases in control groups ranged from 1.5% to 33.8% (the latter being nurses in San Francisco hospitals), whereas between 1.4% and 3.5% (the latter being hospital corpsmen on duty in an influenza ward) of those in the inoculation group became ill with influenza.

Puget Sound Navy Yard (Ely 1919). In all, 4,212 people were vaccinated with a streptococcal vaccine. The investigators reported that the influenza attack rate in the vaccinated ranged from 2% to 57% and in the unvaccinated from 1.8% to 19.6%. However, they noted that no deaths occurred in the vaccinated men. They stated, "We believe that the use of killed cultures as described prevented the development of the disease in many of our personnel and modified its course favorable in others." The investigators concluded that B. influenza played no role in the outbreak.

Dr. Edward Carl Rosenow (Mayo Clinic) reported on the use of a mixed bacterial vaccine in Rochester, Minnesota, where about 21,000 people received three doses of vaccine in his initial study. He concluded that "The total incidence of recognizable influenza, pneumonia, and encephalitis in the inoculated is approximately one-third as great as in control uninoculated. The total death rate from influenza or pneumonia is only one-fourth as great in the inoculated as in the uninoculated." He would go on to test his vaccine in nearly 100,000 people.

~~~

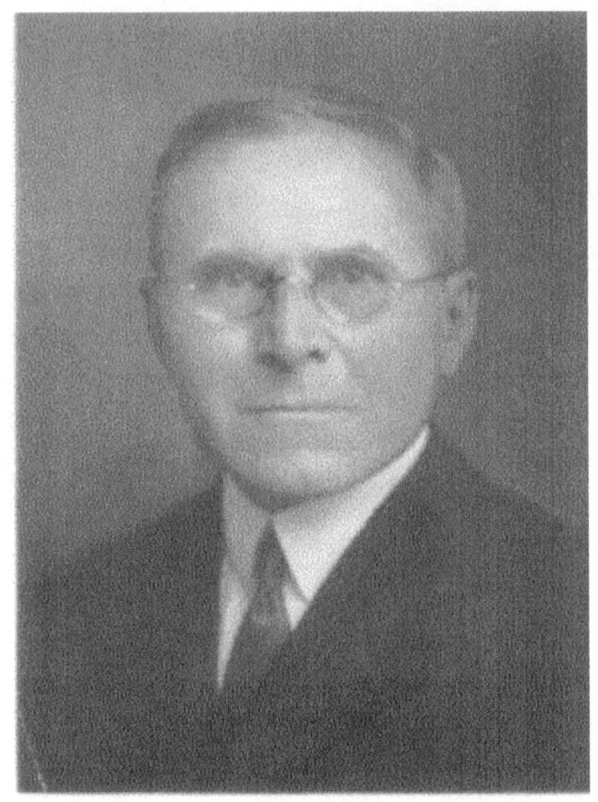

EDWARD CARL ROSENOW, M.D.

THE END

ABOUT THE AUTHOR

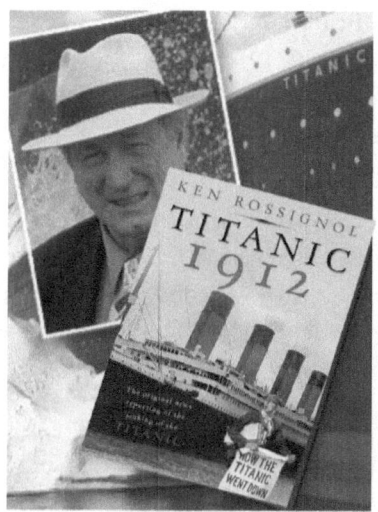

Author, publisher and newsman, Ken Rossignol has appeared on dozens of ships in the Pacific, Atlantic, Mediterranean, and the Caribbean discussing the stories of the history of the Panama Canal, the heroes of the Titanic, the explorations of the new world voyagers, the Bermuda Triangle and the history of piracy, among other maritime history topics.

Rossignol has appeared at the Titanic Museum Attractions in Pigeon Forge, Tennessee and Branson, Missouri for book signings and to talk with visitors about the RMS Titanic.

Appearing at the International Book Fair 2016 in Panama as one of the United States Delegation of authors and entertainers Rossignol enjoyed telling the stories of the History of the Panama Canal, Piracy, and of the heroes of the Titanic.

Rossignol has appeared live on Good Morning America, and in news productions in ABC 20/20; ABC

World News Tonight and in a 2012 production of Discovery Channel Investigation Motives & Murders Series, A Body in the Bay.

In 2018, Rossignol was selected for the Serenbe Fellows program as a guest speaker on the voyage of RMS Titanic before their dramatic Serenbe Playhouse presentation of Titanic the Musical.

Rossignol's landmark First Amendment case, represented by Levine Sullivan Koch & Schulz (Ballard-Spahr), re United States Fourth Circuit Court of Appeals *Rossignol v Voorhaar*, 2003, spelled out that public officials cannot retaliate against a publisher for criticism of their official acts.

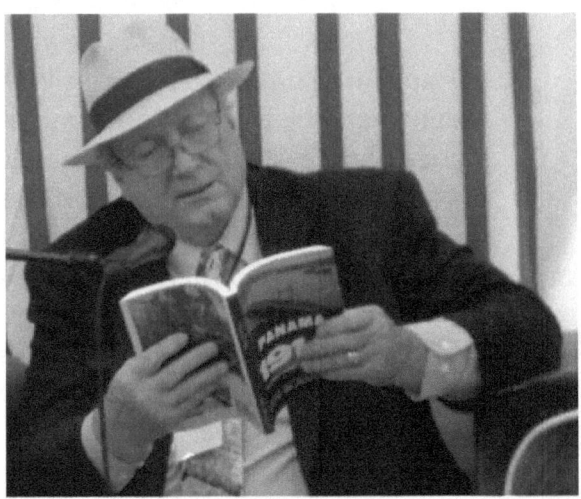

SIGN UP for notices of new releases, prizes and special presentations at ThePrivateerClause.com

Books by Ken Rossignol
All books are in Kindle, paperback and Audible formats
SPANISH INFLUENZA
TITANIC 1912
TITANIC POETRY, MUSIC & STORIES
KLAN: KILLING AMERICA
WRECK OF THE WHALE SHIP ESSEX
PANAMA 1914: The Early Years of the Big Dig
LEOPOLD & LOEB: Killed Bobby Franks
BATTLE OF SOLOMON'S ISLAND
COKE AIR – Chesapeake Crime Confidential Book 1
CRUISE FACTS
FIRE CRUISE
NINETY-NINE CENT TOUR OF BAR HARBOR MAINE
CRUISING THE WATERFRONT RESTAURANTS
OF THE LOWER POTOMAC
BANK OF CROOKS & CRIMINALS
CHESAPEAKE 1850
CHESAPEAKE 1880
CHESAPEAKE 1910
PIRATE TRIALS: Dastardly Deeds & Last Words
PIRATE TRIALS: Hung by the Neck Until Dead
PIRATE TRIALS: Famous Murderous Pirates
PIRATE TRIALS: The Three Pirates
THE CHESAPEAKE: Tales & Scales
THE CHESAPEAKE: Legends, Yarns & Barnacles
THE CHESAPEAKE: Oyster Buyboats, Ships & Steamed Crabs
THE CHESAPEAKE: A Man Born to Hang Can Never Drown
THE CHESAPEAKE: Country Cornpone Cornucopia
THE CHESAPEAKE: Tidewater Sagas
ST. MARY'S TODAY NEWSPAPER: THE STORY OF THE RAG
MURDER USA: True Crime, Real Killers
CHESAPEAKE TRUE CRIME:
Top Stories from THE CHESAPEAKE TODAY
THE CHESAPEAKE TODAY – All Crime, All The Time (Books 1-30)
SINS OF HER FATHER
The Marsha & Danny Jones Thrillers
THE PRIVATEER CLAUSE
RETURN OF THE SEA EMPRESS
FOLLOW TITANIC
FOLLOW TRIANGLE – VANISH
CRUISE KILLER
BEHEADED
WHO COLLECTS THE SOULS
PANAMA GOLD
Six Killer Thriller Novels (Books 1-6

SPANISH INFLUENZA – THE STORY OF THE EPIDEMIC THAT SWEPT
AMERICA FROM THE NEWSPAPER REPORTS OF 1918

SPANISH INFLUENZA – THE STORY OF THE EPIDEMIC THAT SWEPT AMERICA FROM THE NEWSPAPER REPORTS OF 1918

SPANISH INFLUENZA – THE STORY OF THE EPIDEMIC THAT SWEPT
AMERICA FROM THE NEWSPAPER REPORTS OF 1918

www.ingramcontent.com/pod-product-compliance
Lightning Source LLC
Chambersburg PA
CBHW030605220526
45463CB00004B/1170